Third Edition

Review of
Diagnosis,
Oral Medicine,
Radiology and
Treatment Planning

Norman K. Wood, D.D.S., M.S., Ph.D.

Professor of Oral Biology and Stomatology
Dean, Faculty of Dentistry, University of Alberta
Edmonton, Alberta, Canada

with 915 illustrations

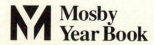
Mosby
Year Book

St. Louis Baltimore Boston Chicago London Philadelphia Sydney Toronto

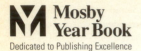

Editor: Robert W. Reinhardt
Assistant Editor: Melba Steube
Project Manager: Victoria Hoenigke
Book Design: Jeanne Wolfgeher

THIRD EDITION

Printed in the United States of America

Mosby–Year Book, Inc.
11830 Westline Industrial Drive
St. Louis, Missouri 63146

Library of Congress Cataloging in Publication Data

Wood, Norman K. (Norman Kenyon), 1935-
    Review of diagnosis, oral medicine, radiology and treatment
planning / Norman K. Wood.—3rd ed.
        p.   cm.
    ISBN 0-8016-6523-X : $33.95
    1. Mouth—Diseases—Examinations, questions, etc. I. Title.
    [DNLM: 1. Mouth Diseases—problems. 2. Tooth Diseases—problems.
WU 18 W877r]
RC815.W67 1993
617.5′22′0076—dc20
DNLM/DLC
for Library of Congress   92-12906
                                                                         CIP

93 94 95 96 97 GW/MY 9 8 7 6 5 4 3 2 1

▪ Contributors

Patricia G. Benca, D.D.S., M.S.
Lecturer
Department of Hospital Dentistry
University of Washington School of Dentistry
Seattle, Washington

Vickyann Chrobak, D.D.S., M.S.
Director of Clinics and Associate Professor
Department of Operative Dentistry
Loyola University School of Dentistry
Maywood, Illinois
Private Practice: General Dentistry
Elmwood Park, Illinois

Donald B. Doemling, M.S., Ph.D.
Professor and Chairman
Department of Physiology and Pharmacology
Loyola University School of Dentistry
Maywood, Illinois

Alphonse V. Gargiulo, D.D.S., M.S.
Clinical Assistant Professor
Department of Stomatology—Division of Periodontics
Northwestern University Dental School
Chicago, Illinois

William R. Groetsema, D.D.S.
Associate Professor
Department of Removable Prosthodontics
Loyola University School of Dentistry
Maywood, Illinois

Peter S. Hasiakos, D.D.S.
Associate Professor
Director of Operative Dentistry
Loyola University School of Dentistry
Maywood, Illinois

Kirk C. Hoerman, D.D.S., M.S.D.
Clinical Professor
Department of Preventive Dentistry/Community
  Health
Loyola University School of Dentistry
Maywood, Illinois

Joseph J. Keene, Jr., D.D.S., M.S.
Chairperson
Department of Periodontics, Microbiology,
  Biochemistry, and Dental Hygiene
Loyola University School of Dentistry
Maywood, Illinois

Martin F. Land, D.D.S., M.S.D.
Associate Professor and Chairman
Director, Postdoctoral Combined Prosthodontics
Department of Fixed Prosthodontics
Loyola University School of Dentistry
Maywood, Illinois

James F. Lehnert, D.D.S.
Associate Professor and Director
Division of Oral Diagnosis
Department of Oral Diagnosis, Radiology, and
  Pathology
Loyola University School of Dentistry
Maywood, Illinois

William McElroy, D.D.S.
Clinical Assistant Professor
Department of Pediatric Dentistry
Loyola University School of Dentistry
Maywood, Illinois
Private Practice: Pediatric Dentistry
Bloomingdale, Illinois

Roger G. Noonan, D.M.D., M.S.
Director, Postgraduate Education
Department of Pediatric Dentistry
Loyola University School of Dentistry
Maywood, Illinois

Larry J. Pierce, D.D.S.
Director
Department of Oral Diagnosis
Northwestern University Dental School
Chicago, Illinois

James M. Plecash, D.D.S., M.Sc.
Professor and Chairman
Division of Oral Diagnosis
Department of Stomatology
Faculty of Dentistry
University of Alberta
Edmonton, Alberta
Canada

Edward A. Rothman, D.D.S.
Private Practice: Pediatric Dentistry
Skokie, Illinois

Contributors

Danny R. Sawyer, D.D.S., Ph.D.
Professor and Chairman
Department of Oral Diagnosis, Pathology, Radiology
Loyola University School of Dentistry
Maywood, Illinois

E. Steven Smith, D.D.S.
Division Director of Oral Diagnosis/Medicine
Department of Oral Diagnosis
Northwestern University Dental School
Chicago, Illinois

Gary N. Taylor, D.D.S., M.S.
Professor and Chairman
Department of Endodontics, Operative Dentistry,
    Pediatric Dentistry, and Preventive
    Dentistry/Community Health
Loyola University School of Dentistry
Maywood, Illinois
Private Practice: Endodontics
LaGrange, Illinois

■ Preface

This edition includes the important new information that has come forward during the last several years in oral diagnosis, oral medicine, oral radiology, oral pathology, and treatment planning. Also, minor corrections and adjustments have been made on some of the previous questions. Specifically, questions regarding use of prophylactic antibiotics to preclude subacute bacterial endocarditis have been rewritten in order to be consistent with the new guidelines established by the American Heart Association in 1990. Likewise, information relative to non-A, non-B hepatitis and hepatitis C has been updated.

Most important, a completely new section has been added on the subject of AIDS and Infection Control. Questions in this section reflect the current literature concerning diagnosis, clinical aspects, and management considerations. A new section, "Pitfalls in Treatment Planning," has also been added to Part 2 (Comprehensive Treatment Planning) in this third edition.

I am pleased to express my appreciation to my very pleasant and competent secretary, Mrs. Arlene Bradley, for so carefully typing the several drafts of the new material. In addition, I have received helpful suggestions from colleagues and users of the second edition and have been pleased to include these in writing the third edition. Please keep these suggestions coming!

Norman K. Wood

■ Acknowledgments

These listed illustrations were received by courtesy of the following persons or institutions.
The numerals refer to the question numbers that accompany the illustration mentioned.

PART 1
Diagnosis, oral medicine, and radiology

101 Custodian of Dr. A.C.W. Hutchinson's Collection, Northwestern University Dental School Library, Chicago, Illinois
106 Dr. Orion Stuteville, Saint Joe, Arkansas
107 Dr. Dennis Boyer, Bloomingdale, Illinois
111 Custodian, see ack. 101
126 Custodian, see ack. 101
127 Dr. R. Averback, Denver, Colorado
150 Dr. Richard Lee, Findley, Ohio
162 Custodian, see ack. 101
175 Dr. Joseph Romano, Hinsdale, Illinois
178 Dr. Orion Stuteville, Saint Joe, Arkansas
182 Dr. Paul Akers, Evanston, Illinois
201 Dr. Steve Smith, Chicago, Illinois
234 Dr. Stephen Raibley, Oak Park, Illinois
235 Dr. Wilson Heaton, Oak Lawn, Illinois
236 Dr. Thomas Ahnger, Spring Valley, Illinois
239 Dr. Michael Lehnert, Minneapolis, Minnesota
243 Dr. Michael Lehnert, Minneapolis, Minnesota
244 Dr. Steve Smith, Chicago, Illinois
260 Dr. Eugene Seklecki, Tucson, Arizona
295 Dr. Wilson Heaton, Oak Lawn, Illinois
297 Dr. Michael Lehnert, Minneapolis, Minnesota
301 Dr. Rolley Bateman, Palatine, Illinois

302 Dr. Wilson Heaton, Oak Lawn, Illinois
304 Dr. Richard Lee, Findley, Ohio
305 Dr. Dean Skuble, Hinsdale, Illinois
325 Dr. Orion Stuteville, Saint Joe, Arkansas
327 Dr. Stephen Svalina, Palos Heights, Illinois
328 Dr. Patrick Toto, Maywood, Illinois
331 Dr. Robert Goepp, Chicago, Illinois
322 Custodian, see ack. 101
330 Custodian, see ack. 101
335 Custodian, see ack. 101
347 Dr. Frank Mourshed, Washington, D.C.
356 Dr. Rocco Latronica, Albany, New York
368A Dr. Kenneth Giedt, Aberdeen, South Dakota
370 Dr. Stephen Raibley, Oak Park, Illinois
371 Dr. Robert Goepp, Chicago, Illinois
374 Dr. Richard Lee, Findley, Ohio
375 Dr. William Schoenheider, Oak Lawn, Illinois
380 Dr. Wilson Heaton, Oak Lawn, Illinois
381 Custodian, see ack. 101
383 Dr. Orion Stuteville, Saint Joe, Arkansas
384 Custodian, see ack. 101
385A Dr. Nabil Barakat, Beirut, Lebanon
394 Dr. Lamar Byrd, Dallas, Texas
398 Dr. Richard Lee, Findley, Ohio
399 Dr. William Schoenheider, Oak Lawn, Illinois
400 Dr. Vernon Saunders, Richmond, Virginia
448 Custodian, see ack. 101

453 Dr. Vernon Saunders, Richmond, Virginia
461 Dr. Leslie Heffez, Chicago, Illinois
469 Dr. Regelio Moncada, Maywood, Illinois
472 Dr. Joseph Canzona, Chicago, Illinois
477 Dr. Wilson Heaton, Oak Lawn, Illinois
478 Dr. Michael Lehnert, Minneapolis, Minnesota
479 Dr. Patrick Toto, Maywood, Illinois
480 Custodian, see ack. 101
484 Dr. Michael Lehnert, Minneapolis, Minnesota
485 Dr. Thomas Emmering, Wheaton, Illinois
487 Dr. Sol Silverman, San Francisco, California

PART 2
Comprehensive treatment planning

2 Dr. Donald Bonomo, Flossmoor, Illinois
14 Custodian, see ack. 101
15 Custodian, see ack. 101
20 Dr. Michael Lehnert, Minneapolis, Minnesota
21 Dr. Patrick O'Flaherty, Downers Grove, Illinois
26 Dr. Richard Lee, Findley, Ohio
32 Dr. Drew Smith, Farmington, Connecticut
42 Custodian, see ack. 101
43 Dr. Michael Lehnert, Minneapolis, Minnesota
46 Dr. Wilson Heaton, Oak Lawn, Illinois
67 Dr. Joseph Canzona, Chicago, Illinois

106 Custodian, see ack. 101
184 Dr. Stephen Rosenstiel, Columbus, Ohio
187 Dr. Stephen Rosenstiel, Columbus, Ohio
207 Dr. Robert Mroz, Hines, Illinois
209 Dr. Robert Mroz, Hines, Illinois
210 Dr. Robert Mroz, Hines, Illinois
217 Dr. Robert Mroz, Hines, Illinois
218 Dr. Robert Mroz, Hines, Illinois
219 Dr. Robert Mroz, Hines, Illinois
223 Dr. Robert Mroz, Hines, Illinois

PART 3
AIDS and infection control

1. Dr. Joel Epstein, Vancouver, British Columbia, Canada
3. Dr. Joel Epstein, Vancouver, British Columbia, Canada

■ Contents

PART 1

Diagnosis, oral medicine, and radiology

1. A. Which *one* of the following bones is indicated by *1*?
   a. premaxillary bone.
   b. palatine bone.
   c. palatal process of maxillary bone.
   d. palatal process of the vomer bone.
   e. palatal process of the inferior turbinate bone.

B. Which *one* of the following is indicated by the arrows?
   a. incisive fissure.
   b. palatomaxillary suture.
   c. intermaxillary suture.
   d. sphenomaxillary suture.
   e. pterygomaxillary suture.

C. Which *one* of the following is indicated by *2*?
   a. anterior palatine foramen.
   b. posterior palatine foramen.
   c. incisive foramen.
   d. greater palatine foramen.
   e. pterygopalatine foramen.

2. A. Which *one* of the following is indicated by the white arrow?
   a. hamulus.
   b. medial pterygoid plate.
   c. lateral pterygoid plate.
   d. posterior nasal spine.
   e. pterygoid spine.

B. What muscle is associated with the structure indicated in Question 2A?
   a. levator palati.
   b. tensor palati.
   c. medial pterygoid.
   d. lateral pterygoid.
   e. palatoglossus.

C. What structure is indicated by *1*?
   a. nasopalatine foramen.
   b. anterior palatine foramen.
   c. posterior palatine foramen.
   d. lesser palatine foramen.
   e. sphenopalatine foramen.

D. Which *one* of the following structures is associated with the entity indicated in Question 2C?
   a. nasopalatine nerve.
   b. sphenopalatine nerve.
   c. anterior palatine nerve.
   d. posterior palatine nerve.
   e. nasopalatine artery.

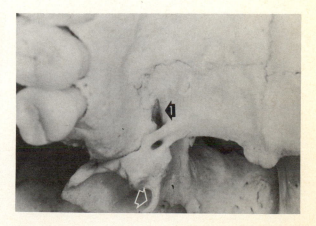

3. A. Which *one* of the following structures is indicated by the white arrow?
   a. vomer bone.
   b. vertical process of maxillla.
   c. vertical process of sphenoid bone.
   d. medial pterygoid plate.
   e. posterior nasal spine.

B. Which *one* of the following structures is indicated by *1*?
   a. vertical process of sphenoid bone.
   b. vomer bone.
   c. lateral pterygoid plate.
   d. medial pterygoid plate.
   e. hamular process.

C. Which *one* of the following structures is indicated by the black arrow?
   a. posterior palatine foramen.
   b. sphenoid palatine foramen.
   c. foramen spinosum.
   d. jugular foramen.
   e. foramen ovale.

4. A. Which *one* of the following structures is indicated by *1*?
   a. maxillary bone.
   b. zygomatic bone.
   c. temporal bone.
   d. pterygoid process of the sphenoid bone.

B. Which *one* of the following structures is intimately associated with the structure indicated in Question 4A?
   a. lateral pterygoid muscle.
   b. medial pterygoid muscle.
   c. temporal muscle.
   d. masseter muscle.
   e. buccinator muscle.

C. Which *one* of the following structures is indicated by the arrow?
   a. temporal ridge.
   b. mylohyoid ridge.
   c. external oblique ridge.
   d. masseter ridge.
   e. pterygoid ridge.

D. The structure indicated in Question 4C is produced by which *one* of the following?
   a. occlusal forces of molar teeth.
   b. function of the medial pterygoid muscle.
   c. function of the masseter muscle.
   d. function of the temporal muscle.
   e. function of the buccinator muscle.

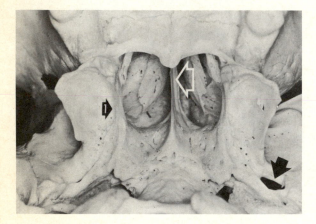

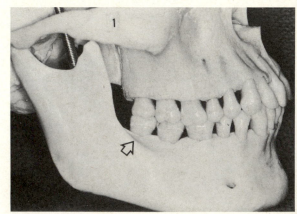

5. A. What anatomic structure is indicated by
   1?
   a. vomer bone.
   b. vertical process of the maxilla.
   c. incisive crest.
   d. anterior nasal spine.
   B. What anatomic structures are indicated
   by *2* and *3*?
   a. infranasal fossa and incisive ridge.
   b. incisive fossa and zygomatic process of
   maxillary bone.
   c. maxillary fossa and canine eminence.
   d. infraorbital fossa and zygomatic process of maxillary bone.
   e. canine eminence and incisive fossa.
   C. What anatomic structure is indicated by
   4?
   a. inferior turbinate bone.
   b. turbinate process of zygomatic bone.
   c. lateral process of the nasal bone.
   d. lateral nasal spine.

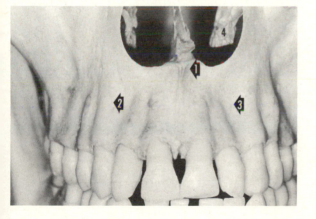

6. A. What anatomic structures are closely associated with **A** and **B**?
   a. hyoglossus muscle and sublingual salivary gland.
   b. medial pterygoid muscle and submandibular salivary gland.
   c. sphenomandibular ligament and digastric muscle.
   d. mylohyoid muscle and submandibular
   salivary gland.
   e. pterygomandibular ligament and submandibular gland.
   B. What anatomic structures are indicated
   by **C** and **D**?
   a. lingual and genial tubercles.
   b. antegonial notch and mental protuberance.
   c. mandibular foramen and genial tubercles.
   d. submandibular fossa and progonion.
   e. mandibular foramen and mental protuberance.
   C. The roughened region outlined by the dot-
   ted line represents:
   a. the origin of the medial pterygoid muscle.
   b. the insertion of the medial pterygoid
   muscle.
   c. the origin of the lateral pterygoid muscle.
   d. the attachment of the deep segment of
   the temporal muscle.
   e. the attachment of the sphenomandibular ligament.

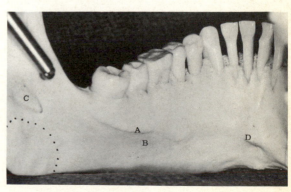

7. A. The anatomic structures indicated by **A** and **B** are:
   a. the zygomatic bone and posterior aspect of the maxilla.
   b. the zygomatic bone and the tuberosity.
   c. the condylar fossa and the lateral pterygoid plate.
   d. the articular eminence and the medial pterygoid plate.
   e. the articular eminence and the lateral pterygoid plate.
   B. The anatomic structures indicated by **C** and **D** are:
   a. the maxillary process of the zygoma and the lateral pterygoid plate.
   b. the zygomatic process of the maxilla and the tuberosity.
   c. the canine eminence and the tuberosity.
   d. the zygomatic process of the maxilla and the hamulus.
   e. the canine eminence and the hamulus.
   C. The arrow indicates the suture between:
   a. the maxilla and the zygoma.
   b. the zygoma and the sphenoid bone.
   c. the zygomatic process and the zygomatic arch.
   d. the zygomatic process of the maxillary bone and the zygomatic bone.
   e. the zygomatic bone and the temporal bone.

8. A. Which *one* of the following pairs of anatomic regions is indicated by **A** and **B**?
   a. mental protuberance and mental fossa.
   b. genial tubercle and incisive fossa.
   c. genial tubercle and mental fossa.
   d. mental protuberance and incisive fossa.
   e. mental protuberance and submental fossa.
   B. Which *one* of the following anatomic regions is indicated by **C**?
   a. incisive foramen.
   b. mental foramen.
   c. mandibular foramen.
   d. round foramen.
   e. inferior dental foramen.

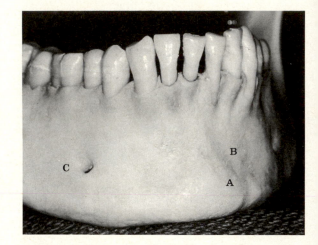

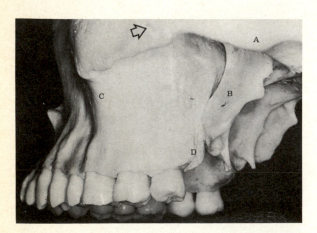

9. A. Which *one* of the following pairs of anatomic structures correctly identifies the entities marked **A** and **B**?
  a. temporal muscle and median pterygoid muscle.
  b. lateral pterygoid muscle and masseter muscle.
  c. lateral pterygoid muscle and medial pterygoid muscle.
  d. levator palati muscle and medial pterygoid muscle.
  e. lateral pterygoid muscle and superior constrictor muscle.

B. The anatomic region indicated by the open-faced arrow serves as the origin of which *one* of the following muscles?
  a. anterior belly of the digastric.
  b. trapezius.
  c. stylohyoid.
  d. sternocleidomastoid.
  e. superior constrictor muscle.

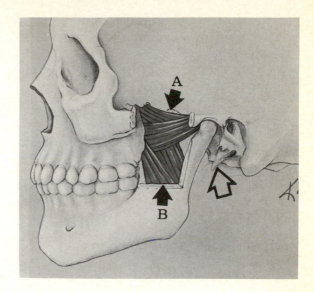

10. In this view of the medial aspect of the mandible, the entity identified by the arrows is *most* likely:
  a. the submandibular fossa.
  b. the area of insertion of the medial pterygoid muscle.
  c. an unusually large mandibular foramen.
  d. a lingual salivary gland depression (Stafne's cyst).

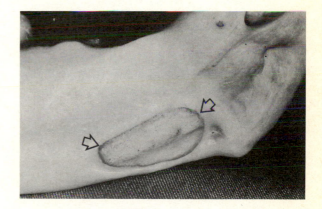

11. Which *one* of the following options is correct?
  a. Patient's head position is incorrect.
  b. Tube design is incorrect.
  c. Film position is incorrect.
  d. Vertical angulation is incorrect.
  e. All is in correct order.

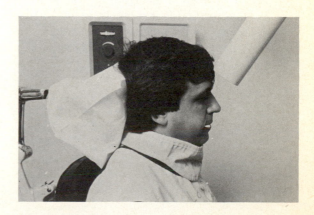

12. Which *one* of the following is true?
   a. Patient's head position is incorrect.
   b. Tube design is incorrect.
   c. Radiation protection to patient is inadequate.
   d. Vertical angulation is incorrect.
   e. Horizontal angulation is incorrect.

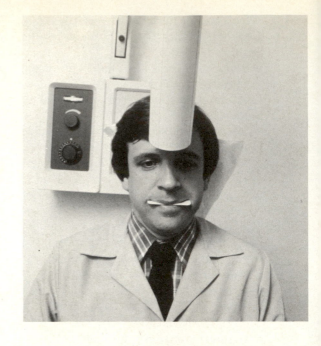

13. Which *one* of the following is true concerning this view that shows a periapical radiograph being taken of the mandibular right first molar tooth? Parallel technique is being used.
   a. Patient's head position is incorrect.
   b. X-ray cone is of incorrect design.
   c. Vertical angulation is incorrect.
   d. Patient protection is inadequate.
   e. Film holder is being improperly used.

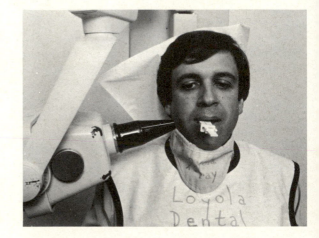

14. Which *one* of the following is true?
   a. Cone design is incorrect.
   b. Film position is incorrect.
   c. Patient's head position is incorrect.
   d. Horizontal angulation is incorrect.
   e. Patient protection is inadequate.

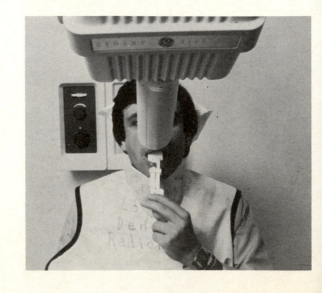

15. This view illustrates a periapical radiograph being taken of the mandibular first molar tooth. The parallel technique is being employed. Which *one* of the following options is true?
a. Film position is incorrect.
b. Horizontal angulation is incorrect.
c. There is a problem with the patient protection materials.
d. Tube design is incorrect.

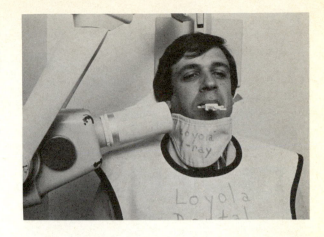

16. This view illustrates a maxillary first molar periapical radiograph being taken. The parallel technique is being employed. Which *one* of the following options is true?
a. Vertical angulation is incorrect.
b. Horizontal angulation is incorrect.
c. Patient's head position is incorrect.
d. Patient protection is inadequate.
e. Tube design is incorrect.

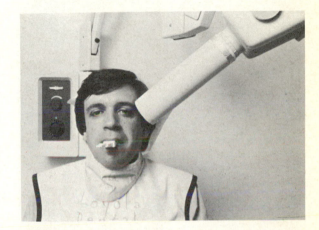

17. This radiograph is:
a. a submental vertex projection of the skull.
b. a Waters' projection.
c. a posteroanterior projection of the mandible and skull.
d. a zygomatic arch projection.
e. a cephalometric projection.

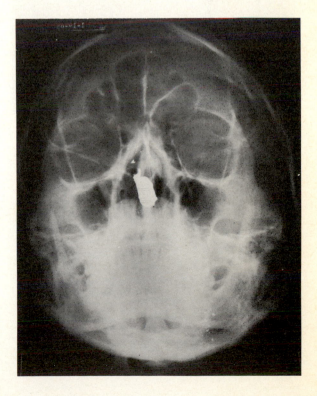

18. This radiograph is:
- a. a Towne's projection.
- b. a Waters' projection.
- c. a posteroanterior projection of the skull.
- d. a transcranial projection of the temporo-mandibular joint.
- e. a submental vertex projection.

19. This radiograph is:
- a. a Towne's projection.
- b. a Waters' projection.
- c. a transcranial projection of the temporo-mandibular joints.
- d. a submental vertex projection.
- e. an inferior cephalometric projection.

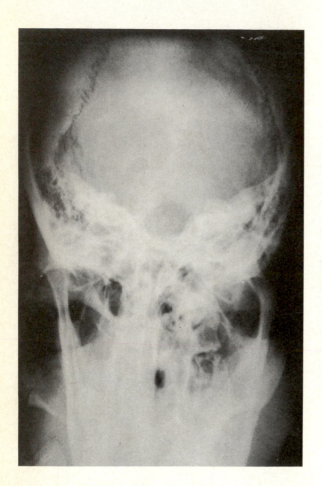

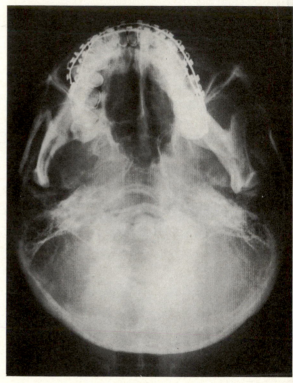

20. This radiograph is:
 a. a Towne's projection.
 b. a Waters' projection.
 c. an inferior cephalometric projection.
 d. a projection of the zygomatic arches.

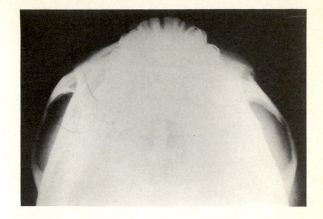

21. This radiograph is:
 a. a lateral oblique view of the mandible.
 b. a panoral view.
 c. a posteroanterior view of the mandible.
 d. a Waters' view.

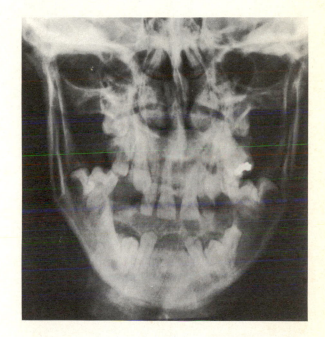

22. A. This radiograph is:
 a. a submental vertex projection.
 b. a Towne's projection.
 c. a lateral Waters' projection.
 d. a lateral cephalometric projection.
 e. a lateral oblique projection.
 B. Numerals *1* and *2* identify which *one* of the following pairs of anatomic structures?
 a. sphenoid sinus and frontal sinus.
 b. frontal sinus and maxillary sinus.
 c. frontal sinus and sphenoid sinus.
 d. ethmoid sinus and maxillary sinus.

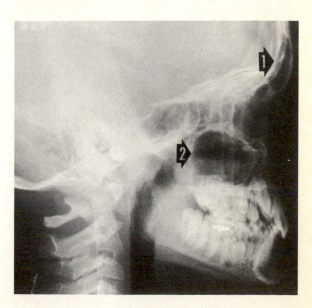

23. This radiograph is:
   a. a right lateral oblique projection.
   b. a left lateral oblique projection.
   c. a lateral projection of the jaws.
   d. a Waters' projection.

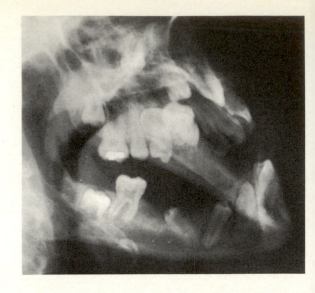

24. The most serious problem associated with this bite-wing radiograph is due to:
   a. film position.
   b. improper horizontal angulation.
   c. improper vertical angulation.
   d. overexposure.

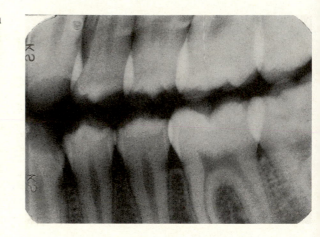

25. A. This is:
   a. a bilateral lateral oblique projection.
   b. an Orthopantomogram.
   c. a Panorex film.
   d. a Panelipse film.
   B. Which age group does this radiograph best depict?
   a. 6 to 7 years.
   b. 4 to 5 years.
   c. 1 to 3 years.
   d. 8 to 9 years.

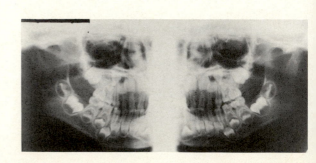

26. What age group is depicted in this radiograph?
a. 6 to 7 years.
b. 4 to 5 years.
c. 8 to 9 years.
d. 11 to 12 years.

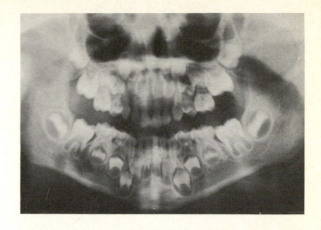

27. What age group is depicted in this radiograph?
a. 6 to 7 years.
b. 4 to 5 years.
c. 9 to 10 years.
d. 11 to 12 years.

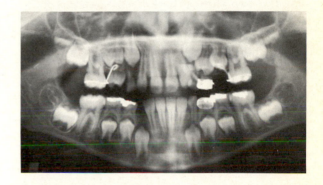

28. A. The solid white arrows indicate:
a. external oblique ridges.
b. mylohyoid ridges.
c. ghosting of ear rings from the opposite sides.
d. artifacts produced by darkroom error.
B. The open-face white arrows indicate:
a. ghosting of the inferior border of the rami of the opposite sides.
b. external oblique ridges.
c. mylohyoid ridges.
d. that the film has been double-exposed.

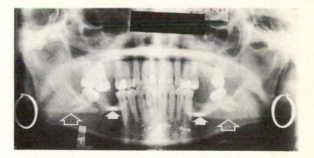

29. The alternate radiolucent/radiopaque linear pattern seen over the images of the second molar tooth in this radiograph:
a. is an example of reticulation.
b. is caused by static electricity.
c. is due to patient movement.
d. is due to movement of the x-ray head.
e. could be avoided by wearing cotton gloves in the darkroom.

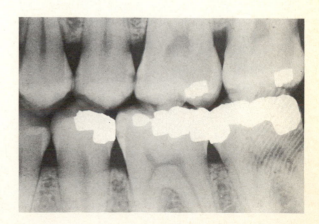

30. The pattern in this periapical radiograph is:
   a. referred to as tire tracks.
   b. referred to as reticulation.
   c. caused by static electricity.
   d. due to darkroom error.

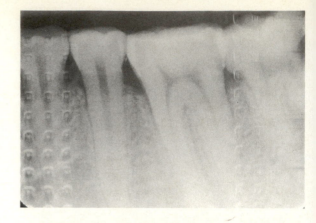

31. The two vertical dark lines extending inferiorly from the root end regions of the two incisor teeth are *most* likely:
   a. nutrient canals.
   b. fractures of the bone.
   c. caused by bending of the film.
   d. caused by darkroom error.

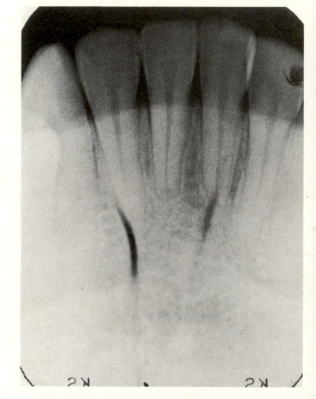

32. This radiographic error is *most* likely a result of:
   a. two films contacting each other in the developer.
   b. double exposure.
   c. the film being placed with the wrong side to the tooth surface.
   d. reticulation.

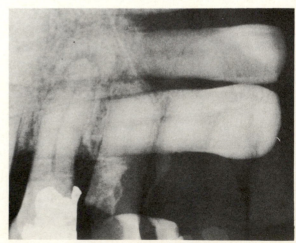

33. What has produced the *most* serious error in this canine film?
   a. horizontal angulation.
   b. vertical angulation.
   c. depleted developer.
   d. film position.

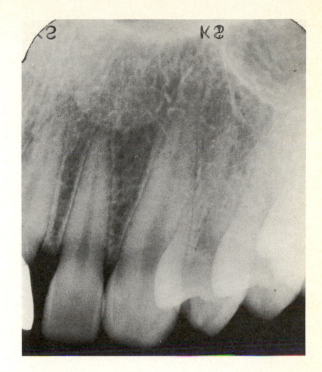

34. In this lateral cephalometric radiograph, *1* and *2* identify, respectively:
   a. the oropharyngeal airway and the tongue.
   b. the nasopharyngeal airway and the soft palate.
   c. the posterior pharyngeal wall and the tongue.
   d. the adenoids and the palatine tonsils.

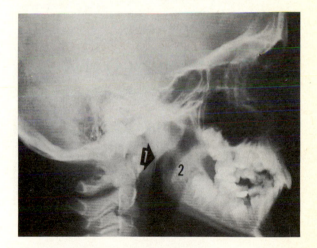

Dr. Patricia Benca authored questions 35 through 53.

35. A panoramic film taken in a 5-year-old child for evaluation of the developing dentition shows a bilateral mandibular radiopacity. This radiopacity *most* likely represents:
   a. distortion of the image due to a malformation of the patient's spine.
   b. an artifact due to a fixed orthodontic appliance.
   c. an artifact due to a piece of jewelry remaining around the patient's neck.
   d. an artifact due to an improperly positioned lead protector.
   e. an intrinsic artifact seen in this type of panoramic machine.

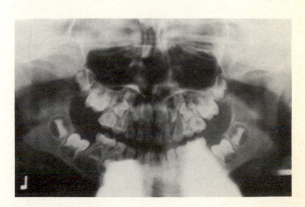

36. This maxillary occlusal film of an asymptomatic adult shows multiple, well-defined radiolucencies.
   A. The central palatal radiolucency *most* likely represents:
      a. the nasal fossa.
      b. a median palatal cyst.
      c. the sphenoid sinus.
      d. the ethmoid sinus.
      e. the frontal sinus.
   B. The radiolucencies located both medially and laterally to the maxillary first molar represent:
      a. periapical lesions associated with one of the molars.
      b. the greater and lesser palatine foramina.
      c. the sphenoid sinuses.
      d. the orbits.
      e. the maxillary sinuses.

37. The curved radiopaque band superimposed over the apices of the canine and premolars is *most* likely due to the presence of:
   a. a partial denture.
   b. eye glasses.
   c. a glass eye
   d. a cone cut.
   e. a fixed orthodontic appliance.

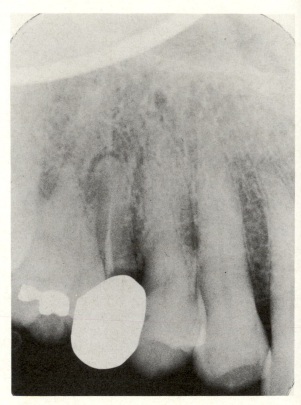

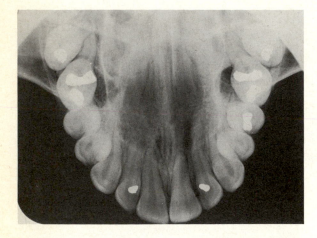

38. The premolar periapical film is technically correct in all respects except that:

a. there is interproximal overlap.
b. the teeth are elongated.
c. the teeth are foreshortened.
d. the film is malpositioned.
e. the film is cone cut.

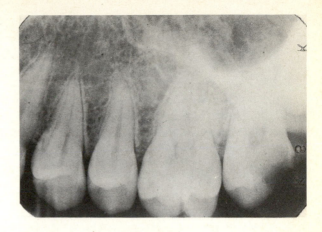

39. The striking anatomic anomaly found in this 14-year-old boy's molar teeth is the height of the pulp chambers and necks of these teeth. This condition is:

a. associated with dentinogenesis imperfecta.
b. assciated with amelogenesis imperfecta.
c. known as fusion.
d. known as cynodontism.
e. known as taurodontism.

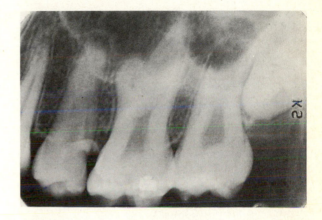

40. The small, round radiolucency in the maxilla located in the area of missing No. 7 *most* likely represents:

a. a surgical defect.
b. the lateral fossa.
c. the incisive foramen.
d. a globulomaxillary cyst.
e. a residual cyst.

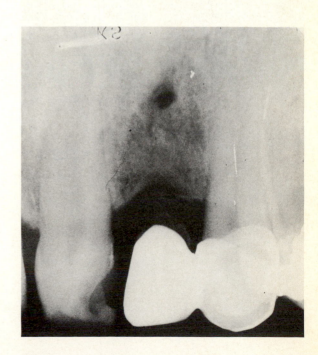

41. The supernumerary tooth situated between the maxillary permanent central incisors is called:
   a. a paramolar and is the most common of the supernumerary teeth.
   b. a microdont and is the most common of the supernumerary teeth.
   c. a microdont and is the least common of the supernumerary teeth.
   d. a mesiodens and is the most common of the supernumerary teeth.
   e. a mesiodens and is the least common of the supernumerary teeth.

42. This premolar periapical film shows a loss of the image just below the apices of the posterior teeth. This is *most* likely caused by:
   a. an underexposed film.
   b. cone cutting the film.
   c. improper film fixation.
   d. the thyroid shield.

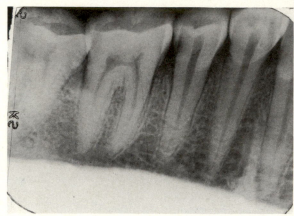

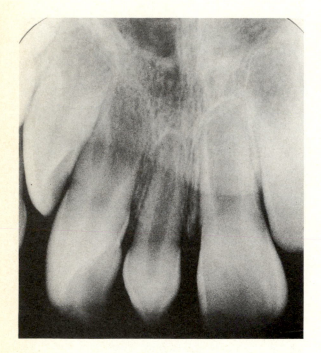

43. This maxillary canine periapical film shows which *one* major technique error?
   a. elongation.
   b. foreshortening.
   c. malpositioning.
   d. underexposure.
   e. overexposure.

44. The blackness of the superior aspect of this periapical film is *most* likely a result of:
   a. overexposure of the film.
   b. underexposure of the film.
   c. the film not being fully immersed in fixing solution.
   d. the film not being fully immersed in developing solution.
   e. two films being overlapped during processing.

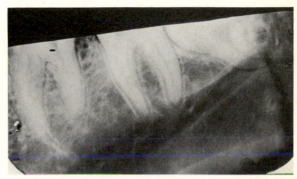

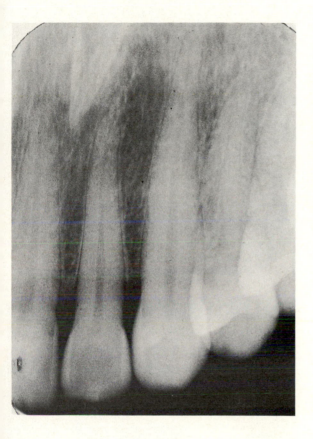

45. The primary technique error demonstrated in this canine periapical film is:
a. gross interproximal overlapping.
b. elongation.
c. foreshortening.
d. film position.

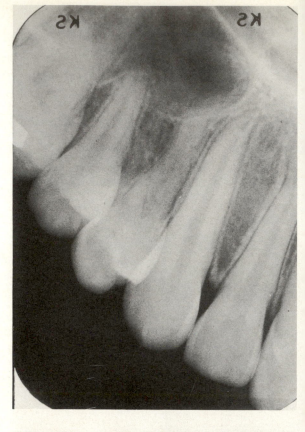

46. The alternating dark and light vertical patterns seen on this film can be attributed to:
a. overexposure of the film.
b. underexposure of the film.
c. double exposure of the film.
d. the film being caught or delayed in the automatic processor.
e. the film being rushed through the automatic processor.

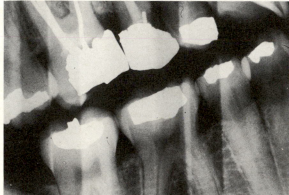

47. The technique used in taking this premolar bite-wing is *correct* in all respects *except*:
a. the vertical angulation of the cone.
b. the horizontal angulation of the cone.
c. the film position.
d. that the film is overexposed.
e. that the film is underexposed.

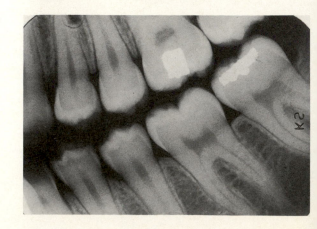

48. The "spots" on this film are caused by which processing error?
   a. fixer splashed on the film prior to developing.
   b. developer splashed on the film prior to developing.
   c. water splashed on the film prior to processing.
   d. water splashed on the film after processing.
   e. film overlap during processing.

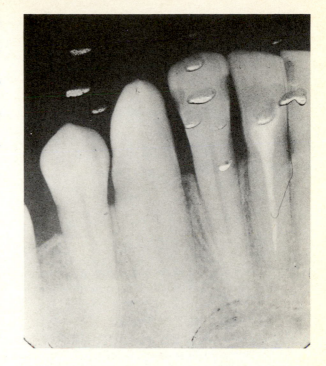

49. The *best* description of the root and periapical tissues of this mandibular premolar is:
   a. loss of lamina dura and associated periapical radiolucency.
   b. loss of lamina dura with internal/external root resorption.
   c. pulpal involvement and associated periapical radiolucency.
   d. pulpal involvement and associated periapical condensing osteitis.
   e. pulpal involvement and a widened periodontal ligament space.

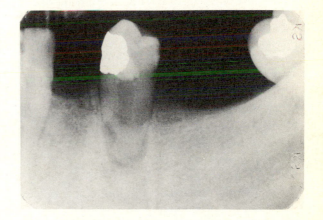

50. The radiopacity located in the alveolar bone in the area of the missing first mandibular molar is *most* likely:
   a. a root fragment.
   b. a foreign body.
   c. condensing osteitis.
   d. irregular, but not pathologic, alveolar bone formation.
   e. associated with chronic osteomyelitis.

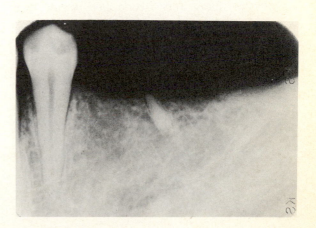

51. The technique error that caused this film to appear light was:
a. overdeveloping.
b. underfixing.
c. overexposure.
d. underexposure.
e. increased temperature of the developer.

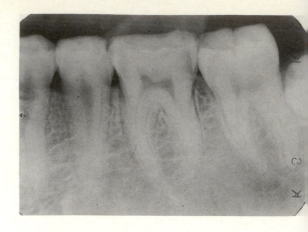

52. The loss of image on the superior aspect of this film is due to which technique error?
a. Overexposure of the film.
b. Underexposure of the film.
c. The film was not fully immersed in fixing solution during developing.
d. The film was not fully immersed in developing solution during developing.
e. Two films were overlapped during developing.

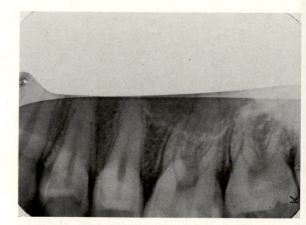

53. The defect on the anterior portion of this film is due to which developing error?
a. Overexposure.
b. Underexposure.
c. The film was not fully immersed in fixer during processing.
d. The film was not fully immersed in the developer during processing.
e. Two films were overlapped during processing.

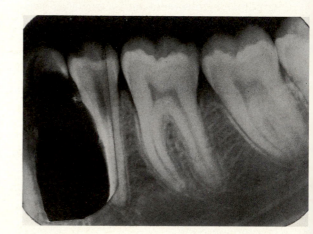

54. The mixed radiolucent-radiopaque region posterior to the second molar tooth was *most* likely:

a. a compound odontoma.
b. a developing crown of a permanent tooth.
c. a cementoma.
d. an adenomatoid odontogenic tumor.
e. a calcifying odontogenic cyst.

55. The large cystlike radiolucency in this radiograph of a 58-year-old woman was *most* likely:

a. a residual cyst.
b. a primordial cyst.
c. the maxillary sinus.
d. an ameloblastoma.
e. a traumatic bone cyst.

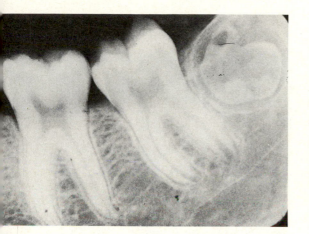

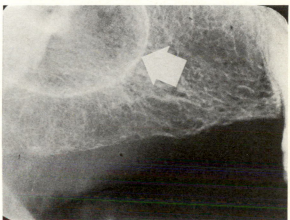

56. A. Arrow *1* points to a curved radiopaque band that is correctly identified as:

   a. the zygomatic arch.

   b. the inferior aspect of the zygomatic process of the maxillary bone and the maxillary process of the zygomatic bone.

   c. the horizontal process of the palatine bone.

   d. the posterior aspect of the vomer bone.

   e. the sigmoid notch.

   B. Arrow *2* indicates the radiopaque shadow of:

   a. the cheek.

   b. the malar process of the maxillary bone.

   c. the lateral pterygoid plate.

   d. the zygomatic bone.

   e. an antrolith.

   C. Arrow *3* indicates:

   a. a calcified blood vessel.

   b. a nutrient canal.

   c. the floor of the nasal cavity.

   d. the junction of the alveolar process and the basal bone.

   e. the floor of the maxillary sinus.

   D. Arrow *4* correctly identifies:

   a. the bony tuberosity.

   b. the gingival tissue.

   c. the coronoid process.

   d. the lateral pterygoid plate.

   e. the horizontal process of the palatine bone.

57. This honeycombed appearance was observed in the full-mouth radiographs of a 22-year-old woman who had presented for dental care. This appearance is:

   a. pathognomonic of thalassemia.

   b. pathognomonic of sickle cell anemia.

   c. pathognomonic of hyperparathyroidism.

   d. pathognomonic of intraosseous hemangioma.

   e. within normal limits.

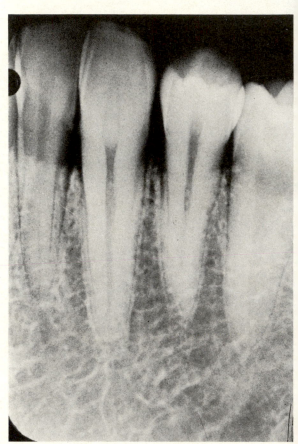

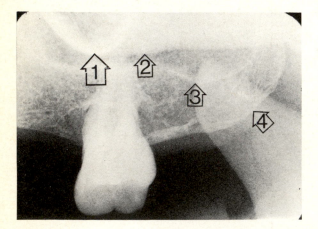

58. What is the *most* likely diagnosis of the asymptomatic periapical radiolucency associated with the asymptomatic second molar tooth?
   a. dental granuloma.
   b. periapical cementoma.
   c. dental papilla.
   d. marrow pattern.
   e. mental foramen.

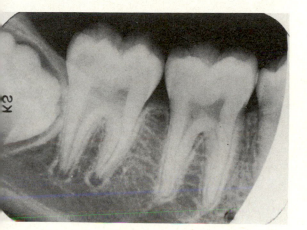

59. This asymptomatic radiolucency *(arrow)* was found during the routine examination of a 15-year-old girl. The lateral incisor and canine teeth were both asymptomatic and tested vital. This radiolucency is *most* likely:
   a. a globulomaxillary cyst.
   b. a lateral radicular cyst.
   c. an anterior cleft.
   d. the crypt of a developing supernumerary tooth.
   e. caused by a valley in the labial alveolar plate (incisive fossa).

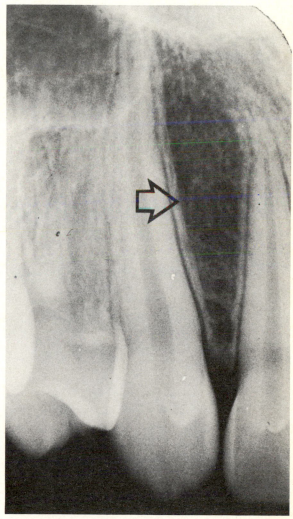

60. The multilocular radiolucent pattern shown in this radiograph is *most* likely produced by:
a. the maxillary sinus.
b. the nasal chamber.
c. a combination of the maxillary sinus and the nasal chamber.
d. an ameloblastoma.
e. a central hemangioma.

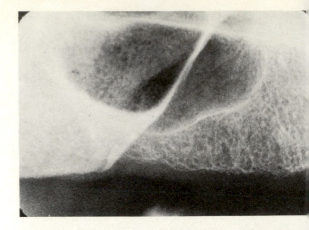

61. The radiolucency posterior to the second molar was *most* likely:
a. a primordial cyst.
b. an ameloblastoma.
c. a cystlike marrow pattern.
d. a residual cyst.
e. the crypt of a developing permanent tooth.

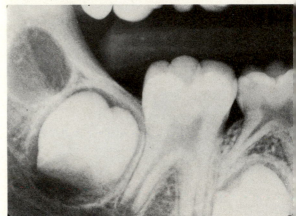

62. A. The open-faced white arrow identifies:
a. the tip of the nose.
b. the singulum of the incisor teeth.
c. the lipline.
d. the extent of abrasion on the lingual aspects of the incisor teeth.
B. The solid black arrow identifies:
a. the tip of the nose.
b. the nares.
c. the lipline.
d. the anterior nasal spine.
C. The solid white arrow indicates:
a. the presence of significant periodontal bone loss.
b. the incisive fossa.
c. the midline suture.
d. the incisive foramen.
D. The open-faced black arrow indicates:
a. the floor of the maxillary sinus.
b. the floor of the nasal fossa.
c. the anterior nasal spine.
d. the soft tissue shadow of the nose.

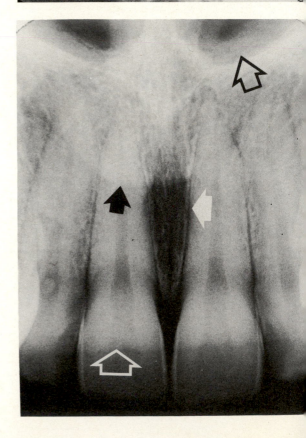

63. The arrow indicates:
  a. a blood vessel with calcified walls.
  b. a nutrient canal.
  c. an abscess tract within bone.
  d. an artifact.
  e. a vertical section of the mental foramen.

64. The arrows indicate:
  a. the nasal chambers.
  b. periapical pathology.
  c. twin incisive canals.
  d. the nares.

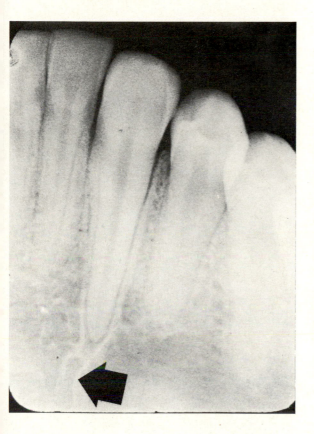
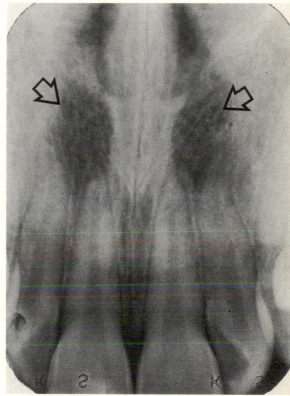

65. The open-faced white arrow and the solid white arrow indicate, respectively:
   a. the temporal crest and the mylohyoid (internal oblique) ridge.
   b. the external oblique ridge and the mental ridge.
   c. the external oblique ridge and mylohyoid (internal oblique) ridge.
   d. the pterygoid ridge and the mylohyoid (internal oblique) ridge.

66. The radiopaque shadow over the apex of the lateral incisor tooth is *most* likely:
   a. a condensing osteitis.
   b. the projected image of a palatal torus.
   c. the ala of the right side of the nose.
   d. a cementoma.
   e. the shadow of the incisive papilla.

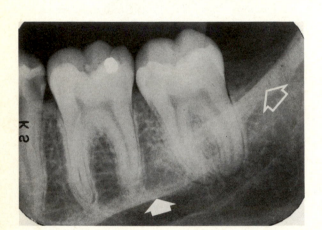

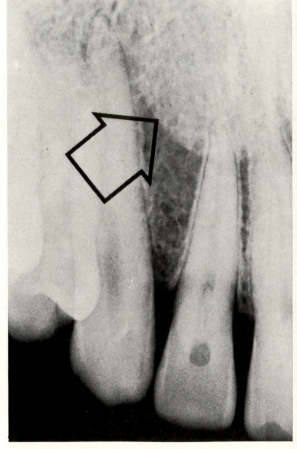

67. The arrows indicate:
  a. the canals of Scarpa.
  b. the common incisive canal.
  c. a subclinical anterior cleft.
  d. an abnormally wide midline suture.

68. The asymptomatic radiolucencies at the apices of this asymptomatic third molar tooth are *most* likely:
  a. caused by the presence of the dental papillae alone.
  b. produced by periapical granulomas.
  c. caused by the presence of the mandibular canal alone.
  d. caused by the presence of periapical scars.
  e. produced by the combined effects of the dental papillae, the mandibular canal, and the submandibular fossa.

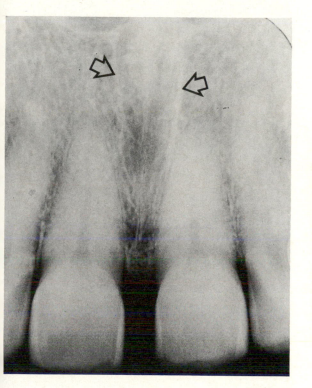

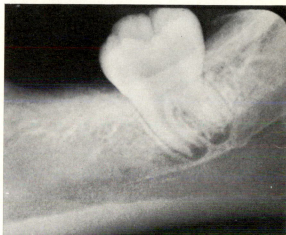

69. A. The solid arrow indicates:
   a. the floor of the maxillary sinus.
   b. the inferior margin of the bony tuber-osity.
   c. the buccal mucosa.
   d. the inferior margin of the fibrous tu-berosity.
B. The open-faced arrow indicates:
   a. the lateral pterygoid plate.
   b. the zygomatic process of the maxilla.
   c. the zygomatic bone.
   d. the zygomatic arch.

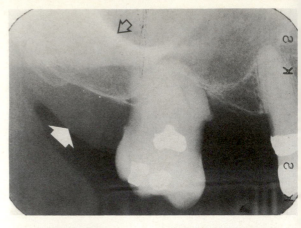

70. The radiolucency, indicated by the arrow, at the apices of this asymptomatic first molar tooth is *most* likely:
   a. a periapical granuloma.
   b. bone marrow pattern within normal limits
   c. the mental foramen.
   d. a cementoma.
   e. suggestive of serious systemic disease.

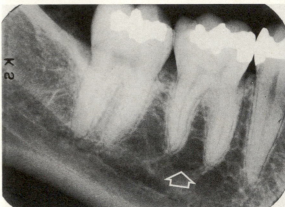

71. A. *1* identifies:
   a. the maxillary sinus.
   b. the nasal chamber.
   c. the hard palate.
   d. the superior turbinate bone.
   e. the naris.
B. *2* identifies:
   a. the nasal chamber.
   b. the maxillary sinus.
   c. the orbit.
   d. the naris.
   e. the malar process of the zygomatic bone.
C. The arrow indicates the radiopaque shadow produced by:
   a. the coronoid process.
   b. the commissure.
   c. the anterior border of the cheek where it terminates in the nasolabial groove.
   d. the side of the nose.
   e. the soft palate.

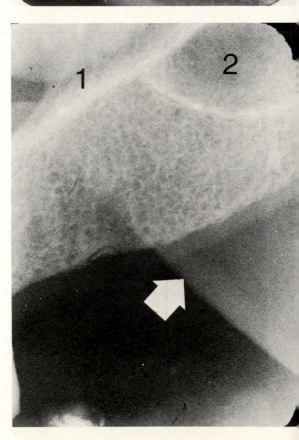

72. This asymptomatic radiolucent-radiopaque area found on a routine radiographic survey was *most* likely:

a. a complex odontoma.

b. a cementoma.

c. a sialolith.

d. a developing torus.

e. the calcifying crown of a supernumerary tooth.

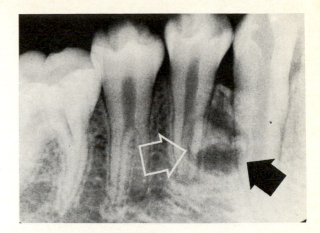

73. The small radiolucency indicated by the arrow is *most* likely:

a. the incisive canal.

b. a remnant of the midline suture.

c. a nutrient canal.

d. the result of a surgical procedure.

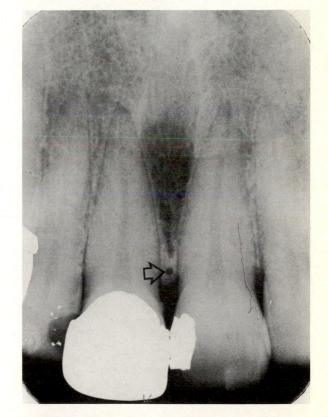

74. The black arrow and the white arrow indicate, respectively:

a. the external oblique line and the mylohyoid (internal oblique) line.

b. the superior and inferior borders of the mandibular canal.

c. condensing osteitis and the external oblique line.

d. the mylohyoid (internal oblique) line and inferior border of the mandibular canal.

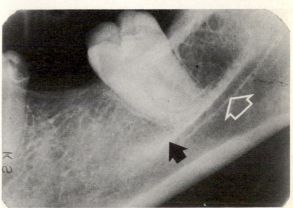

75. The radiolucency indicated by the arrow is *most* likely:
   a. a nutrient canal.
   b. a fracture.
   c. the midline suture.
   d. an artifact.

76. This asymptomatic radiolucency was found at the apex of the asymptomatic vital second premolar during the routine examination of a 38-year-old man. This radiolucency *most* likely was:
   a. a traumatic bone cyst.
   b. a cementoma.
   c. a periapical cyst.
   d. an outpouching of the maxillary sinus.
   e. a nutrient canal.

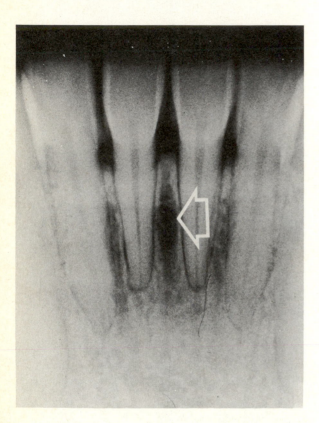

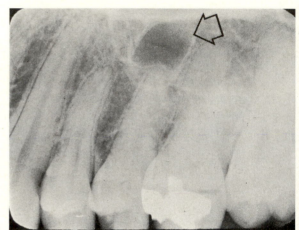

77. This stepladder pattern of the interseptal bone was observed in the routine radiographs of a 16-year-old boy. This appearance is:
a. pathognomonic of sickle cell anemia.
b. pathognomonic of thalassemia.
c. within normal limits.
d. pathognomonic of hypoparathyroidism.
e. indicative of a light occlusal load.

78. A. The radiolucency surrounded by the radiopaque ring indicated by the arrow is correctly identified as:
a. osteomyelitis.
b. the lingual or round foramen.
c. combined rarefying and condensing osteitis.
d. an artifact.
e. a calcified blood vessel.
B. The bony architecture in this radiograph is:
a. highly suggestive of sickle cell anemia.
b. highly suggestive of thalassemia.
c. within normal limits.
d. highly suggestive of hyperparathyroidism.
e. highly suggestive of the presence of a hemangioma.

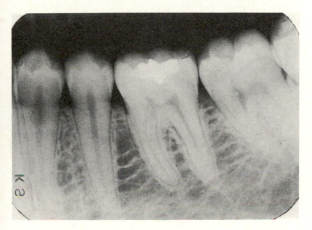

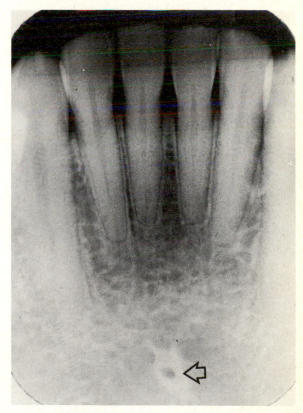

79. A. The radiopacities coded with *1* are correctly identified as:
   a. the alae.
   b. rhinoliths.
   c. inferior turbinates.
   d. nasal polyps.
   e. bilobed palatal tori.

   B. The single (solid black) arrow points to a linear radiolucency that is correctly identified as:
   a. a nutrient canal.
   b. a vertical fracture.
   c. the anterior nasal spine.
   d. the midline suture.
   e. the greater palatine foramen.

   C. The two lower (open-faced) arrows delineate a radiolucency that is correctly identified as:
   a. the incisive foramen.
   b. the greater palatine foramen.
   c. the anterior nasal spine.
   d. a residual cyst.
   e. an extraction socket.

80. The radiopaque line indicated by the arrow is:
   a. the floor of the nasal cavity.
   b. the floor of the maxillary sinus.
   c. a bony septum in the maxillary sinus.
   d. the infraorbital rim.

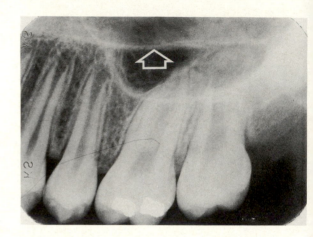

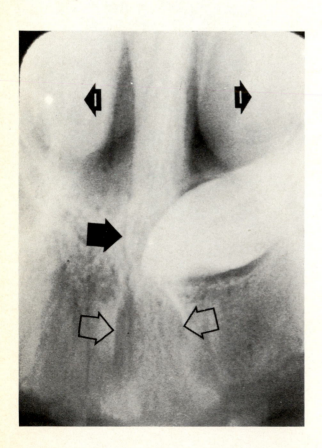

81. The entity marked by the arrow is the image of:
   a. the incisive canal.
   b. the remaining segment of the intermaxillary suture.
   c. a nutrient canal.
   d. a recent fracture of the bone.

82. The arrow correctly identifies:
   a. a palatal torus.
   b. the anterior border of the malar process and the malar bone.
   c. the posterior border of the malar process and the malar bone.
   d. the vomer bone.
   e. the inferior turbinate bone.

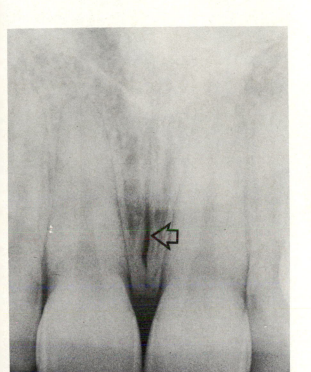

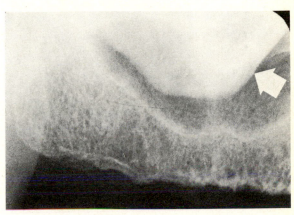

83. The radiopaque structure indicated by the arrow is the image of:
   a. the zygomatic process of the maxilla and the maxillary process of the zygoma.
   b. the zygomatic arch.
   c. the floor of the maxillary sinus.
   d. the sigmoid notch.

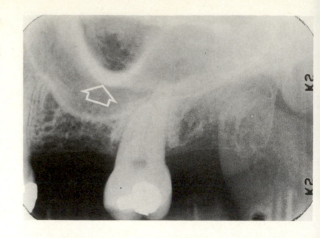

84. The two radiopaque lines, one running horizontally over the apices of the anterior teeth and the curved one near the superior right margin of the film, indicate:
   a. a cyst associated with the nasal cavity.
   b the floor and wall of the nasal cavity only.
   c. the floor and wall of the maxillary sinus only.
   d. the antral Y.

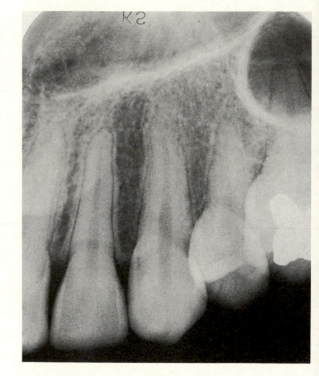

85. A. The more superiorly placed arrow correctly identifies:
   a. the buccal plate.
   b. the base of the alveolar bone.
   c. the mylohyoid line (internal oblique).
   d. the alveolar crest.
   e. the external oblique line.
   B. The more inferiorly placed arrow correctly identifies:
   a. the inferior border of the mandible.
   b. the mylohyoid line (internal oblique).
   c. the base of the alveolar bone.
   d. the external oblique line.
   e. the lingula.

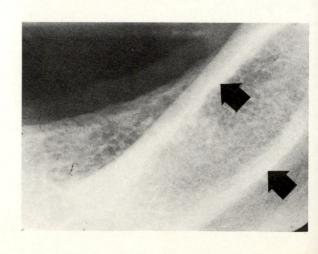

86. The radiolucent band indicated by the arrow correctly identifies:
   a. the tympanic tube.
   b. the sphenopalatine fissure.
   c. the pterygomaxillary suture.
   d. the pterygoid canal.
   e. the shadow between the inferior border of the zygoma and the posterosuperior aspect of the coronoid process.

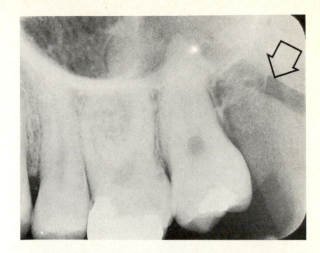

87. A. The black arrow indicates the image of:
   a. the hyoid bone.
   b. the inferior border of the mandible.
   c. the mental ridge.
   d. the mylohyoid ridge.
   B. The white arrow points to:
   a. the lingual process.
   b. the lingula.
   c. a sequestrum.
   d. the genial tubercle.

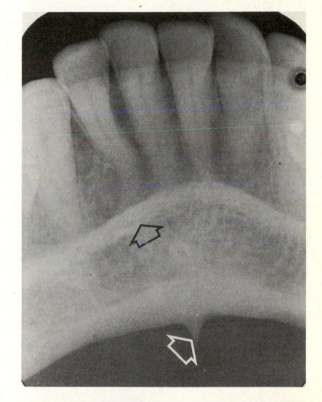

88. This asymptomatic radiolucency observed on routine radiographs of a 44-year-old man, which has not changed in several years, is *most* likely:
   a. a primordial cyst.
   b. a residual cyst.
   c. a previous extraction socket.
   d. an ameloblastoma.
   e. a lingual salivary gland invagination.

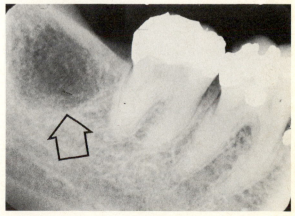

89. The radiolucency indicated by the arrow is *most* likely:
   a. a midpalatal cyst or a radicular cyst.
   b. the incisive canal or a traumatic bone cyst.
   c. the incisive canal or an incisive canal cyst.
   d. the incisive canal or a radicular cyst.

90. A. The large radiolucency is *most* likely:
   a. not pathologic.
   b. a traumatic bone cyst.
   c. a radicular cyst.
   d. a squamous cell carcinoma.
   e. an artifact.

   B. The numerous radiolucent bands running through the region in question *most* likely:
   a. represent multiple comminuted fracture lines.
   b. represent surgical resection sites.
   c. represent nutrient canals.
   d. represent abscess-drainage tracts.
   e. strongly suggest the possibility of an intraosseous hemangioma.

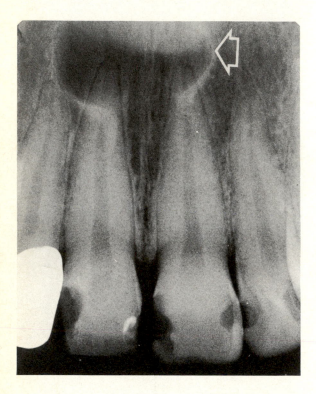

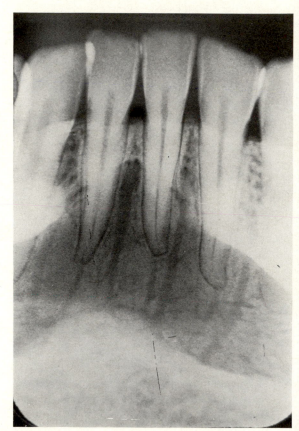

91. This asymptomatic radiopacity located on routine perusal of full-mouth radiographs of this 68-year-old man was *most* likely:
    a. the ala.
    b. a rhinolith.
    c. a torus palatinus.
    d. condensing osteitis.
    e. cementoma.

92. This asymptomatic radiolucency, which was discovered on routine radiographic examination of an asymptomatic 54-year-old woman, is *most* likely:
    a. a residual cyst.
    b. a surgical defect.
    c. an ameloblastoma.
    d. a lingual salivary gland invagination.
    e. a traumatic bone cyst.

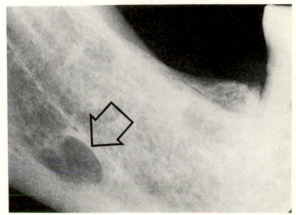

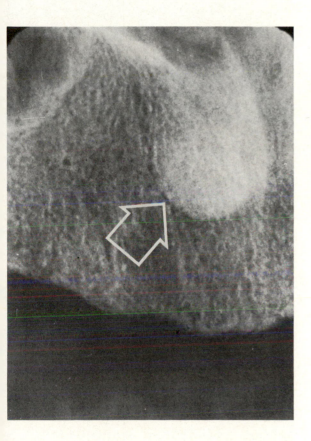

93. The radiolucency indicated by the arrow is *most* likely either:
   a. a section of the maxillary sinus or a residual cyst.
   b. a section of the maxillary sinus or an ameloblastoma.
   c. a residual cyst or a traumatic bone cyst.
   d. a section of the maxillary sinus or a globulomaxillary cyst.

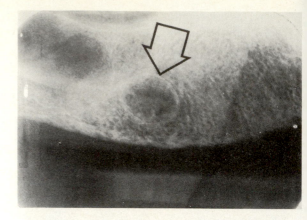

94. These multiple radiopacities were found during the routine radiographic examination of a 43-year-old woman. They were *most* likely:
   a. cementomas.
   b. tori or exostoses.
   c. odontomas.
   d. cotton-wool lesions of Paget's disease.
   e. foreign bodies.

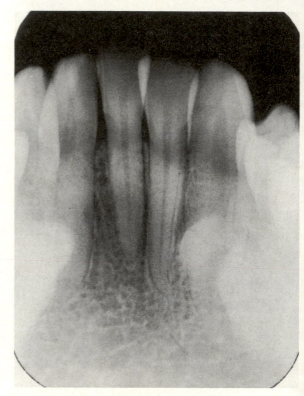

95. A. This radiograph is:
   a. a lateral oblique.
   b. a submental vertex.
   c a mandibular occlusal.
   d. a maxillary occlusal.
   B. The open-faced arrow and the solid arrow identify, respectively, the images of:
   a. the anterior border of the tongue and the genial tubercles.
   b. the soft palate and the hamulus.
   c. the anterior border of the lower lip and the genial tubercle.
   d. the hyoid bone and the genial tubercle.

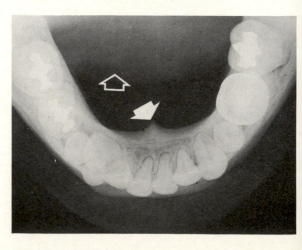

96. This pericoronal radiolucency found during a routine radiographic examination was *most* likely produced by:
a. a dentigerous cyst.
b. an ameloblastoma.
c. an adenomatoid odontogenic tumor.
d. a normal follicle.
e. an odontogenic keratocyst.

97. A. This radiograph is:
a. a panoral projection.
b. a Waters' projection.
c a maxillary occlusal projection.
d. a posteroanterior projection.

B. The paired round radiolucencies indicated by the arrows are:
a. the nasopalatine foramina.
b. the nasolacrimal ducts.
c. the anterior palatine foramina.
d. the posterior palatine foramina.

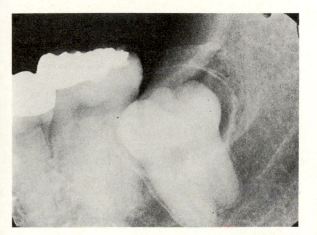

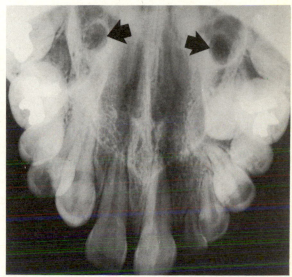

98. This radiopacity *(arrow),* which is cast over the apex of the canine tooth, is *most* likely:
  a. a cementoma.
  b. a rhinolith.
  c. an odontoma.
  d. condensing osteitis.
  e. the projected image of a torus.

99. In this panoral radiograph, the solid arrow and the open-faced arrow indicate, respectively:
  a. the antegonial notch and the mandibular canal.
  b. the articular fossa and the submandibular fossa
  c. the sigmoid notch and the mandibular canal.
  d. the hamular notch and the mandibular canal.

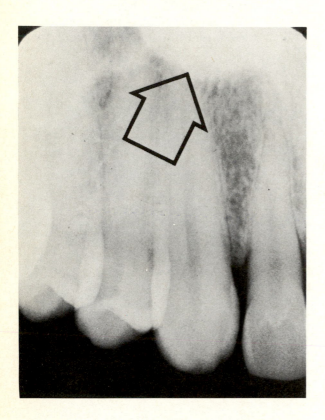

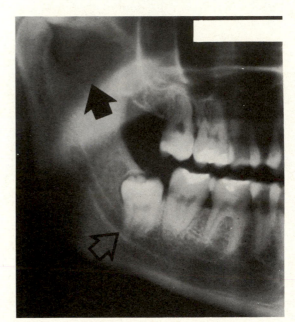

100. In this panoral radiograph, the solid arrow and the open-faced arrow indicate, respectively:

a. the styloid process and the soft palate.

b. the articular eminence and the soft palate.

c. the articular eminence and the lower lip.

d. the articular eminence and the tongue.

101. The radiolucency identified by the arrow is *most* likely:

a. the mental canal.

b. the mental foramen.

c. a bone marrow pattern more prominent than usual but within normal limits.

d. a lytic lesion of bone related to tooth pathology.

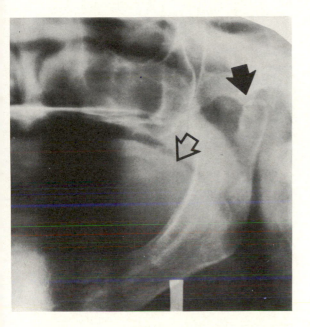

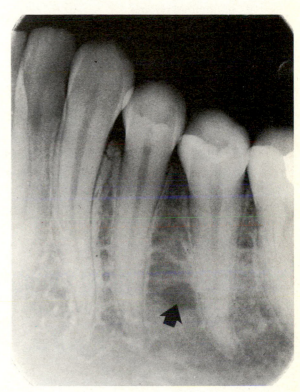

102. This asymptomatic radiolucency associated with the deciduous and permanent canine teeth was found on routine radiographic examination of an 11-year-old boy.
- A. The radiolucency is *most* likely:
  - a. a radicular cyst.
  - b. a follicular cyst.
  - c. an enlarged follicle but within normal limits.
  - d. an adenomatoid odontogenic tumor.
  - e. an ameloblastoma.
- B. The *most* suitable management approach in this case after comparison with the opposite side would be:
  - a. reevaluation with a new radiograph in 3 months.
  - b. a block resection.
  - c. a marsupialization procedure.
  - d. immediate extraction of the deciduous canine, enucleation of the radiolucent lesion, and submission of the specimen for microscopic study.
  - e. radiographs of the chest in order to check for the presence of bifid ribs.

103. This radiolucency *(arrow)* was found in a patient who had undergone jaw surgery approximately 5 years previously in the second premolar–first molar region. The patient has been asymptomatic since the surgery. Clinically, the ridge is markedly narrowed in the region. The radiolucency is *most* likely:
- a. an enlarged mental foramen.
- b. an amputation neuroma.
- c. a surgical defect.
- d. a residual cyst.

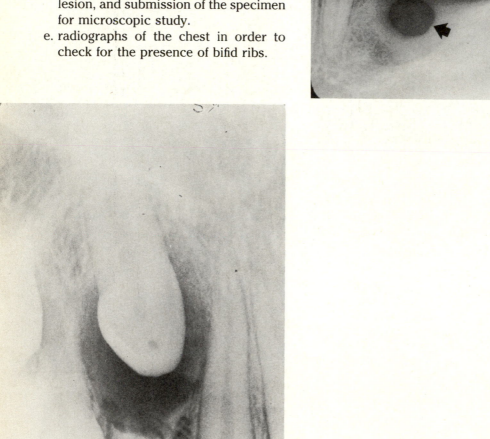

104. This asymptomatic radiopacity *(arrow)* which is not surrounded by a radiolucent rim but image of which can be shifted to some degree on changing the angle of x-ray, is *most* likely:

a. a torus.

b. condensing osteitis.

c. an odontoma.

d. a cementoma.

105. This rounded asymptomatic radiolucency *(arrow)*, positioned interradicularly between asymptomatic lateral incisor and canine teeth that have vital pulps, is *most* likely:

a. a lateral radicular cyst located at the exit of a lateral canal.

b. a residual cyst.

c. a lateral periodontal cyst.

d. a gingival cyst.

e. a globulomaxillary cyst.

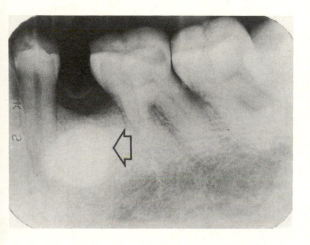

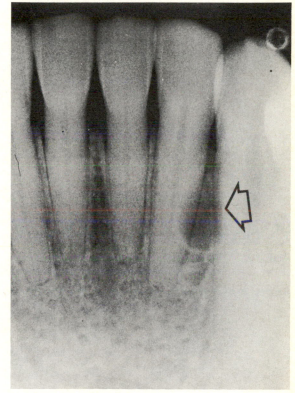

106. The type of border that this lesion has produced *(arrows)* is strongly indicative of:

a. a malignancy.
b. an infective process.
c. an invading lesion.
d. a benign process.
e. osteogenic sarcoma.

107. This asymptomatic radiolucency *(arrow)* was found in a 27-year-old man who had had four impacted third molars removed 6 years previously. On opening the radiolucency, the oral surgeon found it was composed of a waxy substance that could be easily removed, leaving a crater with smooth walls. What is the *most* likely diagnosis?

a. a residual cyst.
b. ameloblastoma.
c. keratocyst.
d. paraffinoma.

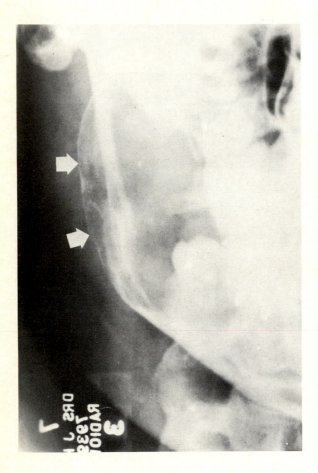

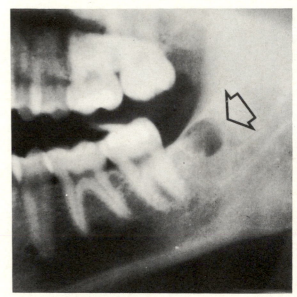

108. This asymptomatic radiopacity *(arrow)* was found on routine radiographs of a 46-year-old man who appeared to be in good health. The radiopacity is *most* likely:
   a. the zygomatic bone.
   b. an antrolith.
   c. a projected image of a palatal torus.
   d. an odontoma.
   e. a rhinolith.

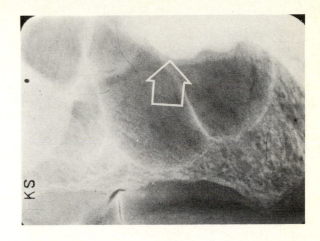

109. This 16-year-old boy *most* likely has:
   a. multiple odontomas.
   b. multiple impacted supernumerary teeth (no syndrome).
   c. cleidocranial dysostosis.
   d. hypothyroidism.
   e. hypoparathyroidism.

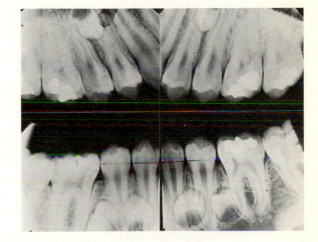

110. This lateral incisor tooth shows an example of:
   a. Turner's tooth.
   b. Hutchinson's tooth.
   c. a dens in dente.
   d. gemination.
   e. fusion.

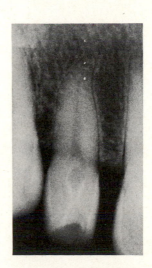

111. The arrows *most* likely indicate:
  a. areas of hypercementosis.
  b. cementomas.
  c. deposits of calculus.
  d. enamel pearls.

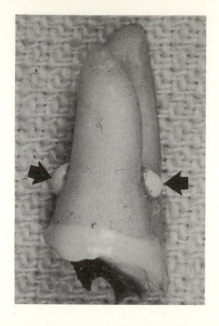

112. This 56-year-old-man had been in a car accident 2 weeks previously. When you ask him to bite on his back teeth, this is how he occludes. On repeated attempts, he closes this way each time. The basic problem is *most* likely:
  a. a malocclusion of long standing.
  b. a muscle spasm.
  c. a cardiovascular accident (stroke).
  d. fracture of the mandible.

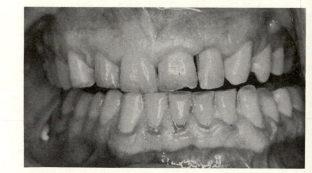

113. The asymptomatic radiopacity *(arrow)* found in this patient is *most* likely:
  a. condensing osteitis.
  b. idiopathic osteosclerosis.
  c. a foreign body.
  d. a retained deciduous molar root fragment.
  e. a small complex odontoma.

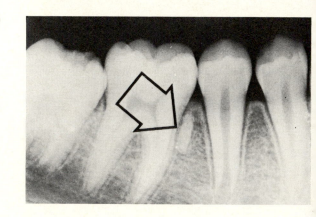

114. The adult patient shown in **A** is most likely suffering from what disease? The radiograph **(B)** is of teeth extracted from a child who is suffering from the same disease.
a. amelogenesis imperfecta.
b. dentinogenesis imperfecta.
c. ectodermal dysplasia.
d. rickets.
e. tetracycline staining.

115. This asymptomatic radiopacity was discovered on routine radiographs of a 33-year-old woman. The radiopacity is *most* likely:
a. an impacted molar tooth.
b. a compound odontoma.
c. a complex odontoma.
d. a cementoma.
e. condensing osteitis.

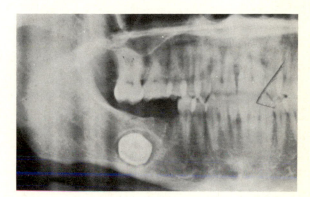

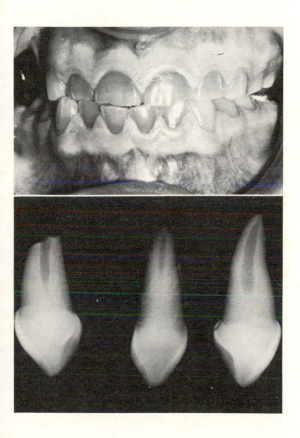

116. The entity to which the arrow points on the maxillary left central incisor is known as:

a. Hutchinson's incisor.

b. talon cusp.

c. dens in dente.

d. transposition.

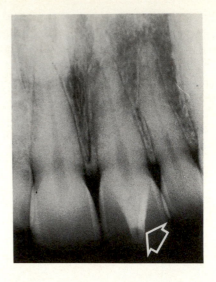

117. These radiographs of the maxillary anterior teeth of a 21-year-old patient demonstrate changes seen in:

a. hyperparathyroidism.

b. irradiation.

c. bulimia.

d. bruxism.

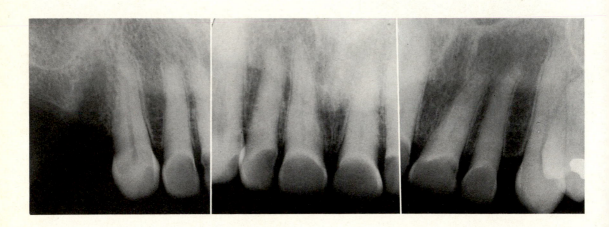

118. The mixed radiolucent-radiopaque lesion that is obviously preventing the eruption of the left central incisor tooth in this 8-year-old boy is *most* likely:
    a. a compound odontoma.
    b. a complex odontoma.
    c. a cementoma.
    d. an osteomyelitis.
    e. an osteogenic sarcoma.

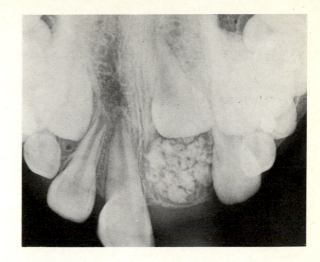

119. This bite-wing radiograph shows the presence of:
    a. pulp stones.
    b. enamel pearls.
    c. congenital anodontia.
    d. dens in dente.
    e. mulberry molars.

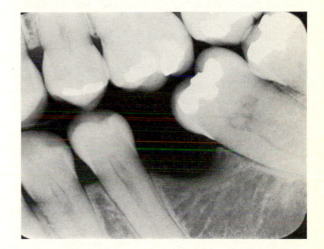

120. The radiopacity *(arrow)* at the end of the root of the posterior molar tooth is *most* likely:
    a. condensing osteitis.
    b. hypercementosis.
    c. cementoma.
    d. an odontoma.
    e. a buccal exostosis.

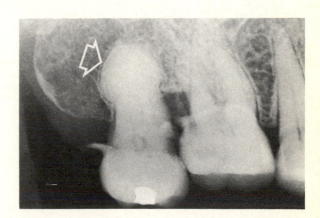

121. The defects identified by the arrows are *most* likely an example of:
  a. irradiation caries.
  b. erosion.
  c. abrasion.
  d. hypoplasia.
  e. gold foil restorations.

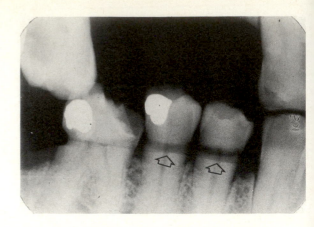

122. These radiopacities, which were found on radiographs of a 55-year-old woman and were taken to investigate the cause of a denture sore, are *most* likely:
  a. sclerosed sockets.
  b. multiple cementomas.
  c. multiple exostoses.
  d. retained root fragments.
  e. complex odontomas.

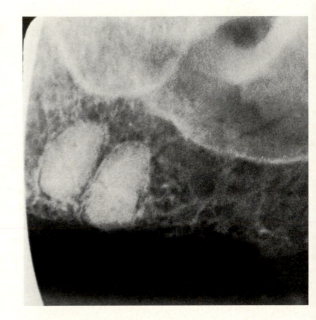

123. This is an example of:
  a. porphyria.
  b. tetracycline staining.
  c. Turner's tooth.
  d. pulpal hemorrhage.
  e. localized fluorosis.

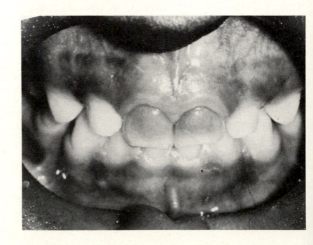

124. Assuming that the radiolucency *(arrow)* at the apex of the lateral incisor tooth is pulpal in origin, which of the following was the *most* likely cause of pulp injury?
   a. dens in dente with a lingual pulpal communication.
   b. Class V caries.
   c. trauma.
   d. infection from the periapical region of the canine tooth.

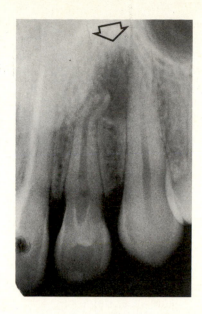

125. The appearance of these teeth is *most* likely attributable to:
   a. tetracycline administration during infancy.
   b. poor oral hygiene.
   c. fluorosis.
   d. severe hypoplasia.
   e. excessive consumption of citric juices.

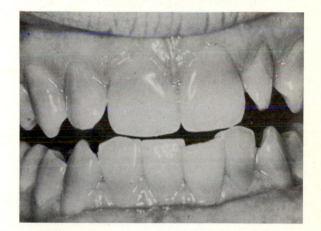

126. The arrow indicates:
   a. a mesiodens.
   b. a paramolar.
   c. transposition.
   d. dilaceration.

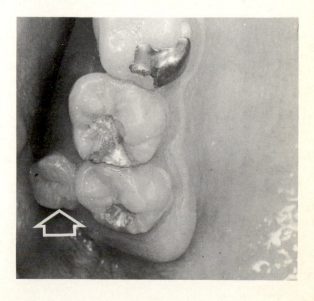

127. The brown staining seen in these teeth is *most* likely a good example of:
  a. tetracycline staining.
  b. extrinsic stain.
  c. porphyria.
  d. fluorosis.
  e. dentinogenesis imperfecta.

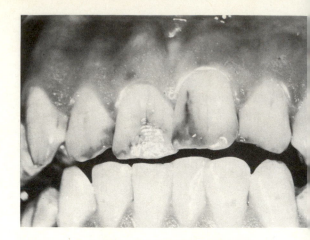

128. The two images indicated by the arrow are *most* likely an example of:
  a. dens in dente.
  b. enamel pearls.
  c. prominent lingual cusps.
  d. areas of enamel hypoplasia.

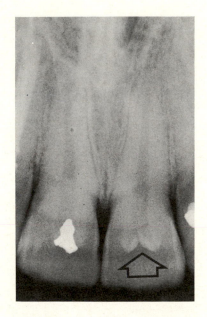

129. The asymptomatic radiopacity between the premolar and molar teeth found during routine examination of a 42-year-old woman is *most* likely:
  a. a cementoma.
  b. condensing osteitis.
  c. a root fragment.
  d. a lingual torus.
  e. a sialolith.

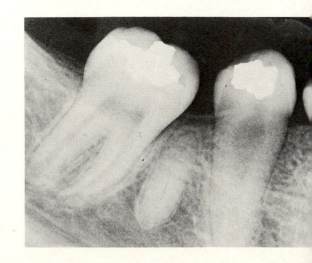

130. The lower left incisor tooth in this 22-year-old male dental student is an example of:
a. fluorosis.
b. Hutchinson's incisor.
c. hypoplasia from systemic disease during infancy.
d. Turner's tooth.
e. tooth mutilation caused by a habit.

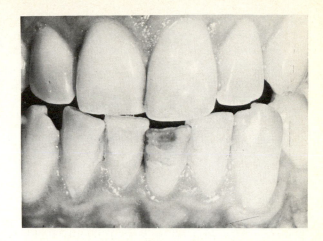

131. This periapical radiograph of a 37-year-old man suggests the presence of:
a. dentinogenesis imperfecta.
b. extensive hypoplasia.
c. Hutchinson's incisors.
d. an anterior open bite.

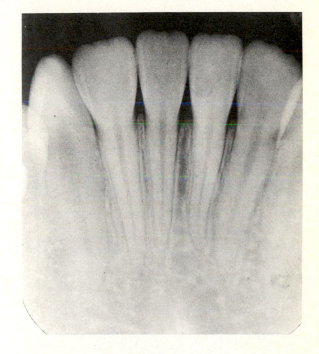

132. These radiopacities were found on routine radiographs of a 52-year-old woman. They *most* likely represent:
a. retained root fragments.
b. socket sclerosis.
c. frequent changes seen in hyperparathyroidism.
d. lesions of fibrous dysplasia.
e. a feature seen in Albright's disease.

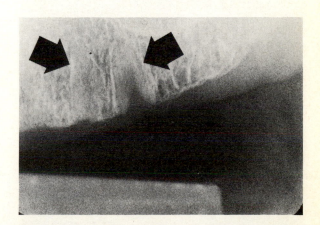

133. The process illustrated here is correctly identified as:
  a. abrasion.
  b. caries.
  c. erosion.
  d. attrition.
  e. a result of poor diet.

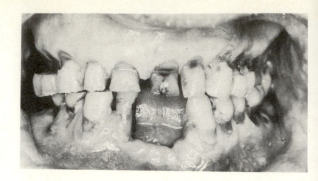

134. The condition shown by the premolar teeth has an increased incidence in:
  a. Paget's disease.
  b. hypoparathyroidism.
  c. hyperparathyroidism.
  e. thalassemia.
  e. sickle cell anemia.

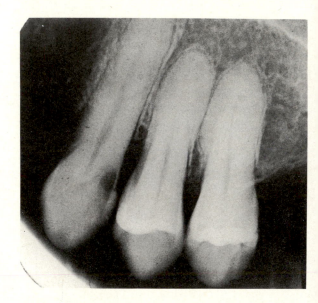

135. This boy (**A** and **B**) is *most* likely suffering from:
  a. cleidocranial dysostosis.
  b. osteogenesis imperfecta.
  c. severe anemia.
  d. rickets.
  e. ectodermal dysplasia.

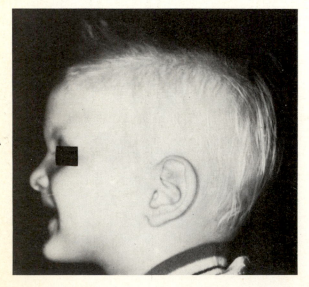

A

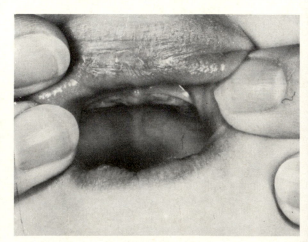

136. The painless radiopaque lesion associated with the crown of the impacted canine tooth in this 20-year-old patient is *most* likely:
a. sclerosed bone.
b. an odontoma.
c. a cementoma.
d. an adenomatoid odontogenic tumor.
e. a calcifying odontogenic cyst.

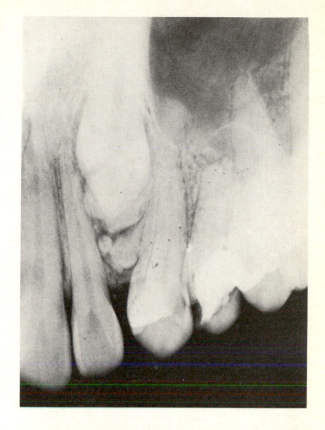

137. A complete examination fails to reveal other significant findings in this patient whose family has been in military service for several generations. As a result of this military background, the family has lived in many places throughout the world. The patient states that this dental problem "runs in the family." This is an example of:
a. dentinogenesis imperfecta.
b. amelogenesis imperfecta.
c. rickets.
d. fluorosis.
e. ectodermal dysplasia.

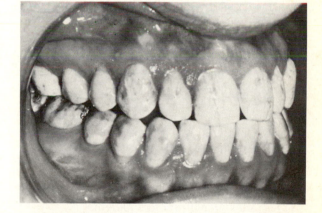

138. The white areas on the labial surfaces of the maxillary central incisors are *most* likely examples of:
a. hypoplasia.
b. hypocalcification.
c. erosion.
d. abrasion.

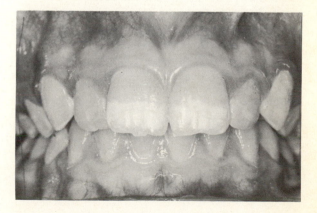

139. This 5-year-old black boy walks with a peculiar gait because his legs are bowed. A skeletal survey reveals that all his bones show a generalized rarefaction. His mother states that he has experienced numerous broken bones, but she describes them as "partial" rather than complete fractures. Radiographs of the teeth show apparently normal pulp chambers. The boy *most* likely has:
   a. fluorosis.
   b. enamel hypoplasia from local causes.
   c. amelogenesis imperfecta.
   d. dentinogenesis imperfecta.
   e. rickets.

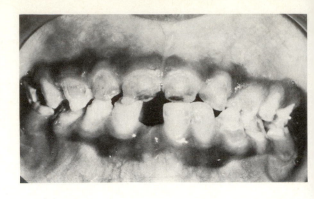

140. This incisor radiograph of a 12-year-old boy that shows the right permanent canine tooth on the extreme right is an example of:
   a. Turner's tooth.
   b. amelogenesis imperfecta.
   c. partial anodontia.
   d. congenital syphilitic teeth.

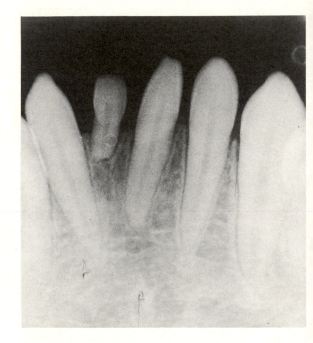

141. It is *most* likely that this patient:
   a. has just had a tooth extracted.
   b. has experienced a long-standing malalignment of the teeth.
   c. has a fractured mandible.
   d. is taking dicumarol.
   e. has none of the above.

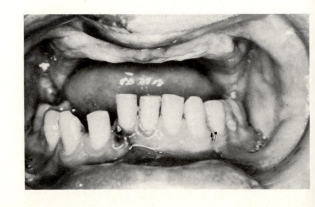

142. The molar tooth indicated by the arrow is an example of:
   a. taurodontism.
   b. fusion.
   c. a mulberry molar.
   d. hypercementosis.

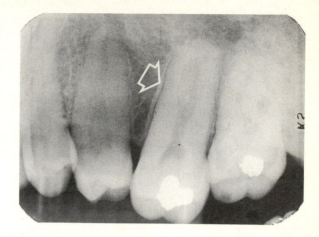

143. This adult patient *most* likely has:
   a. enamel hypoplasia.
   b. acquired deformities caused by a habit.
   c. Hutchinson's incisors.
   d. heavy occlusal wear caused by a peculiar masticatory pattern.
   e. fractured incisor edges as a result of an accident.

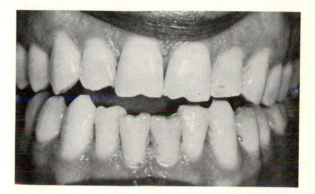

144. The maxillary left lateral tooth *(arrow)* shows an example of:
   a. dens in dente.
   b. Hutchinson's incisor.
   c. supernumerary tooth.
   d. talon cusp.

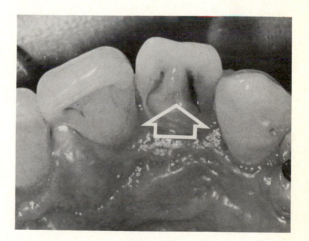

145. The spherical radiopacity indicated by the arrow does not change position significantly when subjected to the shift-shot technique. This radiopacity is *most* likely:
   a. a sialolith.
   b. a pulp stone.
   c. a buccal restoration.
   d. an enamel pearl.
   e. a buckshot pellet.

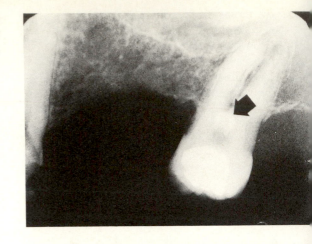

146. This clinical picture **(A)** and bite-wing film **(B)** are of a 14-year-old boy. This condition is:
   a. dentinogenesis imperfecta.
   b. amelogenesis imperfecta.
   c. due to irradiation in the developing years.
   d. an example of severe chemical erosion.

A

B

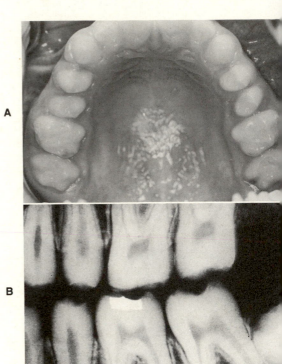

147. The upper central incisor teeth in this patient are examples of:
   a. Hutchinson's incisors.
   b. Turner's tooth.
   c. notching caused by a habit.
   d. attrition.
   e. micrognathia.

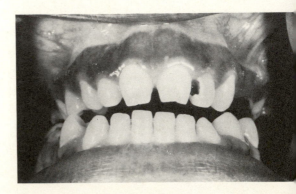

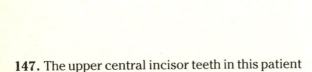

148. Only the labial surfaces of the anterior maxillary and mandibular teeth are affected as shown in this 55-year-old man. The condition is *most* likely:
a. abrasion.
b. enamel hypoplasia.
c. enamel hypocalcification.
d. attrition.

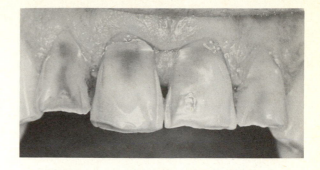

149. This periapical radiograph shows an excellent example of:
a. concrescence.
b. dilaceration.
c. twinning.
d. a mucosal cyst of the maxillary sinus.
e. micrognathia.

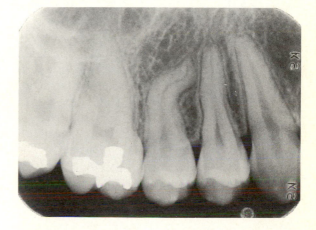

150. This 38-year-old woman has blue sclera. The condition that may be associated with this finding is:
a. dentinogenesis imperfecta.
b. amelogenesis imperfecta.
c. cleidocranial dysostosis.
d. ectodermal dysplasia.

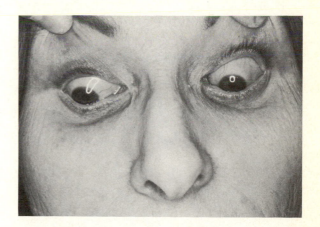

151. A. All the following findings may be seen in this radiograph *except* one:
   a. the fractured incisal edge of the left central incisor.
   b. a supernumerary tooth.
   c. a Hutchinson's tooth.
   d. the composite restoration in the distal aspect of the left lateral incisor.
   e. the midline suture of the maxilla.

   B. If shifts shots are done in an effort to determine the location of the supernumerary tooth, which *one* of the following is correct?
   a. If the supernumerary tooth moves in the same direction as the tube, the tooth is lingual to the central incisor.
   b. If the supernumerary tooth moves in the opposite direction to that of the tube, the tooth is lingual to the central incisor.
   c. If the supernumerary tooth fails to move, it is on the labial aspect.
   d. If the supernumerary tooth fails to move, it is on the lingual aspect.
   e. The maxillary occlusal radiograph will indicate exactly where the supernumerary tooth is.

152. The radiopacity indicated by the arrow is *most* likely:
   a. a cementoma.
   b. a root fragment.
   c. an exostosis.
   d. idiopathic osteosclerosis (enostosis).
   e. an odontoma.

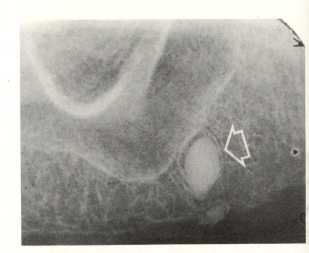

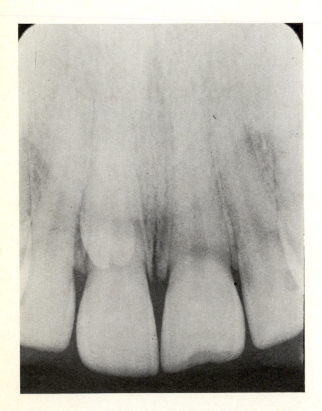

153. This 13-year-old boy (**A** and **B**) *most* likely has:

a. occlusal caries only.
b. Turner's teeth.
c. an acute alveolar abscess.
d. a pulp polyp (hyperplastic pulpitis).
e. gemination.

154. These pictures are of the dentition of a 21-year-old woman. Notice the lack of luster as well as the lack of detail in the teeth shown in the anterior view (**A**). In the palatal view (**B**) notice that the most extensive loss of tooth tissue is on the lingual surfaces of the six anterior teeth. This condition is *most* likely an example of:

a. toothbrush abrasion.
b. amelogenesis imperfecta.
c. bruxism.
d. bulimia.

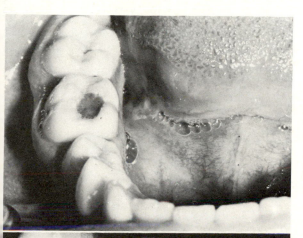
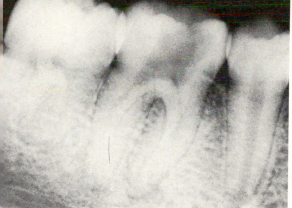

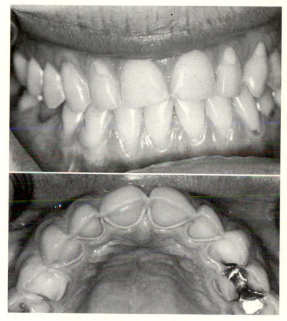

A

B

155. The lesion indicated by the arrow at the cervical line of the maxillary second premolar tooth is *most* likely caused by:
a. decay.
b. chemical erosion.
c. mechanical abrasion.
d. attrition.
e. hypoplasia.

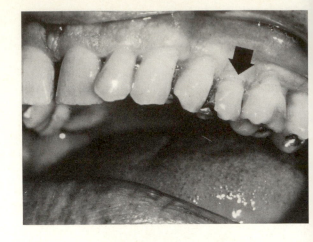

156. This tooth with a porcelain-fused-to-metal crown was finally extracted after the patient complained of pain on biting. Heat applications did not cause pain. The cause of failure is *most* likely:
a. periapical pericementitis.
b. periapical abscess.
c. poor marginal adaptation.
d. tooth fracture.

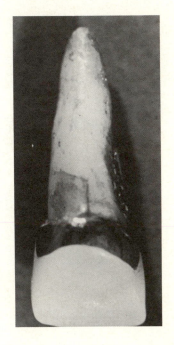

157. This radiograph illustrates a good example of:
a. mulberry molar.
b. dentinogenesis imperfecta.
c. macrodontia.
d. concrescence.
e. a complex odontoma.

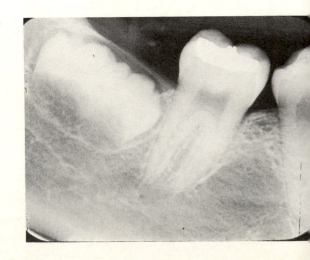

158. The color of this reddish incisor tooth is *most* likely produced by:
   a. blood pigments.
   b. internal resorption.
   c. porphyria.
   d. tetracycline.
   e. extrinsic stain.

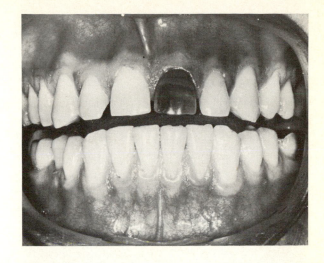

159. This pathologic condition is *most* likely caused by:
   a. severe illness during infancy.
   b. porphyria.
   c. amelogenesis imperfecta.
   d. chemical erosion.
   e. localized insult during infancy.

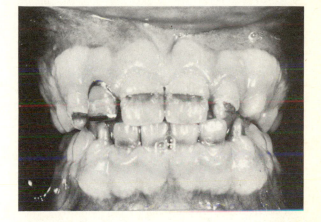

160. The tooth marked *9* is the left lateral incisor, whose distal surface is in contact with the mesial aspect of the permanent left central incisor. This case is *most* likely an example of:
   a. transposition.
   b. mesiodens.
   c. marked hypoplasia.
   d. Hutchinson's incisor.

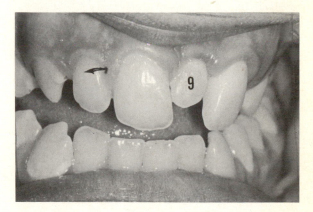

161. The dark lines running horizontally across the crowns of the lower incisor teeth are *most* likely:
   a. an artifact.
   b. caused by congenital syphilis.
   c. indications of a familial disease.
   d. associated with Turner's teeth.
   e. caused by serious systemic illness during infancy.

162. This case *most* likely illustrates:
   a. microdontia.
   b. fusion.
   c. dilaceration.
   d. gemination.
   e. Hutchinson's incisor.

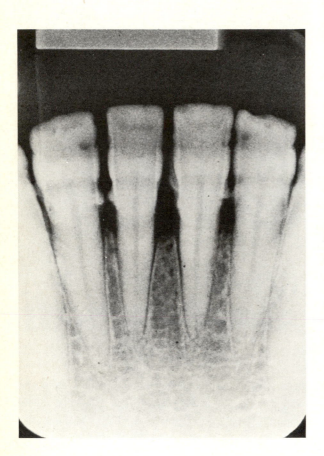

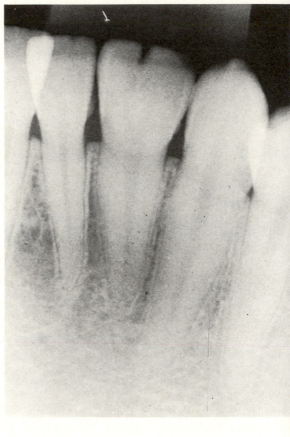

163. This case (**A** and **B**) *most* likely illustrates:
   a. Hutchinson's incisor.
   b. mutilation of a tooth caused by a habit.
   c. fusion.
   d. gemination.
   e. concrescence.

164. The pathology associated with the incisors and the canine tooth is *most* likely the result of:
   a. carious exposure.
   b. deep restoration.
   c. dentinogenesis imperfecta.
   d. dens in dente.
   e. trauma (possibly too rapid orthodontic movement).

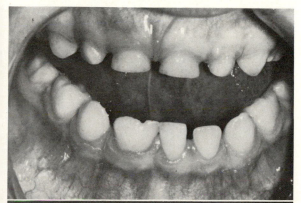

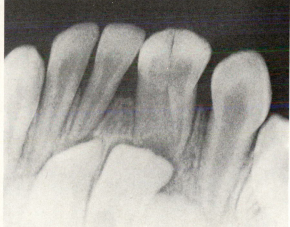

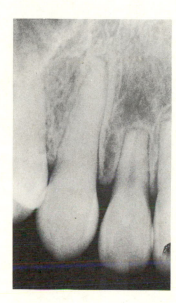

165. The condition associated with the second premolar tooth is called:
  a. micrognathia.
  b. Hutchinson's tooth.
  c. Turner's tooth.
  d. dens in dente.
  e. hypercementosis.

166. This radiograph indicates the presence of:
  a. Class IV periodontics.
  b. supernumerary teeth.
  c. amelogenesis imperfecta.
  d. a severe crossbite.

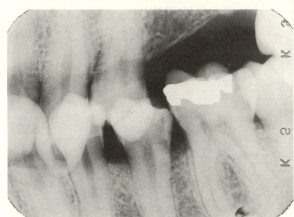

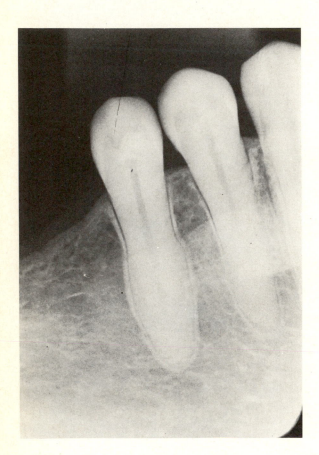

167. This radiograph shows changes in the dentition that you would *most* likely find in an elderly patient who:
   a. drinks a lot of citrus juices.
   b. suffers from gastric regurgitation.
   c. suffers from xerostomia.
   d. has had hyperparathyroidism.
   e. suffers from fluorosis.

168. The entity indicated by the arrow is *most* likely:
   a. osteomyelitis.
   b. a foreign body.
   c. an odontoma.
   d. an antrolith.

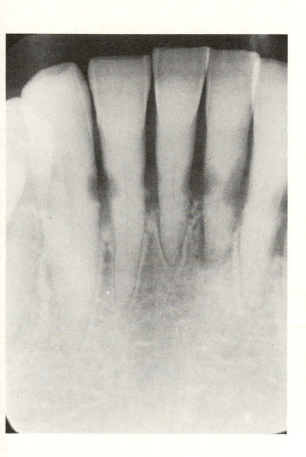

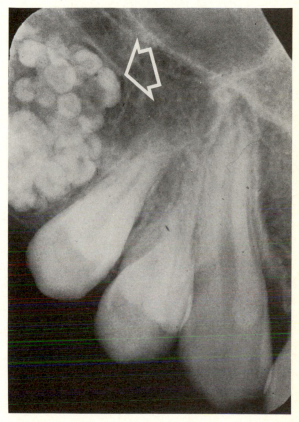

169. The dark area on the facial aspect of the maxillary lateral incisor is quite red and bleeds easily. The exploratory examination reveals that there is continuity of tooth tissue across the superior margins of the red area. This is an example of:

a. gingival hypertrophy.
b. a pulp polyp (hyperplastic pulpitis).
c. erythrodontia.
d. amelogenesis imperfecta.
e. localized porphyria.

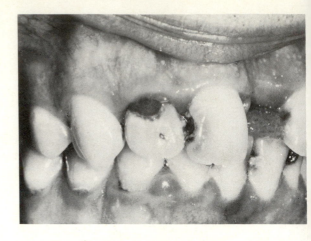

170. The condition associated with the lower molar is referred to as:

a. pulp polyp (hyperplastic pulpitis).
b. an inflammatory hyperplasia of the gingiva.
c. a squamous cell carcinoma.
d. epulis fissurata.
e. dehiscence.

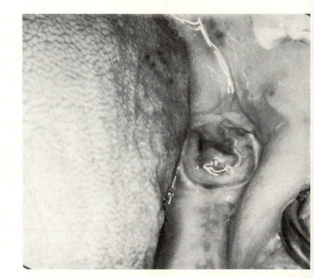

171. If the opposite side of the mouth is similar to what is shown here, one would suspect that the patient has:

a. a bruxism habit.
b. dentinogenesis imperfecta.
c. xerostomia.
d. gastric regurgitation.

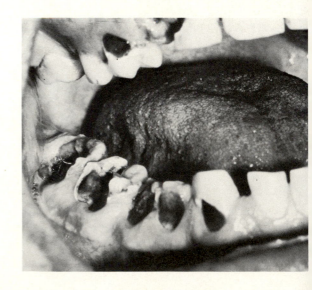

172. The mandibular right second premolar cannot be observed in this radiograph. Which *one* of the following statements is incorrect?
   a. If development is not apparent by this time, we can be sure that the tooth is not going to appear.
   b. The tooth may still develop.
   c. A primordial cyst may develop in its place.
   d. There is room for the second premolar to develop.

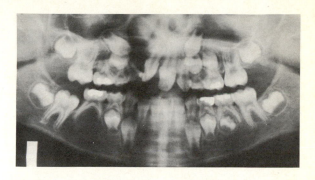

173. What two features are evident in this periapical radiograph?
   a. concrescence and fusion.
   b. concrescence and a missing tooth.
   c. gemination and a missing tooth.
   d. fusion and a missing tooth.

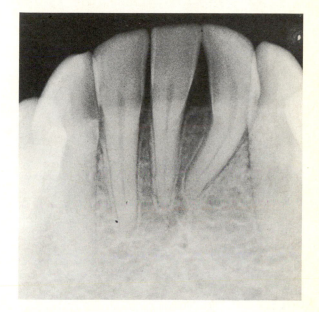

174. This periapical radiograph *most* likely illustrates in association with the left central incisor tooth:
   a. dens in dente.
   b. external resorption.
   c. internal resorption.
   d. metastatic carcinoma to the pulp.
   e. a primary malignant tumor.

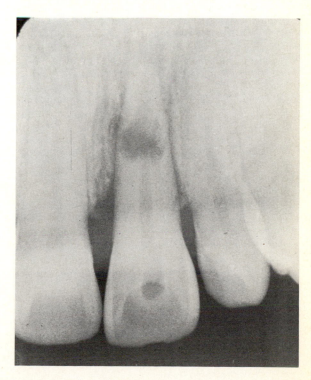

175. An oral surgeon, while removing an impacted maxillary left third molar, saw it suddenly "pop" out of sight. New radiographs (**A** and **B**) show where the tooth lies at present (*arrows*). Where is the tooth?
a. on the palatal side of the ridge.
b. in the maxillary sinus.
c. in the pharynx.
d. just lingual to the condyle.
e. in the infratemporal fossa.

176. The defect shown in this radiograph of the maxillary incisor region of this otherwise healthy 15-year-old boy is *most* likely:
a. congenital in origin.
b. caused by osteomyelitis.
c. traumatic in nature.
d. caused by a pathosis of the nasopalatine duct.
e. caused by a gumma.

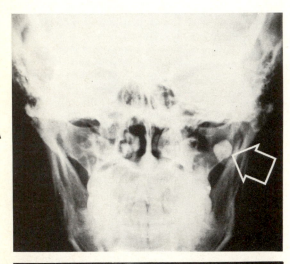

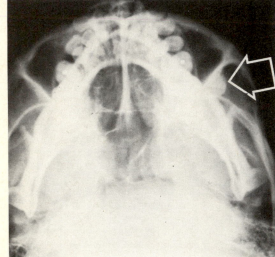

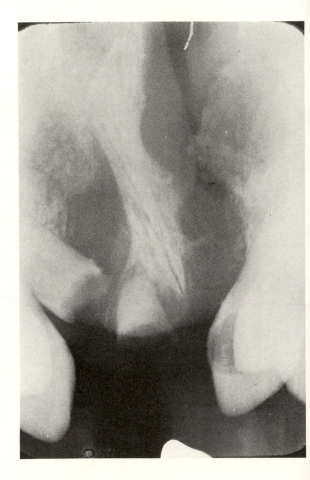

177. This posteroanterior radiograph of a 5-year-old child shows images indicative of:

a. condylar trauma at a very early age.
b. delayed development of the teeth.
c. Paget's disease.
d. osteopetrosis.
e. normal development.

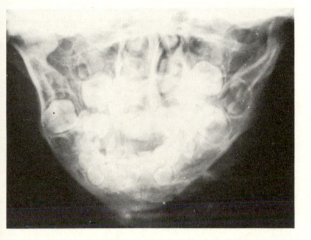

178. A. This radiograph is:

a. a lateral skull view.
b. a lateral oblique view.
c. a Waters' view.
d. a tomograph (laminagram).
e. a posteroanterior view of the temporomandibular joint.

B. The radiograph shows:

a. a normal joint with the condyle in the closed position.
b. a normal joint with the condyle in the open position.
c. osteoarthritis with the condyle in the open position.
d. osteoarthritis with the condyle in the closed position.
e. a fracture of the condyle.

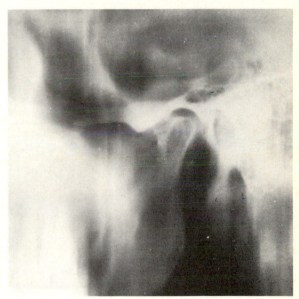

179. This is a microscopic section of a human fetus taken in the frontal plane. Which of the following *most* closely identifies the age of this fetus?
   a. 4 weeks.
   b. 7 weeks.
   c. 10 weeks.
   d. 20 weeks.
   e. 40 weeks.

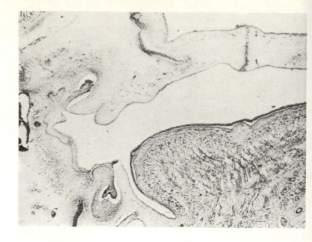

180. This picture demonstrates:
   a. an acquired defect.
   b. a congenital defect.
   c. a papilloma.
   d. a defect that seldom is more extensive.
   e. a defect commonly associated with clubbing of the fingers.

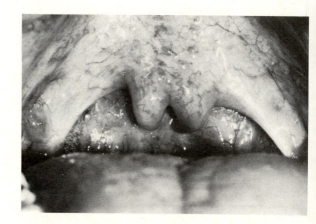

181. Which statement is *most* correct concerning this obvious defect?
   a. It is usually considered to be precancerous.
   b. It is probably congenital.
   c. It is probably iatrogenic.
   d. It usually causes moderate to severe speech defects.
   e. It usually causes a problem in deglutition.

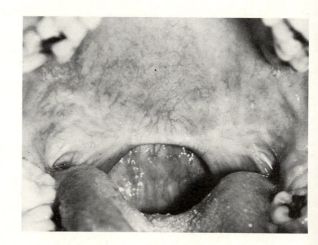

182. A. The obvious facial defect illustrated here results from a malformation that took place in intrauterine life during the:
   a. fifth week.
   b. fifteenth week.
   c. tenth week.
   d. eighth week.
   e. thirty-second week.

   B. The white ligatube seen across the right cheek has been placed in order to hold the tongue forward. The case should be diagnosed as:
   a. bilateral anterior clefts only.
   b. transverse facial cleft.
   c. Down syndrome.
   d. tetralogy of Fallot.
   e. Pierre Robin syndrome.

183. The patient illustrated here has a condition known as:
   a. microglossia.
   b. ankyloglossia.
   c. bifid tongue.
   d. anemia.
   e. avitaminosis.

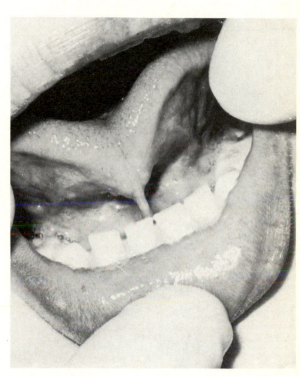

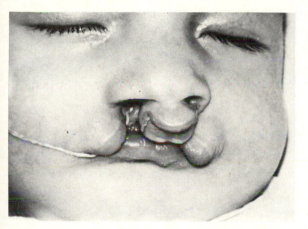

184. From the anterior view of this patient, it is obvious that he:
   a. has a micrognathia of the lower jaw.
   b. is a habitual mouth-breather.
   c. has a flaccid paralysis of the lower lip.
   d. has an abnormally asymmetric face.
   e. has a temporomandibular joint problem on the right side only.

185. The examination modality being demonstrated here is:
   a. percussion.
   b. auscultation.
   c. bilateral palpation.
   d. bimanual palpation.
   e. bidigital palpation.

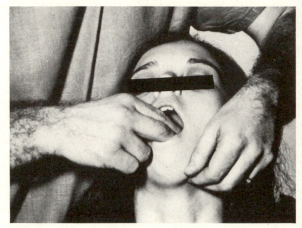

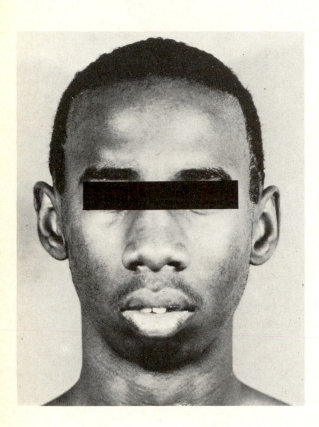

186. This is the examination technique for palpation of:
  a. the masseter muscle.
  b. the medial pterygoid muscle.
  c. the buccinator muscle.
  d. the soft palate.

187. This is the examination technique for the palpation of:
  a. the temporal muscle generally.
  b. the masseter muscle.
  c. the medial pterygoid muscle.
  d. the anteroinferior portion of the temporal muscle near its insertion.

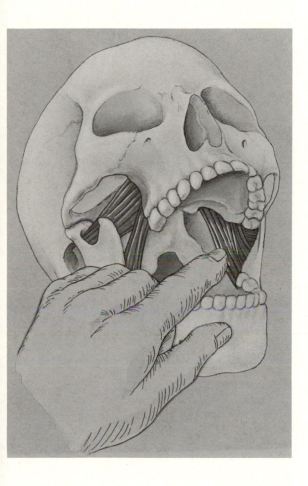

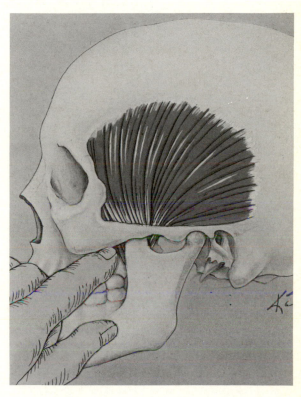

188. This is an attempt to palpate:
  a. the superior constrictor muscle.
  b. the levator palati muscle.
  c. the medial pterygoid muscle.
  d. the lateral pterygoid muscle.

189. The photomicrograph (**B**) is of the small yellowish macules on the mucosa of the upper lip (**A,** *arrow*). The final diagnosis is:
  a. abscess.
  b. Koplik's spots.
  c. xanthomas.
  d. hemosiderin deposits from resolving ecchymosis.
  e. Fordyce's granules.

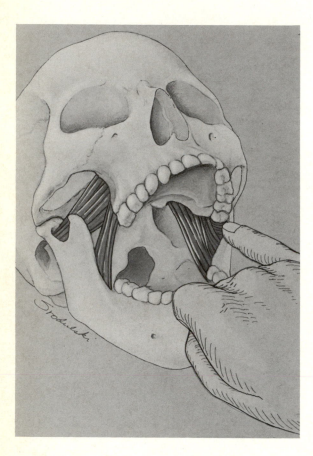

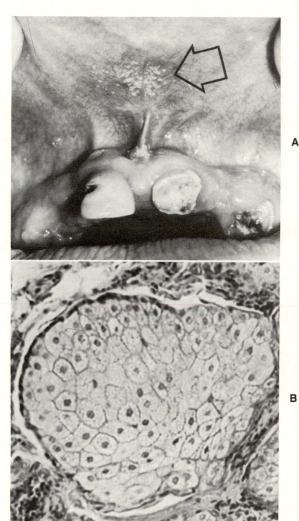

A

B

190. As you examine a 52-year-old patient who smokes 1½ packs of cigarettes per day, you notice this appearance *(arrow)*. Which *one* of the following steps is indicated next?
a. Take a Pap smear of the area.
b. Examine and compare with the opposite side.
c. Perform an incisional biopsy.
d. Make a referral to the proper professional who manages oral tumors.

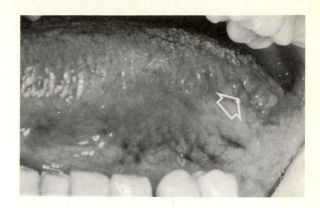

191. This is what you see when you examine the ventral surface of the tongue of a 38-year-old woman. Which *one* of the following is correct?
a. Sublingual varices are present.
b. Ankyloglossia is evident.
c. Geographic tongue is present.
d. The ventral surface appears to be within normal limits.

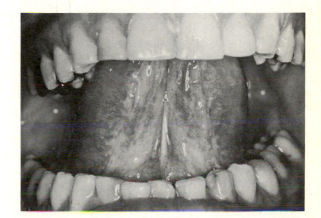

192. The two pits indicated by the arrows are *most* likely:
a. the openings of special salivary gland ducts.
b. draining sinuses.
c. related etiologically to a cleft palate defect.
d. produced by the insertion and pull of the tensor palati muscles.
e. openings of the nasopalatine ducts.

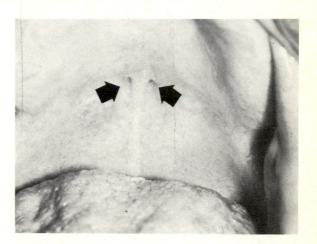

193. This photograph illustrates the basic fact that the attached gingival tissue is usually a paler pink color than the vestibular mucosa. Which *one* of the following statements most completely describes the microscopic structural reason for this difference?
a. The attached gingiva has a thicker keratin layer as well as less vascularity.
b. The attached gingiva has a thinner keratin layer as well as less vascularity.
c. The attached gingiva has a thicker keratin layer but a richer vascularity.
d. The vestibular mucosa functions as lining mucosa rather than as masticatory mucosa; therefore, it has less vascularity.
e. The blood supply of the attached gingiva is just as generous as that of the vestibular mucosa; therefore, the difference in color is attributable only to a thicker layer of keratin on the attached gingiva.

194. The defect illustrated in this 62-year-old man who has been asked to protrude his tongue is *most* likely produced by:
a. an ankylosis of the left temporomandibular joint.
b. a carcinoma in the right side of the floor of the mouth.
c. premature loss of the teeth on the left side of the mandible.
d. a cerebrovascular accident that has affected the facial nerve on the right side.

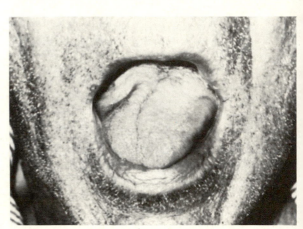

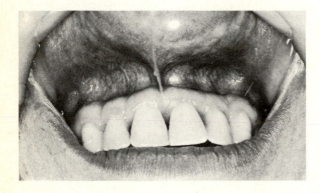

195. This type of scar should suggest the likelihood that this patient has experienced:
a. a radical neck dissection.
b. a thyroidectomy.
c. an emergency tracheotomy.
d. parathyroidectomy.
e. an excision of a sebaceous cyst in the lateral cervical region.

196. This 14-year-old boy has been in an automobile accident and has received a severe blow to the chin. The *most* likely item of severe trauma is:
a. a fracture of the condyle.
b. a tongue laceration.
c. a fracture of the symphysis region.
d. a fracture of the articular fossa.

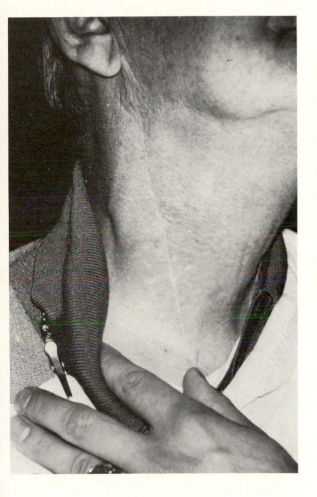

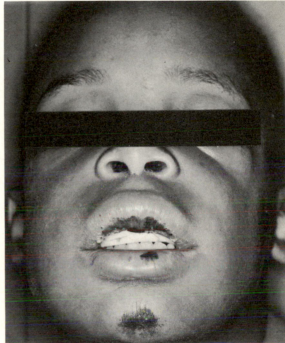

197. On seeing this appliance in place, one may assume that:
   a. a fracture of the jaws is being treated.
   b. maxillary central incisors have been implanted.
   c. an appliance is being used to rotate the maxillary central incisor.
   d. a Caldwell-Luc procedure has been done on the maxillary sinus.

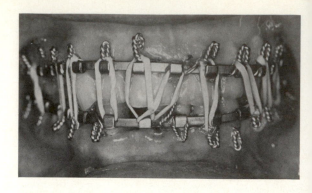

198. The radiolucency indicated by the arrow is *most* likely:
   a. the oropharyngeal airway.
   b. the nasopharyngeal airway.
   c. a fracture of the jaw.
   d. a developmental defect.

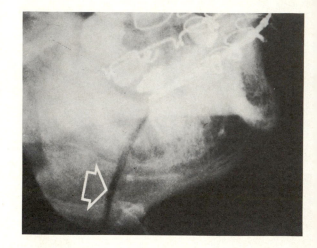

199. When a patient has this appearance, you should be alert to the additional possibility of:
   a. multiple supernumerary teeth.
   b. candidiasis.
   c. hemangiomas.
   d. jaw cysts.
   e. café au lait spots.

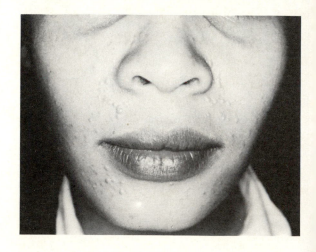

200. A. The patient states that this painful mass has been present for at least 4 weeks. It fluctuates in size and painfulness during the day. Gustatory stimuli seem to make the problem more severe. The diagnosis *most* likely is:

a. space abscess of odontogenic origin.
b. parotid tumor.
c. infected sebaceous cyst.
d. blockage of Stensen's duct.
e. ameloblastoma.

B. All except which *one* of the following steps would be suitable at this point in the workup?

a. Attempt to milk Stensen's duct.
b. Take a panoramic radiograph.
c. Immediately take a sialogram.
d. Take a periapical film of the cheek.
e. If there is purulent drainage, obtain a specimen for culture and sensitivity tests.

201. This bluish lesion (**A,** *arrow*) was found during routine examination of a 47-year-old woman. The microscopic appearance of the lesion is shown in **B.** The final diagnosis is:

a. melanoma.
b. basal cell carcinoma.
c. seborrheic keratosis.
d. nevus.
e. squamous cell carcinoma.

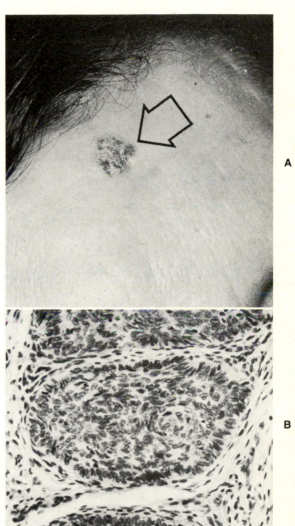

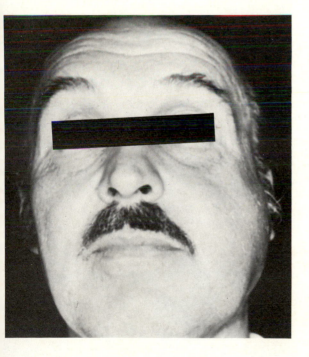

202. This patient denies experiencing recent trauma. She states that this painful swelling began 2 days ago and that it is rapidly growing worse.

A. The working diagnosis is *most* likely:
   a. odontogenic space abscess from maxillary anterior tooth.
   b. odontogenic space abscess from maxillary posterior tooth.
   c. odontogenic space abscess from mandibular anterior tooth.
   d. infected dermoid cyst.
   e. hemangioma.

B. The most dread complication that could occur if this problem is not treated aggressively is:
   a. loss of vision in the left eye.
   b. cavernous sinus thrombosis.
   c. breakdown of the overlying skin.
   d. loss of the causative tooth.
   e. an acute maxillary sinusitis.

C. All the following steps would be suitable except one:
   a. Hospitalize the patient.
   b. Commence high dosages of penicillin immediately if the patient is not allergic to it.
   c. Order a 2-hour postprandial blood glucose test.
   d. Incise and drain the lesion intraorally, provided that the cause is odontogenic.
   e. Wait until the culture and sensitivity test results are known before you begin antibiotics.

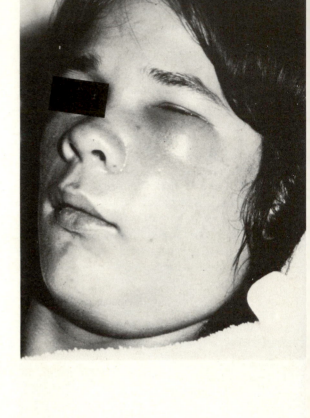

203. This young boy had some dental work done for the first time 2 days previously on the lower right arch. The next morning his mother telephoned the dental office to complain of these painful lesions on the boy's tongue and lower right lip, which were not present prior to the dental appointment. The pain became much less on the following day, and the lesions had completely healed by the fifth day. The lesions were *most* likely:
   a. herpes simplex lesions.
   b. herpes zoster lesions.
   c. allergic manifestations.
   d. traumatic in nature (the boy chewed his tissues while the local anesthetic was in effect).
   e. herpangina.

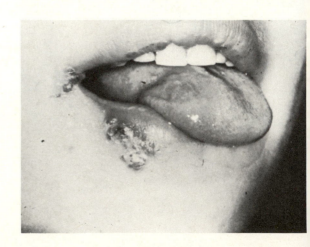

204. This patient complains of a peculiar stiffness in the right side of her face after you have completed some restorations on the mandibular right quadrant. When you ask her to smile, she looks like this. She appeared quite normal prior to the appointment. This patient *most* likely has experienced:

a. a dislocation or subluxation of the right temporomandibular joint.
b. a sudden onset of idiopathic Bell's palsy.
c. a second division block.
d. the injection of local anesthetic solution into the parotid gland region.
e. a cerebrovascular accident.

205. This 34-year-old woman presents to your office complaining of these itching, burning, painful lesions on her face. She tells you that she noticed some itching on her skin about 6 days previously and that soon small blisters appeared. These soon ruptured and became crusted. Her right eye is also involved. This patient *most* likely has:

a. secondary syphilis.
b. herpes simplex.
c. herpes zoster (shingles).
d. erythema multiforme.
e. psoriasis.

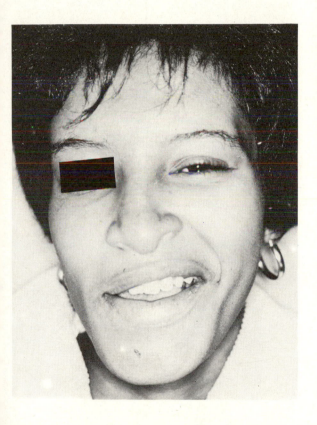

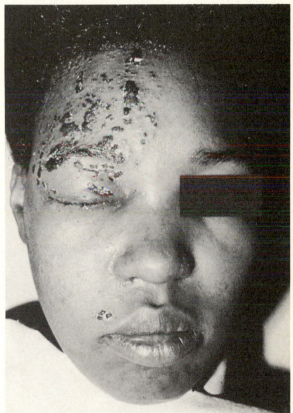

206. This painful, fluctuant mass in front of the ear is *most* likely:

a. a sialadenitis of the parotid.
b. an infected sebaceous cyst.
c. an infected branchial cyst.
d. a parotid tumor.
e. a hemangioma.

207. This man woke up one morning with the condition illustrated here. He has experienced a sudden onset of:

a. tic douloureux.
b. Chvostek's sign.
c. jaw dislocation.
d. Bell's palsy.
e. Horner's syndrome.

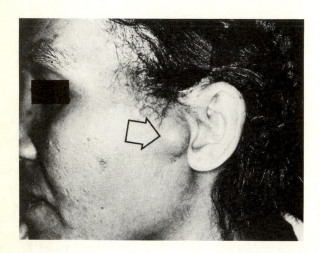

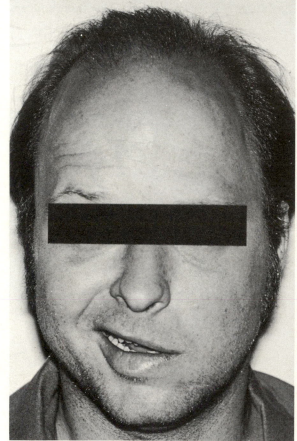

208. This 34-year-old patient presently lives in Chicago, but his company is transferring him to Tennessee. Before he moves permanently, he has to make several trips to Tennessee. Each time he prepares to leave, he finds that his face swells up (as illustrated here) over the eyes and the upper lip on the left side. A careful clinical examination yields no other problems. The swellings are painless but demonstrate pitting edema. This patient is *most* likely showing signs of:

a. electrolyte imbalance.
b. angioneurotic edema.
c. skin abscess from a diabetic condition.
d. hypothyroidism.
e. congestive heart failure.

209. The swelling shown in this patient is painless and radiographs fail to reveal bony destruction. This condition is *most* likely:

a. a nasolabial (nasoalveolar) cyst.
b. a vestibular space abscess.
c. a globulomaxillary cyst.
d. an incisive canal cyst.
e. a radicular cyst.

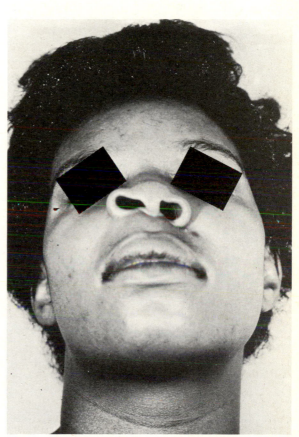

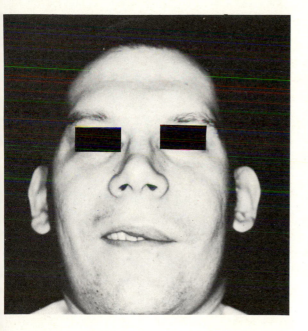

210. This 55-year-old man noticed this lesion, which is partly hidden by the ala, for the first time about 9 months previously. He believes that it is slowly enlarging. The lesion *most* likely is:

a. squamous cell carcinoma.

b. melanoma.

c. basal cell carcinoma.

d. a nevus.

e. seborrheic keratosis.

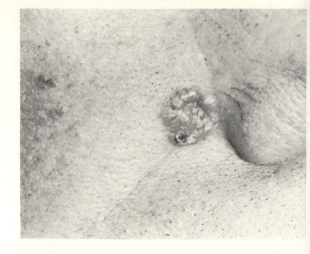

211. This brownish-bluish-black lesion was found during routine examination of a 68-year-old man; it was greasy and crumbly. Small parts of it could be picked off without producing any bleeding. This lesion is *most* likely:

a. seborrheic keratosis.

b. a nevus.

c. melanoma.

d. basal cell carcinoma.

e. squamous cell carcinoma.

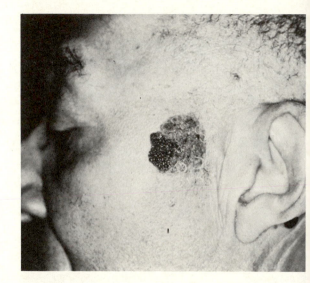

212. This moderately firm, slightly brownish mass was detected during routine examination of a 65-year-old woman who had presented for new dentures. This lesion is *most* likely:

a. seborrheic keratosis.

b. a nevus.

c. melanoma.

d. hemangioma.

e. papular basal cell carcinoma.

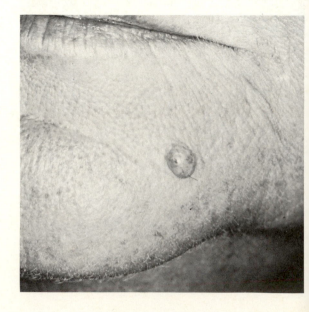

213. This patient is suffering from:
  a. syphilis.
  b. tuberculosis of the nose.
  c. basal cell carcinoma of the nose.
  d. rhinophyma.
  e. squamous cell carcinoma of the nose.

214. A. This painless, solitary lesion on the arm of a 22-year-old man has been present since birth and has remained constant in size. What is the *most* likely diagnosis?
  a. melanoma.
  b. compound nevus.
  c. café au lait spot.
  d. giant hairy nevus.
  B. Which *one* of the following is indicated?
  a. Tell the patient not to worry because it is an innocent lesion.
  b. It should be excised with a suitable margin because a very significant percentage of these lesions become malignant.
  c. Perform a radiographic skeletal survey to check for associated lesions.
  d. Radiograph the jaws to see if there are multiple cysts of the jaws.

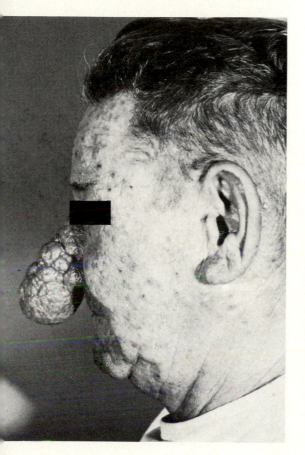

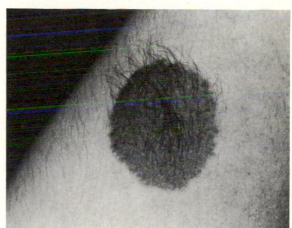

215. According to the patient, this painless, slowly enlarging lesion has been present for 2½ years. The *most* likely diagnosis is:
a. squamous cell carcinoma.
b. traumatic ulcer.
c. basal cell carcinoma.
d. chondrosarcoma (low grade).

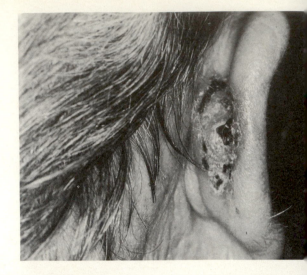

216. This painless, firm mass in the pre- and infra-auricular area has been present for 3 months. The diagnosis is *most* likely:
a. malignant tumor of the parotid gland.
b. benign tumor of the parotid gland.
c. metastatic tumor.
d. sebaceous cyst.

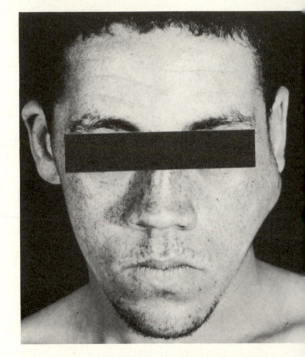

217. You discovered these two firm, painless, freely movable masses on the lateral neck of this healthy 23-year-old woman 6 months ago. Recently you reexamined her, and they are the same. What is the *most* likely diagnosis?
a. lymphomas.
b. two examples of lymphadenitis.
c. two examples of benign lymphoid hyperplasia.
d. sebaceous cysts.

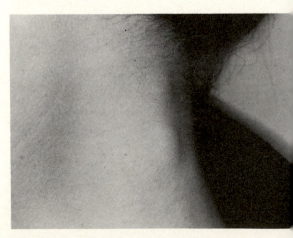

218. Two years previously this 55-year-old man underwent a partial resection of the left side of the tongue. He now presents with a very firm, painless, fixed mass in the left neck. The diagnosis of the neck mass is *most* likely:
a. lymphoma.
b. actinomycosis.
c. metastatic squamous cell carcinoma.
d. a space infection.

219. This 45-year-old man presented with the chief complaint of a painful swelling under the left jaw. He stated that this problem had been bothering him for approximately 4 months and was becoming more severe all the time. It was his impression that the pain became worse during meals. The mass was firm and painful, and the skin could be moved freely over it. The mass is *most* likely:
a. lymphoma.
b. lymphadenitis.
c. an infected sebaceous cyst.
d. a sialadenitis caused by a sialolith.
e. pleomorphic adenoma.

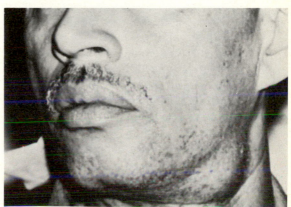

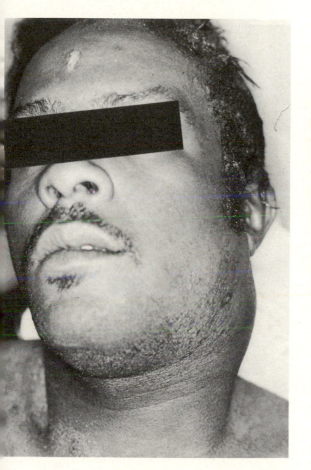

220. This 34-year-old patient presented for treatment of the mass at the inferior border of the mandible. He had noticed the painless mass for the first time about 3 months previously and thought that it was slowly enlarging. The mass was firm and smoothly contoured and was about 3.5 cm in diameter. The skin could be freely moved over it.

A. This mass is *most* likely:

    a. a sebaceous cyst.

    b. lymphadenitis of a cervical node.

    c. pleomorphic adenoma.

    d. sialadenitis.

    e. lymphoma.

B. During the examination, a smaller mass, which the patient was unaware of, was found just inferior to the ear. The mass measured about 1 cm across and was soft, fluctuant, and painless. The mass was fixed to the skin but could be moved freely over the deeper structures. This second mass is *most* likely:

    a. pleomorphic adenoma.

    b. a sebaceous cyst.

    c. a branchial cyst.

    d. benign lymphoid hyperplasia.

    e. a secondary carcinoma.

221. This 55-year-old woman presented with the chief complaint of a dry mouth. An examination revealed tender bilateral parotid swellings that she said had bothered her for a year or so. She also complained of joint pain and burning of the eyes. The parotid swellings in this patient were *most* likely:

    a. a feature of Sjögren's syndrome.

    b. chronic viral parotitis.

    c. sialadenitis secondary to sialoliths.

    d. bilateral pleomorphic adenomas.

    e. a feature of Mikulicz's syndrome.

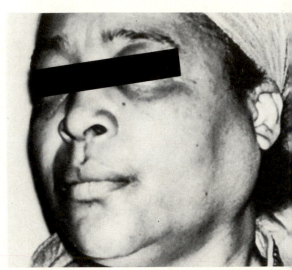

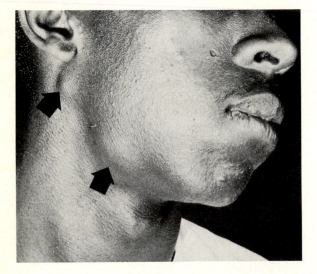

222. This 75-year-old patient presented with this tender mass. She said she had experienced a problem here for about 3 months. When the intraoral examination was being done, it was noted that the mandibular partial denture had not been removed for some months and that there was a tender ulcerated swelling under its lingual border on the right side. The floor of the mouth and neighboring skin were board hard. Clear fluid could be milked from Wharton's duct on that side. The neck lesion was basically firm but contained soft fluctuant regions, some of which were draining to the surface. This patient *most* likely had:

a. an infected sebaceous cyst.
b. an infected lymphoma.
c. a sialadenitis of the submandibular salivary gland.
d. an infected pleomorphic adenoma.
e. actinomycosis.

223. This nontender midline neck mass *(arrows)* was found in this 15-year-old boy during a routine examination. It was doughy in consistency, freely movable in the tissues, and firmly fluctuant. This submental mass is *most* likely:

a. a thyroglossal cyst.
b. benign lymphoid hyperplasia.
c. lymphadenitis.
d. a dermoid cyst.
e. lymphoma.

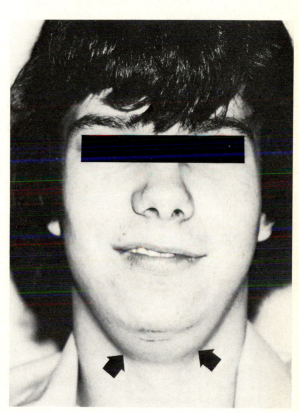

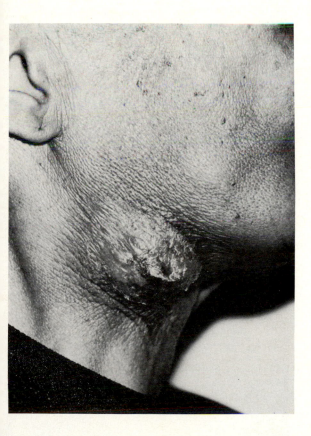

224. This 38-year-old man presented for treatment of this painless, firm, large mass in the region of the left ear. The patient stated that it had been present for at least 1½ years and was slowly becoming larger. The skin could be freely moved over the mass, but the mass could not be moved over the deeper structures. This mass is *most* likely:

a. a retrograde bacterial infection of the parotid gland.
b. pleomorphic adenoma.
c. a fibrosed sebaceous cyst.
d. chronic sialadenitis of the parotid gland.
e. lymphadenitis.

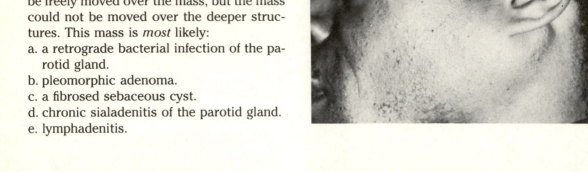

225. This painless mass was found in a 68-year-old man. It was soft and fluctuant and could be moved over the deeper structures, but could not be moved independently of the skin. This mass is *most* likely:

a. a thyroglossal cyst.
b. lymphoma.
c. a sebaceous cyst.
d. benign lymphoid hyperplasia.
e. lipoma.

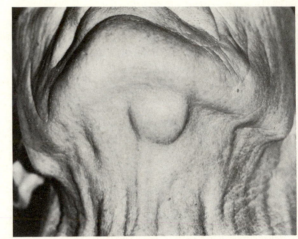

226. This painless, fluctuant mass *(arrow)* had been present for several years. It was soft to rubbery in consistency and elevated when the patient swallowed, and also when he protruded his tongue. The skin could be moved freely over the mass. This mass is *most* likely:

a. a thyroglossal cyst.
b. a dermoid cyst.
c. a thyroid tumor.
d. a branchial cyst.
e. a sebaceous cyst.

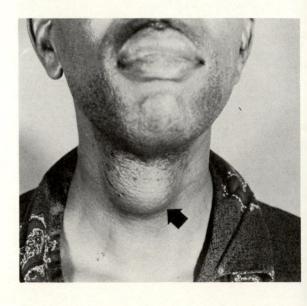

227. This painful, tender midline swelling *(arrow)* in a 12-year-old boy is *most* likely:
a. an infected thyroglossal cyst.
b. sialadenitis.
c. lymphadenitis.
d. a dermoid cyst.
e. benign lymphoid hyperplasia.

228. This long-standing, large, firm, painless mass in the neck of a 55-year-old woman is *most* likely:
a. a thyroglossal cyst.
b. a branchial cyst.
c. a pan-neck infection.
d. a goiter.
e. carcinoma of the thyroid.

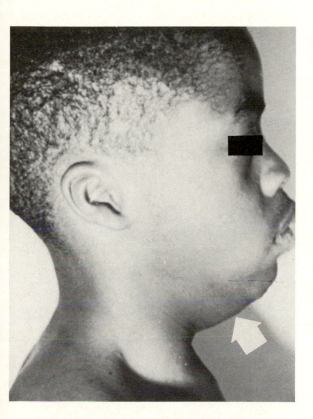

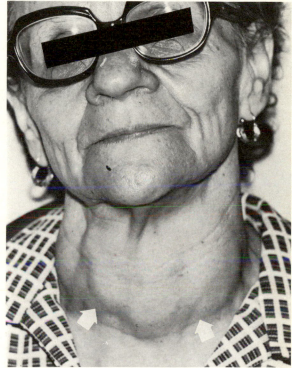

229. This purulent draining lesion *(arrow)* in a man who had received a blow to his jaw 3 weeks previously is *most* likely the sinus opening of:

a. an osteomyelitis.
b. an actinomycosis.
c. a necrotic cervical node.
d. a tubercular infection.
e. an infected branchial cyst.

230. This 35-year-old black man presented with this painful reddish swelling under the tongue **(A)**. The submental and submandibular tissues also demonstrated a very firm type of painful swelling **(B)**. The nostrils were flared and the airway seemed to be partially obstructed. This patient *most* likely has:

a. an anaphylactoid reaction.
b. Ludwig's angina.
c. Vincent's angina.
d. herpangina.
e. actinomycosis.

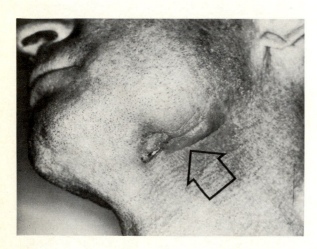

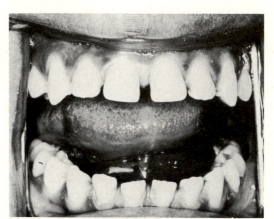

A

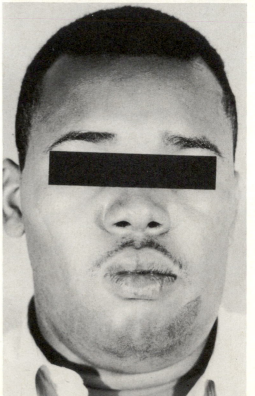

B

231. These two itchy and painful vesicles on the upper lip of this 22-year-old woman have been present for 4 days. The lesions *most* likely are:

a. mucoceles.
b. furuncles.
c. herpes zoster lesions.
d. recurrent herpes simplex lesions.
e. blebs resulting from a burn.

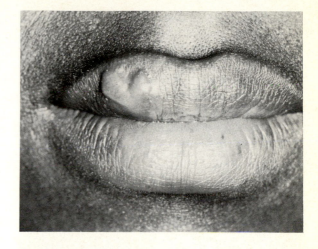

232. This solitary, small, white, painful vesicle on the lip is *most* likely:

a. a herpes simplex lesion.
b. a mucous patch of syphilis.
c. a furuncle.
d. a herpes zoster lesion.
e. a candidal lesion.

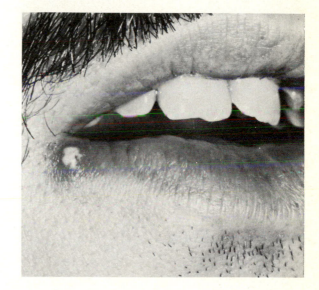

233. This 44-year-old man presented for diagnosis and treatment of this solitary, painless lip lesion. He stated that the lesion had been present for about 2 months and had increased in size very rapidly. The remainder of the examination was unremarkable. The patient was lost to follow-up for a while. He was seen again 6 months later and related that the lesion had started to regress shortly after his initial visit. In summary, the lesion completely disappeared without any treatment whatsoever. The lesion is *most* likely:

a. squamous cell carcinoma.
b. keratoacanthoma.
c. a persistent traumatic ulcer.
d. a chancre.
e. a gumma.

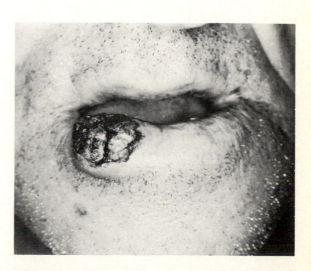

234. During examination, this painless and solitary ulcer was noted on the upper lip. The patient said it had been present for at least a year. This lesion is *most* likely:
   a. squamous cell carcinoma.
   b. a traumatic ulcer.
   c. basal cell carcinoma.
   d. a recurrent herpetic lesion.
   e. a chancre.

235. This 65-year-old farmer presented for examination and treatment of this lip lesion (**A**). He said he noticed it first about 6 months previously and that it was painless, but that it had steadily increased in size. The findings from the remainder of the examination were noncontributory. **B** shows the microscopic anatomy of the lesion. The final diagnosis is:
   a. basal cell carcinoma.
   b. chancre.
   c. squamous cell carcinoma.
   d. traumatic ulcer.
   e. keratoacanthoma.

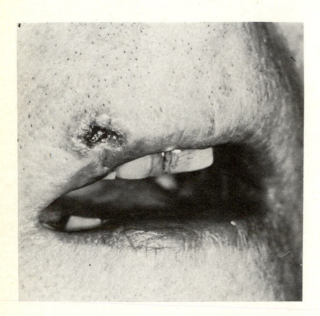

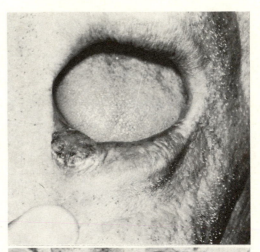

A

B

236. This painful vesiculoulcerative lesion at the angle of the mouth in this 23-year-old man is *most* likely:
a. a recurrent aphthous lesion.
b. a herpes simplex lesion.
c. a herpes zoster lesion.
d. caused by a burn.
e. a chancre.

237. A dentist had been following this bluish-black macule on the lip for the last 2 years in this 15-year-old white boy. The macule was solitary and painless and did not blanch on pressure. This macule is *most* likely:
a. a petechia.
b. a telangiectatic lesion.
c. an amalgam tattoo.
d. a hematoma.
e. a melanotic macule of the lower lip.

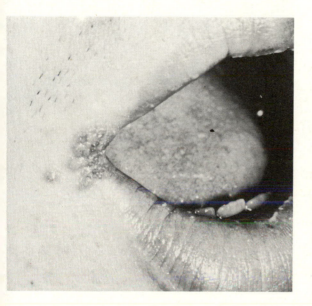

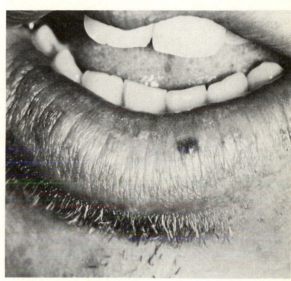

238. This 42-year-old man presented for diagnosis and treatment of this solitary, painful, ulcerated lesion of the lower lip of 2 weeks' duration. He denied using tobacco and alcohol, and although he had been born and raised on a farm, he had been working indoors for the last 20 years of his life.

  A. This lesion is *most* likely:
  - a. a traumatic ulcer.
  - b. a recurrent herpetic lesion.
  - c. squamous cell carcinoma.
  - d. keratoacanthoma.
  - e. a chancre.

  B. The best approach to this lesion would be to:
  - a. culture it.
  - b. excise the ulcer and submit it for microscopic study.
  - c. use intralesional injections of corticosteroids.
  - d. work the patient up for the presence of systemic disease.
  - e. advise the patient to lubricate continually with Vaseline and reexamine in 2 weeks.

239. This asymptomatic lesion detected on the lip of a 65-year-old farmer is *most* likely:
  - a. keratoacanthoma.
  - b. squamous cell carcinoma.
  - c. basal cell carcinoma.
  - d. related to a vitamin B deficiency.
  - e. a herpes simplex infection.

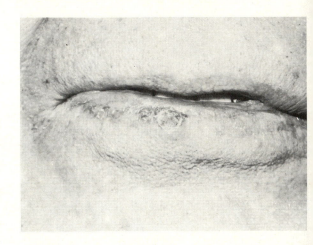

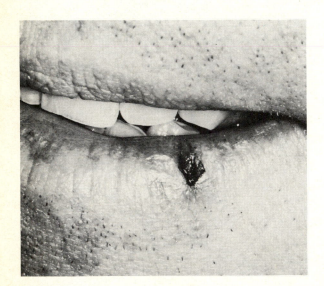

240. This solitary, asymptomatic, pale lesion was noticed on the lip of this patient when he presented for a routine dental examination. The lesion was firmer than the surrounding skin and also had a smoother surface. When questioned about the lesion, the patient related it to an incident some 20 years previously when a dentist burnt his lip with a hot handpiece. The white condition is *most* likely:

a. leukoplakia.
b. scar tissue.
c. a syphilitic rhagade.
d. angular cheilitis.
e. lichen planus.

241. The bilateral reddish areas at the commissures of this woman who smokes heavily are *most* likely:

a. erythroplakia lesions.
b. syphilitic rhagades.
c. traumatic erythemas.
d. angular cheilitis lesions.
e. capillary hemangiomas.

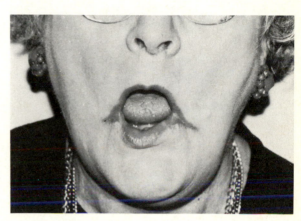

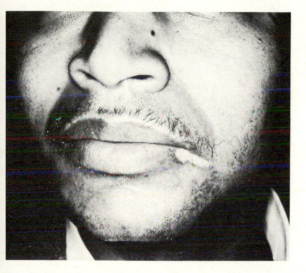

242. A. What is the *most* likely diagnosis of the solitary white lesion indicated by the arrow in **B** in this pipe smoker? It cannot be readily scraped off.
   a. benign leukoplakia.
   b. lichen planus.
   c. candidiasis.
   d. squamous cell carcinoma.
   e. white sponge nevus.
   B. What is the best approach to the management of this lesion?
   a. exfoliative cytology.
   b. incisional biopsy.
   c. excisional biopsy.
   d. have the patient discontinue use of the pipe and reexamine in 2 weeks.
   e. cortisone ointment.

243. A dentist noticed this perioral pigmentation when a mother brought her young child in for a dental examination. The child had experienced some intestinal cramps and melena. This child *most* likely has:
   a. Addison's disease.
   b. Peutz-Jeghers syndrome.
   c. von Recklinghausen's disease.
   d. Albright's syndrome.
   e. hereditary telangiectasia.

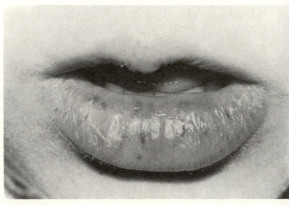

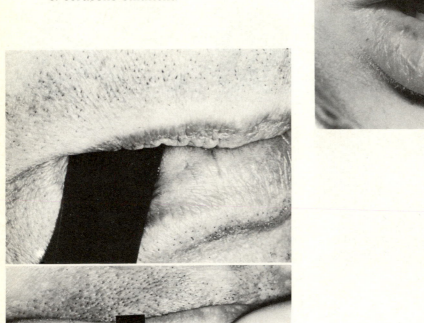

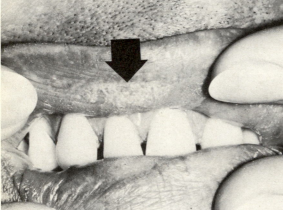

244. These unblanchable, brownish-black macules were found during a routine dental examination of this 54-year-old patient. The patient had enjoyed exceptionally good health until the previous year, when fatigue and malaise were experienced. Lately, the patient recounted experiencing emotional letdowns in difficult situations. No particular gastrointestinal or skeletal problems had been encountered. This patient *most* likely has:
a. Addison's disease.
b. Peutz-Jeghers syndrome.
c. hereditary telangiectasia.
d. Albright's syndrome.
e. secondary melanomas.

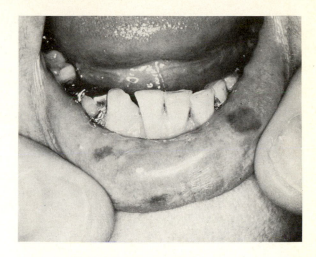

245. The entities indicated by the arrows are *most* likely:
a. syphilitic rhagades.
b. angular cheilosis.
c. bilateral commissural lip pits.
d. accessory salivary gland ducts.

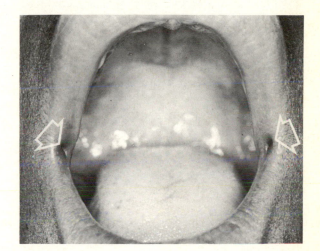

246. A. The lesions at the commissures in this 65-year-old man are *most* likely:
a. syphilitic rhagades.
b. angular cheilosis (perlèche).
c. bilateral squamous cell carcinomas.
d. commissural lip pits.
e. bilateral basal cell carcinoma.
B. Another obvious finding in the picture is:
a. geographic tongue.
b. bald appearance of the tongue.
c. abnormal free-way space.
d. fissured tongue.
e. microglossia.

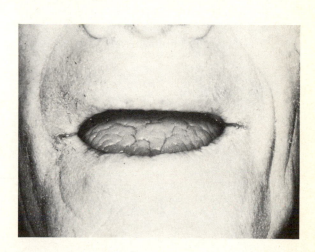

247. These multiple lesions on the lower lip of this 22-year-old man are *most* likely:
a. verrucae.
b. squamous cell carcinomas.
c. mucoceles.
d. fibromas.
e. papular basal cell carcinomas.

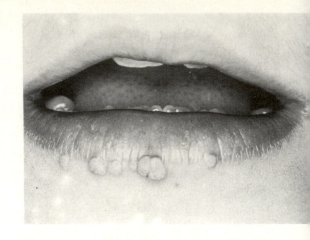

248. These two moderately soft asymptomatic masses *(arrow)* found during a routine dental examination were *most* likely:
a. fibromas.
b. papillomas.
c. pyogenic granulomas.
d. squamous cell carcinomas.
e. the foliate papillae.

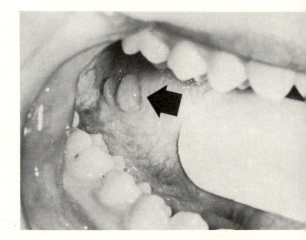

249. This soft, slightly pedunculated mass with a painful surface ulcer *(arrow)* is *most* likely:
a. a pyogenic granuloma.
b. an ulcerated Stensen's papilla.
c. a fibroma.
d. a verrucous carcinoma.
e. a papilloma.

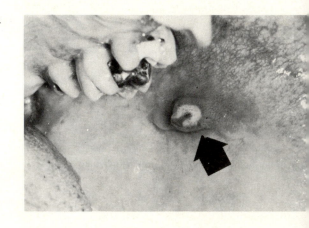

250. This bosselated, very firm, asymptomatic mass was found during routine examination of a 35-year-old woman. Two other similar masses were found on the facial aspect of the dental arches. The mass *most* likely is:
a. exostosis.
b. fibroma.
c. osteogenic sarcoma.
d. lipoma.
e. papilloma.

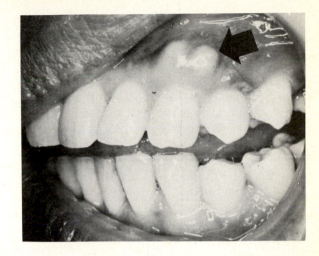

251. These two asymptomatic red areas were found in a 55-year-old man during a periodic dental examination. The patient was unaware of their presence. He admitted to smoking 1 pack of cigarettes per day and to considerable intake of alcohol. He had been under treatment for diabetes during the previous 8 years and had been able to keep it under control so far. The remainder of the examination was unremarkable. These non-tender red areas are *most* likely:
a. areas of erythroplakia.
b. related to trauma from oral sex (traumatic erythemas).
c. atrophic candidiasis.
d. streptococcal inflammatory lesions.
e. within the spectrum of normal appearance for this region.

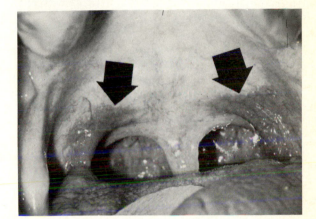

252. This 25-year-old woman informs you that this red-and-white pattern on her tongue changes from week to week. This condition is:
a. erosive lichen planus.
b. an early manifestation of pernicious anemia.
c. migratory glossitis.
d. atrophic and hypertrophic candidiasis.
e. related to avitaminosis B.

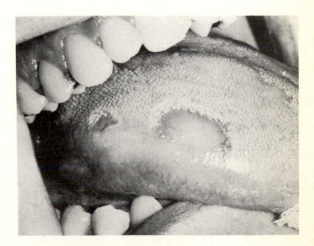

253. This asymptomatic white condition of the dorsal surface of the tongue was found during a routine dental examination. The white material cannot be scraped off.
- A. This condition:
    - a. indicates that the patient is dehydrated.
    - b. is called geographic tongue.
    - c. is called white hairy tongue.
    - d. is called hairy leukoplakia.
    - e. is highly suggestive of anemia.
- B. Correct treatment would be to:
    - a. perform exfoliative cytology.
    - b. perform an incisional biopsy.
    - c. work up the patient for systemic disease.
    - d. use nystatin ointment.
    - e. instruct the patient in proper tongue hygiene.

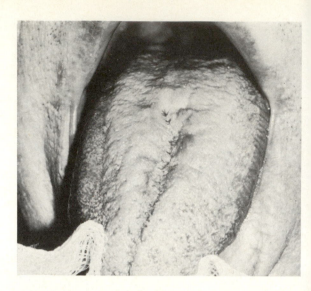

254. You have been looking after the dental needs of this patient for several years. The pinhead black spots have not changed in appearance during this time. This condition is *most* likely:
- a. related to a blood dyscrasia.
- b. related to Addison's disease.
- c. normal pigmentation.
- d. pigmentation related to Peutz-Jeghers syndrome.
- e. caused by an allergy.

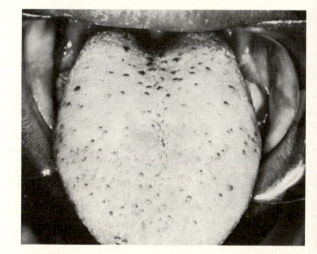

255. This asymptomatic red lesion in a 34-year-old man who smokes and drinks heavily is *most* likely:
- a. erythroplakia.
- b. a capillary hemangioma.
- c. a classic red patch of migratory glossitis.
- d. related to anemia.
- e. median rhomboid glossitis.

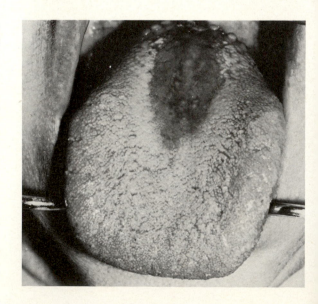

256. This solitary, painless, reddish patch was found on routine examination of a 56-year-old man. When the patient was reexamined after 1 month the area appeared to be the same. Blood studies revealed hyperchromatic macrocytic anemia. This condition is *most* likely:

a. associated with pernicious anemia.
b. geographic tongue.
c. atrophic candidiasis.
d. traumatic erythema.
e. erythroplakia.

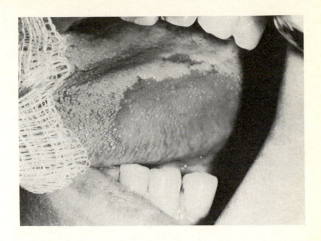

257. This asymptomatic red patch on the dorsal surface of the tongue was seen in a 50-year-old man. Two weeks later, it had changed its shape and was smaller. The diagnosis *most* likely is:

a. changes related to pernicious anemia.
b. geographic tongue.
c. median rhomboid glossitis.
d. erythroplakia.

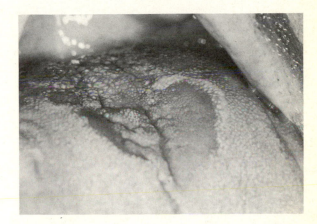

258. This painless condition is known as:

a. fissured tongue.
b. syphilitic glossitis.
c. geographic tongue.
d. lichen planus.

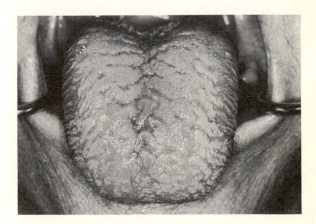

259. The bluish condition of the ventral surface of the tongue of this 73-year-old man is:
   a. most frequently caused by congestive heart failure.
   b. most frequently caused by a tumor in the upper mediastinum.
   c. pathognomonic of Addison's disease.
   d. most likely a harmless condition known as phlebectasia linguae.
   e. a usual feature of the Peutz-Jeghers syndrome.

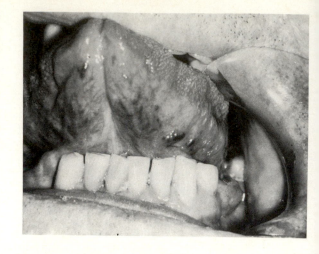

260. This 55-year-old woman complained of lassitude. The painless tongue condition illustrated here is *most* likely:
   a. an atrophic candidal infection.
   b. median rhomboid glossitis.
   c. compatible with pernicious anemia or avitaminosis.
   d. an example of geographic tongue.
   e. related to local chronic trauma.

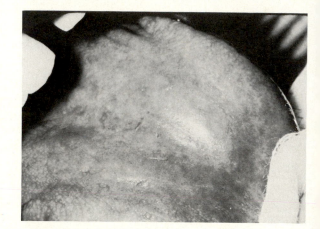

261. This 45-year-old woman presented with the chief complaint of this painful red area of her tongue. She thought it had been present for 6 weeks. The lesion feels soft to palpation, is painful, and blanches somewhat on digital pressure. Tooth No. 29 has a fractured lingual cusp. The solitary lesion is *most* likely:
   a. related to geographic tongue.
   b. a traumatic erythema.
   c. an atrophic candidiasis.
   d. an erythroplakia.
   e. an early sign of anemia.

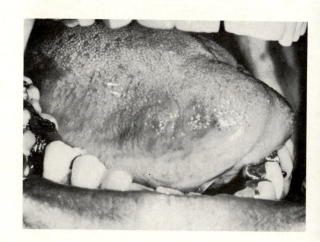

262. The procedure illustrated here is:
  a. an excisional biopsy.
  b. a needle biopsy.
  c. an incisional biopsy.
  d. a toluidine-staining procedure.
  e. an exfoliative cytology.

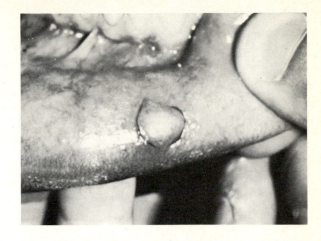

263. This liquid *(arrow)* is *most* likely drainage from:
  a. a buccinator space abscess.
  b. a buccal space abscess.
  c. a retrograde bacterial infection of the parotid gland.
  d. a viral parotitis.
  e. a ruptured epidermoid cyst of the cheek.

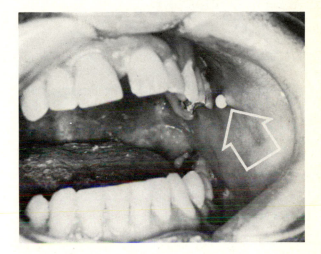

264. This 19-year-old man presents with a complaint of a painful swelling on the ridge just posterior to the second molar tooth with the occlusal amalgam. What is the *most* likely diagnosis?
  a. pericoronitis involving the unerupted third molar tooth.
  b. a deep periodontal pocket distal to the second molar tooth.
  c. an infected dentigerous cyst.
  d. a traumatic neuroma.

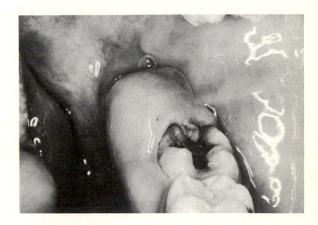

265. The reddish condition of the gums in this 24-year-old woman *most* likely is:
   a. gingivosis.
   b. acute necrotizing ulcerative gingivitis.
   c. marginal gingivitis.
   d. indicative of the presence of leukemia.
   e. medication induced.

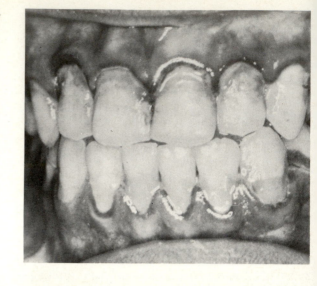

266. This 38-year-old woman presented for treatment of this tender lesion *(arrow),* which she claimed to have noticed for the first time about 1 week previously. The lesion was soft to rubbery in consistency and fluctuant and painful to palpation. The pulps of the teeth in the region tested vital. The mass is *most* likely:
   a. a mucocele.
   b. a lipoma.
   c. a pyogenic granuloma.
   d. a parulis from a draining periapical abscess.
   e. a periodontal abscess.

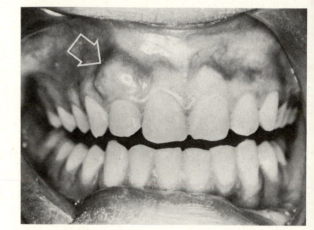

267. The gingival defects seen interproximally in this asymptomatic patient are highly suggestive of:
   a. prior gingivectomy surgery.
   b. leukemic involvement of the gingiva.
   c. active acute necrotizing ulcerative gingivitis (ANUG).
   d. a prior bout with ANUG.

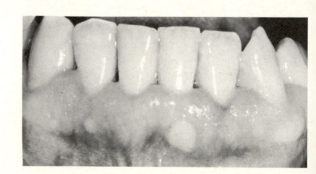

268. The periodontal problem pictured here is:
   a. a gingival pocket.
   b. a McCall's festoon.
   c. a Stillman's cleft.
   d. a gingival fenestration.
   e. a common complication of ANUG.

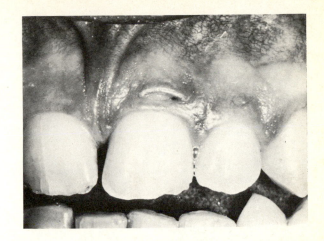

Dr. Alphonse Gargiulo authored questions 269 through 291.

269. This gingival condition was identified 1 week after the patient began brushing with a new brand of toothpaste. The gingival color was fiery red, and the tissue was negative Nikolsky's sign. Cessation of brushing with the new toothpaste resulted in a healthy gingival condition. What is the *most* likely diagnosis?
   a. acute gingivitis.
   b. allergic gingivitis.
   c. periodontitis.
   d. acute periodontitis.
   e. ANUG.

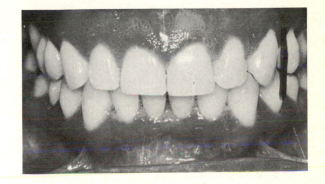

270. A. What type of bone loss pattern is seen in this histologic section?
   a. horizontal.
   b. vertical.
   c. no bone loss; the section represents a healthy anterior dentition.
   d. periapical.
   e. a and b.
   B. In the histologic section, what type of pocket formation is seen?
   a. suprabony.
   b. intrabony.
   c. gingival pockets.
   d. a and b.
   e. all the above.
   C. In the same histologic section, the tooth associated with the widened periodontal ligament space may be due to:
   a. primary occlusal trauma.
   b. secondary occlusal trauma.
   c. periodontal disease.
   d. chronic pulpitis.
   e. none of the above.

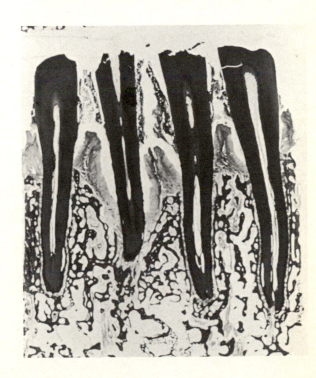

271. A. What tissues can be observed in this histologic section?
   1. dentin.
   2. cementum.
   3. junctional epithelium.
   4. sulcular epithelium.
   5. pulp.
      a. 1.
      b. 1, 2.
      c. 1, 2, 3.
      d. 1, 2, 3, 4.
      e. 1, 2, 3, 4, 5.
   B. What is the calcified mass associated with this root surface?
      a. calculus.
      b. cortical bone.
      c. plaque.
      d. stain.
      e. pulp stone.

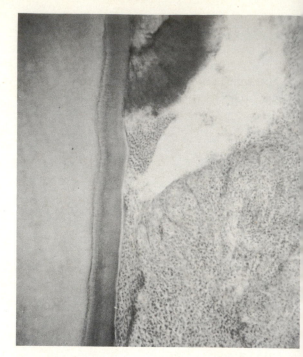

272. What is the clinical term for the condition associated with the lower left canine tooth?
   a. fenestration.
   b. gingival pocket.
   c. dehiscence.
   d. desquamative gingivitis.
   e. toothbrush abrasion.

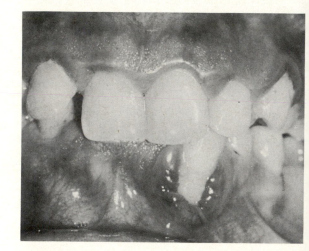

273. This bite-wing x-ray film is representative of a 16-year-old female who upon clinical examination demonstrated gingival pockets, 3 to 4 mm in depth, with bleeding upon gentle probing. What is the American Dental Association classification of the above condition?
   a. Type I.
   b. Type II.
   c. Type III.
   d. Type IV.
   e. juvenile periodontitis.

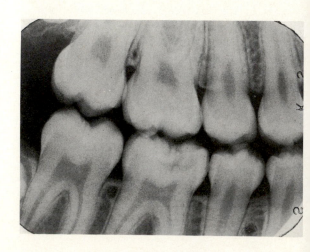

274. This lower right posterior periapical view demonstrates vertical bone loss. Clinically, 6- to 7-mm pockets are found, and Class I mobility on a scale of 0 to 3. What is the American Dental Association classification of this condition?
a. Type I.
b. Type II.
c. Type III.
d. Type IV.
e. juvenile periodontitis.

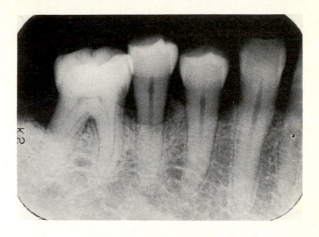

275. This periapical view of the maxillary right first molar demonstrates a bone loss pattern associated with which American Dental Association classification?
a. Type I.
b. Type II.
c. Type III.
d. Type IV.
e. none of the above.

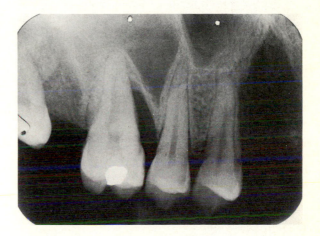

276. This periapical view of the maxillary right molar and premolars is an example of:
a. healthy bone level.
b. vertical bone loss.
c. horizontal bone loss.
d. normal bone height.
e. none of the above.

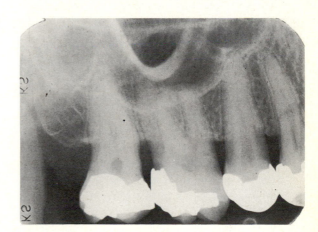

277. What normal radiographic structure is absent in this bite-wing x-ray?
a. lamina dura.
b. crestal lamina dura.
c. alveolar bone.
d. cementoenamel junction.
e. pulp chamber.

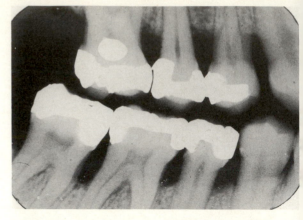

278. A. This 47-year-old woman presented with a chief complaint of loose teeth and bleeding gums **(A)**. A representative periapical film of the lower incisors is seen in **B**. What is your diagnosis?
a. chronic early periodontitis.
b. chronic moderate periodontitis.
c. chronic advanced periodontitis.
d. juvenile periodontitis.
e. ANUG.

B. What is the *most* probable cause of the bone loss associated with the lower anteriors?
a. stain.
b. calculus and microbial plaque.
c. occlusion.
d. toothbrush abrasion.
e. mobility.

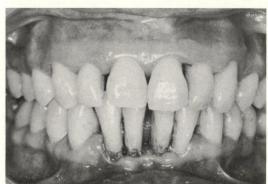

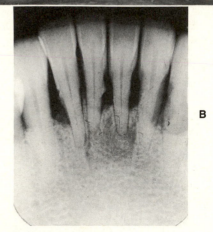

279. This 29-year-old black man is presently medicated with 400 mg of phenytoin (Dilantin) daily for control of epileptic seizures. What is your diagnosis of this gingival condition?
a. Dilantin hyperplasia.
b. familial fibromatosis.
c. gingival hyperplasia.
d. hyperplastic gingivitis.
e. gingivosis.

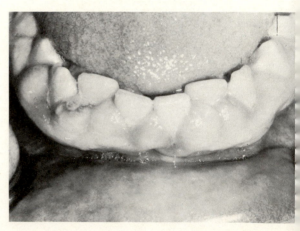

280. This 29-year-old white man presented with acute discomfort, bleeding gums, and bad breath. From this clinical picture, what is your diagnosis?
a. gingivitis.
b. periodontitis.
c. desquamative gingivitis.
d. ANUG.
e. acute gingivitis.

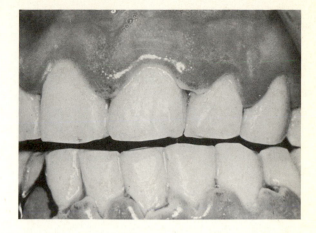

281. The maxillary anterior labial frenum is the probable cause of the loss of papillary gingival height between the maxillary central incisors.
a. true.
b. false.

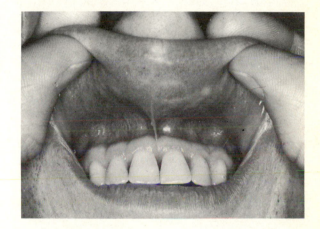

282. What is the defect termed in the buccal cortical bone *(arrow)*?
a. bony fenestration.
b. bony dehiscence.
c. soft tissue fenestration.
d. denuded root.
e. window.

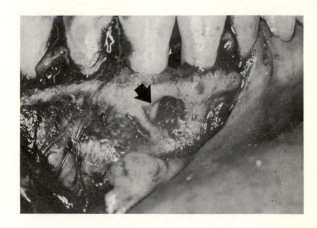

283. These two blunt-ended instruments are used in this manner to measure:
   a. the width of the incisal edge.
   b. the tooth mobility.
   c. the thickness of dentin.
   d. the percussion sensitivity.
   e. all the above.

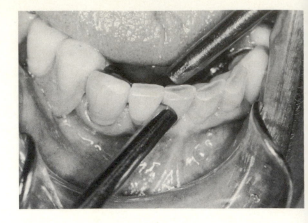

284. This bony defect is best described as an:
   a. intrabony, circumferential defect.
   b. suprabony defect.
   c. intraosseous lesion.
   d. horizontal bone defect.
   e. vertical bone defect.

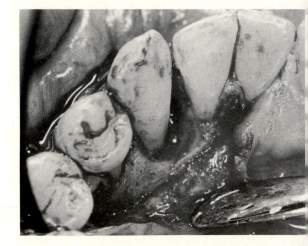

285. Describe the clinical condition in this area of the mouth in this 67-year-old white man.
   a. severe periodontal destruction.
   b. acutely inflamed gingiva.
   c. post–trench mouth.
   d. healthy gingival tissues and recession.
   e. periodontosis.

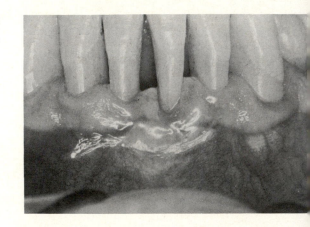

286. This 35-year-old white woman presented with sore and bleeding gums. What is the best term to describe the condition causing the splaying of the anterior teeth?
a. diastemata
b. pathologic migration.
c. buccal version.
d. lingual crossbite.
e. periodontal pocket formation.

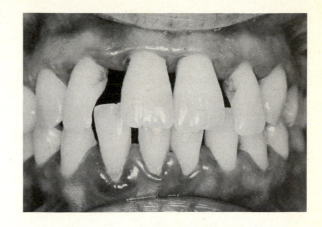

287. The clinical condition of this patient may be best described as:
a. clinically healthy in appearance.
b. juvenile periodontitis.
c. desquamative gingivitis.
d. acute gingivitis.
e. chronic periodontitis.

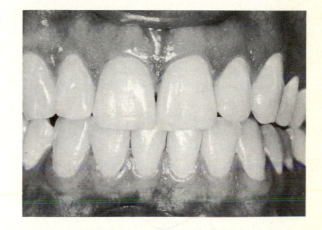

288. This 43-year-old white woman has the following gingival condition: generalized rolled gingival margins, swollen papillary gingiva, and inflamed 3-mm pocket depths that elicit bleeding upon gentle probing. What is your diagnosis?
a. early periodontitis.
b. chronic periodontitis.
c. juvenile periodontitis.
d. desquamative gingivitis.
e. gingivitis.

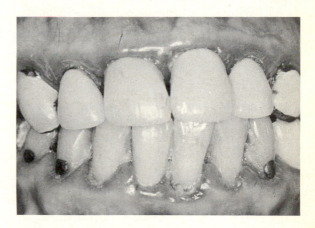

289. This 35-year-old woman has a chief complaint of heavy bleeding while brushing her teeth. Maxillary and mandibular teeth are splayed labially; pocket depths range from 3 mm to 11 mm; and Class II and III mobility is evident. All molar teeth have at least a Grade I furcation involvement. From the above history, what is your diagnosis?
a. advanced periodontitis.
b. localized advanced periodontitis.
c. chronic necrotizing ulcerative periodontitis.
d. juvenile periodontitis.
e. adult periodontitis.

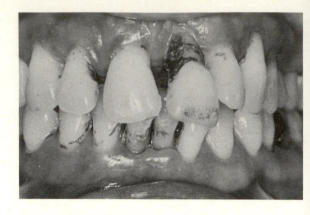

290. This 39-year-old black woman presents with sore, bleeding gums. Clinical examination reveals maxillary and mandibular papillary and marginal gingiva boggy and magenta. Periodontal pocket probing ranges from 3 mm to 7 mm anteriorly and 4 mm to 6 mm posteriorly. Radiographic analysis shows loss of crestal lamina dura and approximately 10% to 25% horizontal bone loss throughout the mouth. The mandibular anteriors demonstrate Class I mobility. What is your diagnosis?
a. chronic gingivitis.
b. chronic adult periodontitis.
c. acute necrotizing ulcerative periodontitis.
d. chronic advanced periodontitis.
e. chronic hyperplastic gingivitis.

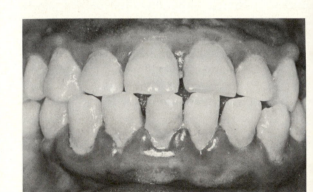

291. What is the etiology of the gingival inflammation seen in this patient?
a. supragingival calculus.
b. bacterial plaque.
c. calculus.
d. calculus and bacterial plaque.
e. none of the above.

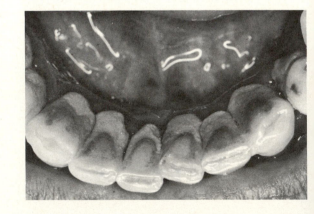

292. This 35-year-old pregnant woman came to the dental office to obtain treatment for this lesion *(arrow)*. The lesion was firm in some areas and softer in others. There was a distal amalgam restoration on the canine tooth, which was overcontoured. The lesion is *most* likely:

a. a papilloma.

b. an osteogenic sarcoma.

c. an inflammatory hyperplasia lesion (pregnancy tumor, pyogenic granuloma).

d. a squamous cell carcinoma.

e. a neurofibroma.

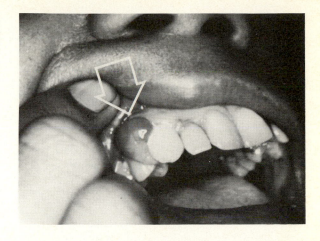

293. This 35-year-old woman presented for treatment of this moderately firm, painless lesion, which she had noticed first about 5 months previously. There was a large carious lesion in the mesial aspect of the left central incisor tooth. Radiographs revealed a few small radiopaque foci within the soft tissue mass. The interseptal bone showed a small, cupped-out defect at the crest. This lesion is *most* likely:

a. a pyogenic granuloma.

b. an inflammatory hyperplasia lesion with calcification (a peripheral odontogenic fibroma).

c. an osteogenic sarcoma.

d. a chondrosarcoma.

e. an exostosis.

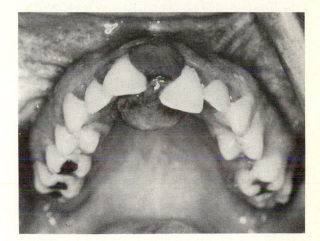

294. Two days after extensive dental procedures were accomplished in this quadrant, the patient experienced burning, tenderness, and pain of the labial gingiva. The correct diagnosis of this ulcerative condition is:

a. allergic mucositis.

b. recurrent aphthous ulceration.

c. traumatic ulceration.

d. a recurrent herpetic lesion.

e. erythema multiforme.

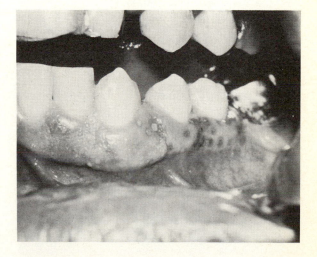

295. This patient is in good health except for the gingival problem. He is likely suffering from:
a. hereditary gingival fibromatosis.
b. phenytoin (Dilantin) gingival hyperplasia.
c. ANUG.
d. mouth-breathing gingivitis.
e. generalized periodontics.

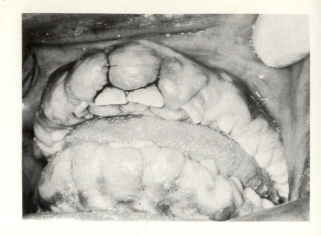

296. This firm, pedunculated, solitary, asymptomatic mass is *most* likely:
a. a papilloma.
b. a pyogenic granuloma.
c. a neurofibroma.
d. a fibroma.
e. an exostosis.

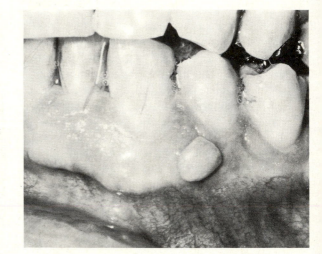

297. A concerned mother brought her 10-year-old daughter for diagnosis and treatment of this solitary, painless pedunculated mass **(A)**. **B** shows the surgical specimen. This lesion is *most* likely:
a. a verrucous carcinoma.
b. a papilloma.
c. a fibroma.
d. a parulis.
e. a pyogenic granuloma.

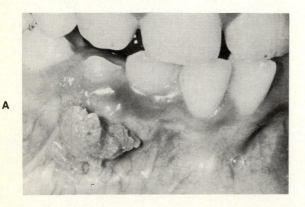

A

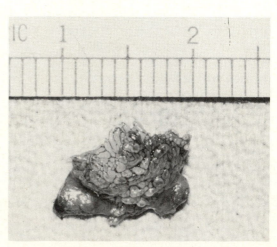

B

298. The yellowish red mass on the gingival surface above the incisor teeth is *most* likely:
   a. an epulis fissurata.
   b. an exostosis.
   c. an abscess.
   d. a lipoma.
   e. a squamous cell carcinoma.

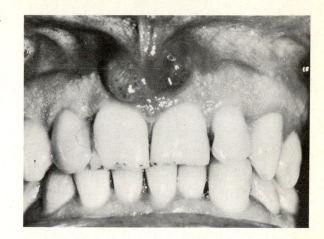

299. This 17-year-old girl presented with a 102°F fever and tender, sore gums of 6 days' duration. Note the vesicles and small ulcers distributed widely over the gingiva. Several of the cervical nodes were enlarged and tender. The diagnosis is *most* likely:
   a. herpangina of the gingiva.
   b. primary herpetic gingivostomatitis.
   c. ANUG.
   d. juvenile periodontitis.

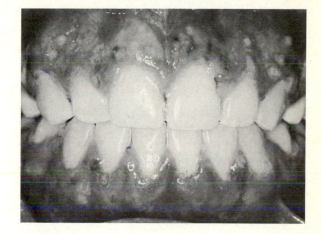

300. This 45-year-old woman presented with a complaint of tender gums. On examination, the appearance in **A** was seen on various places on the gums. This interesting appearance in **B** was seen in the buccal and retromolar areas bilaterally. What is the *most* likely diagnosis?
   a. pemphigus.
   b. ANUG.
   c. lichen planus.
   d. gingivosis.

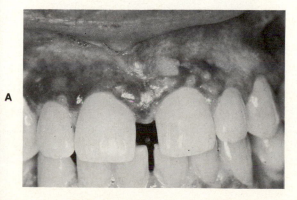

A

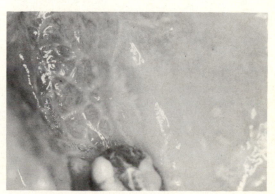

B

301. Worry about this solitary, painless mass **(A)** brought this 35-year-old woman to the dental office. The mass was bluish in color, moderately soft, and blanched somewhat on digital pressure. The patient noticed the mass for the first time about 6 months previously. **B** shows the essential histopathology of the lesion. The final diagnosis of this lesion is:
a. hemangioma.
b. pyogenic granuloma.
c. squamous cell granuloma.
d. giant cell granuloma.

302. This solitary, firm, painless mass **(A)** was found during the examination of a 65-year-old man who was treated for cancer of the large bowel 2 years previously. He stated that he noticed the mass first about 1 month previously and that it is continuing to increase in size at a rapid rate. **B** shows the bony aspect of the lesion. This lesion is *most* likely:
a. a periapical cyst.
b. an exostosis.
c. metastatic carcinoma.
d. osteolytic sarcoma.
e. osteomyelitis.

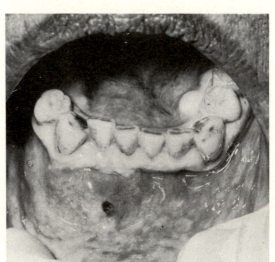

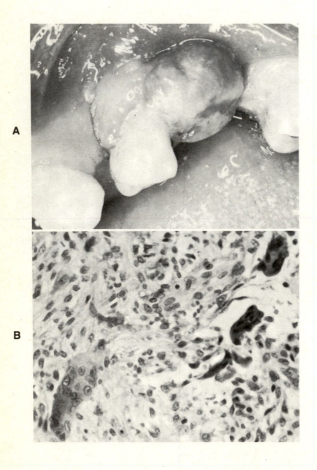

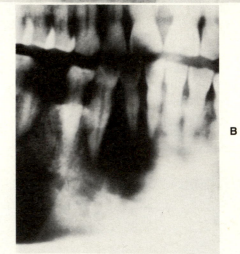

303. A. During routine examination of this 45-year-old black man, a bluish nodular mass *(arrow)* was noticed with two irregularly shaped black macules on either side of it. The nodular mass had a light bluish color and was rubbery and fluctuant, and could not be emptied. Radiographs revealed no bony changes. The patient was unaware of these conditions. The nodular mass is *most* likely:
   a. a mucocele.
   b. a hemangioma.
   c. a gingival abscess.
   d. a gingival cyst.
   e. a parulis.

   B. The two bluish-black macules in the above photo are *most* likely:
   a. indications of Addison's disease.
   b. patches of melanoplakia.
   c. junctional nevi.
   d. malignant melanomas.
   e. associated with Peutz-Jeghers syndrome.

304. This asymptomatic firm mass was found on the gingiva just lingual to the lower central incisors. The patient was unaware of its presence. She had surgery for cancer of the left lung 2 years previously. In this case, primary consideration should be given to the possibility of this lesion being:
   a. a metastatic tumor.
   b. squamous cell carcinoma.
   c. a lingual torus.
   d. verrucous carcinoma.

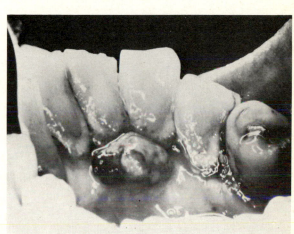

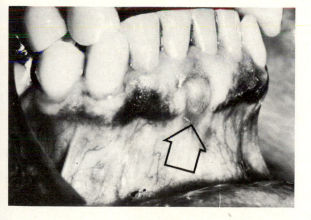

305. This 48-year-old white man underwent treatment for skin cancer last year and is currently on chemotherapy. The dark lesion of the gingiva associated with the lower right second premolar tooth recently appeared and doubled its size during the last month. The lesion is firm and painless. The lesion is *most* likely:

a. a pyogenic granuloma.
b. a nevus.
c. giant cell granuloma.
d. metastatic melanoma.
e. hemangiosarcoma.

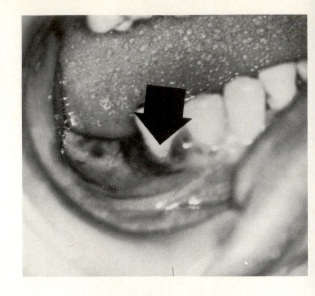

306. The peculiar large radiolucency *(arrow)* in the left central incisor tooth is *most* likely:

a. dens in dente.
b. internal resorption.
c. external resorption.
d. due to metastatic tumor.
e. produced by a bur.

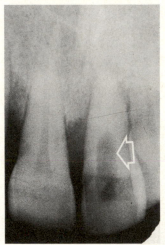

307. The roundish radiolucency *(arrow)* in the distal root of the molar tooth is *most* likely:

a. external resorption.
b. internal resorption.
c. produced by a bur.
d. due to a metastatic tumor.
e. produced by a pulp polyp.

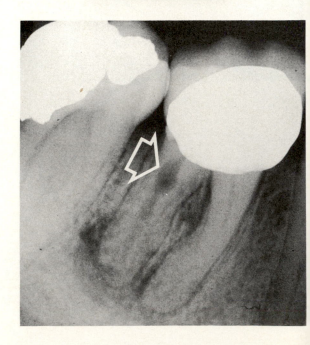

308. The radiolucency in the second premolar tooth is *most* likely:
  a. internal or external resorption.
  b. produced by a bur.
  c. normal pulp chamber.
  d. a result of pulp death.

309. The radiopacity *(arrow)* at the periapex of the distal root of the first molar tooth is *most* likely:
  a. a cementoma.
  b. idiopathic osteosclerosis.
  c. condensing osteitis.
  d. a result of occlusal trauma.

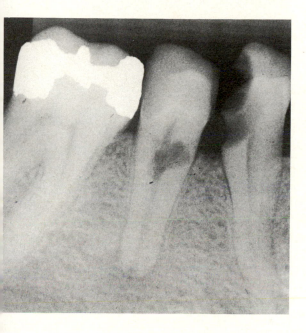
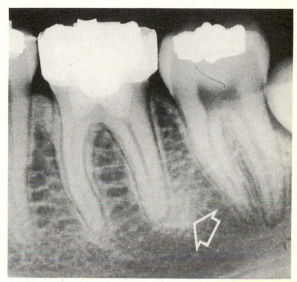

310. The asymptomatic radiolucencies at the apices of the first molar roots **(A)** were found on routine radiographic examination. If the photomicrograph **(B)** represents the histologic appearance of these lesions:

A. the final diagnosis is:
    a. multiple myeloma.
    b. cementomas.
    c. dental granulomas.
    d. radicular cysts.
    e. periapical scars.
B. the radiolucency at the apex of the second premolar *most* likely is:
    a. myeloma.
    b. dental papilla.
    c. dental granuloma.
    d. attributable to hyperparathyroidism.
    e. a marrow design.

311. This patient presented with the chief complaint of pain in this upper second premolar tooth. The *present* complaint is *most* likely directly produced by:
a. acute pulpitis.
b. a periapical cyst.
c. a periapical abscess.
d. a pulp exposure.
e. acute maxillary sinusitis.

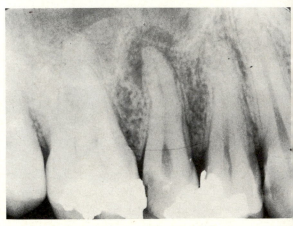

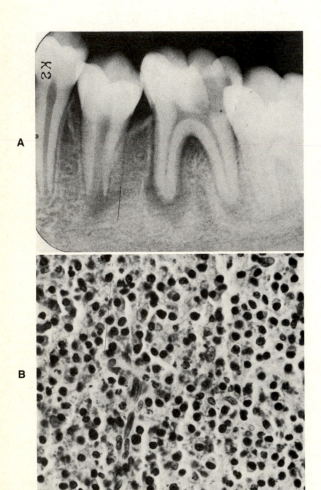

312. This asymptomatic radiolucency at the apex of the lateral incisor and canine teeth was found on routine radiographs **(A)**. If photomicrograph **B** is of this lesion, the final diagnosis is *most* likely:
a. odontogenic keratocyst.
b. radicular cyst.
c. globulomaxillary cyst.
d. the nasal chamber.
e. dental granuloma.

313. Radiograph **B** was taken 9 months after the conservative root canal filling of the central incisor tooth shown in **A**. The periapical radiolucency associated with the asymptomatic central incisor tooth in **A** *most* likely is:
a. a dental granuloma.
b. a periapical scar.
c. an acute periapical abscess.
d. a cementoma.
e. a traumatic bone cyst.

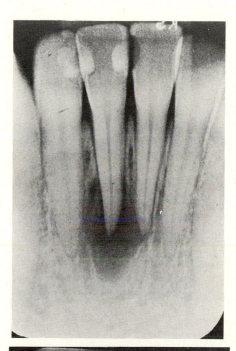

A

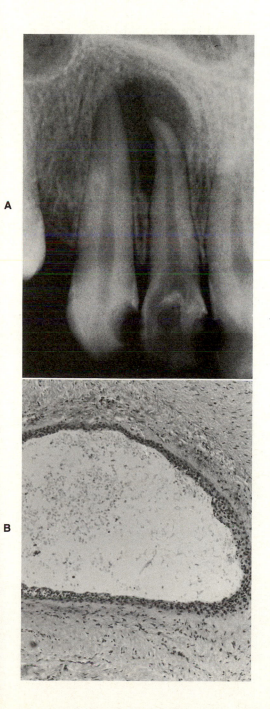

A

B

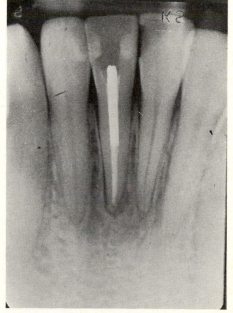

B

314. This asymptomatic radiolucency *(arrow)* was found at the apex of the asymptomatic lateral incisor during routine examination of a new patient. The radiolucency *(arrow)* is *most* likely:

a. a periapical scar.
b. a surgical defect.
c. a periapical granuloma.
d. a radicular cyst.
e. a normal marrow design.

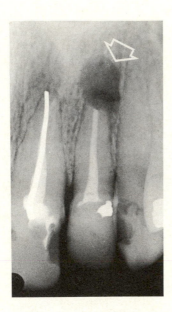

315. The asymptomatic radiolucency at the apex of the mesial root of the asymptomatic first molar tooth was found on the routine radiograph **A.** Radiographs taken at the time of the root canal filling showed a much larger radiolucency *(arrow)* at that time. The tooth had been asymptomatic since that time.

A. If the photomicrograph **B** revealed the microscopic view of the lesion, the final diagnosis is:

a. periapical granuloma.
b. periapical scar.
c. a myeloma lesion.
d. periapical cementoma.
e. a surgical defect.

B. The *most* suitable management approach to the lesion would be to:

a. redo the root canal fillings, making sure that you instrument beyond the apical foramen.
b. perform an apicoectomy.
c. advise the patient that the tooth will very probably become abscessed within a year or two.
d. radiograph the area occasionally.
e. perform a fenestration procedure.

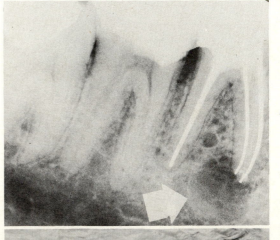

A

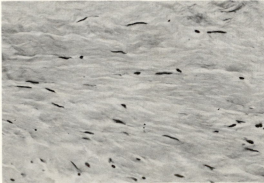

B

316. The mixed radiolucent-radiopaque lesions at the apices of the first molar are *most* likely:
a. cementomas.
b. odontomas.
c. rarefying and condensing osteitis lesions.
d. indicative of heavy occlusal trauma.
e. idiopathic osteosclerosis lesions.

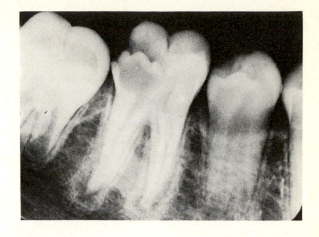

317. The radiolucency in **A** and **B** may be correctly identified as:
a. the incisive foramen.
b. a pulpoperiapical lesion.
c. a foramen of Scarpa.
d. the greater palatine foramen.
e. a median alveolar cyst.

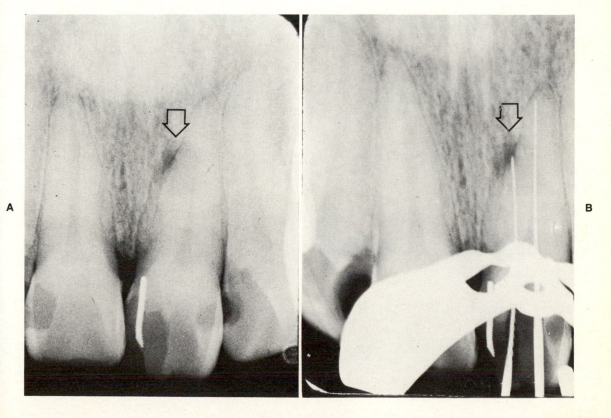

318. A. The *most* serious problem illustrated in this radiograph is the:
   a. presence of cervical decay.
   b. diastema between the central incisors.
   c. prominent lingual ridges on the central incisors.
   d. deep lingual pits.
   e. dens in dente in the right central incisor.
B. The problem identified in Question A will very likely precipitate:
   a. the need for orthodontic closure of the diastema.
   b. the development of caries in the lingual pits.
   c. the death of the pulp of the right central incisor if it is not already dead.
   d. occlusal problems.
   e. the need for cl. 3 gold-foil restorations.

319. This asymptomatic periapical radiolucency was seen during routine examination of radiographs of a 46-year-old woman. From the evidence seen in the radiograph, it is *most* likely that the working diagnosis should have been:
   a. dental granuloma.
   b. periapical cementoma.
   c. traumatic bone cyst.
   d. radicular cyst.
   e. the mental fossa.

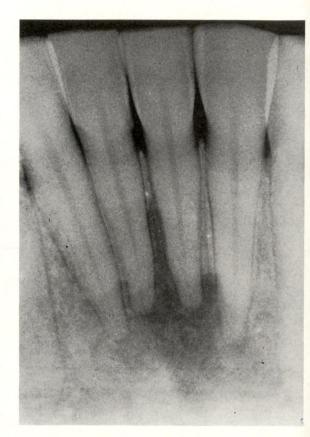

320. This asymptomatic radiolucency overlying the apices of the central incisors was detected on this film. The incisor teeth were asymptomatic and tested vital. The radiolucency is *most* likely:

a. a radicular cyst.
b. a primordial cyst.
c. the incisive canal.
d. a midline palatal cyst.
e. a nasolabial (nasoalveolar) cyst.

321. It is *most* likely that this 15-year-old boy who presents for treatment of a painful mandibular left molar tooth has:

a. a pulp polyp.
b. a mulberry molar.
c. a carious lower molar tooth and a "boil" on the skin.
d. a malignancy of the jawbone.
e. an abscessed molar tooth that is draining onto the skin surface.

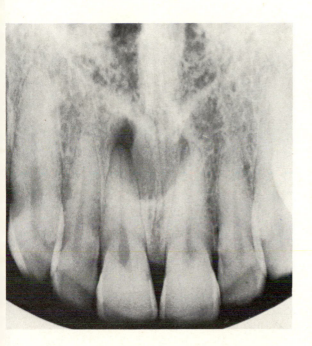

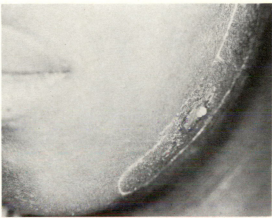

A

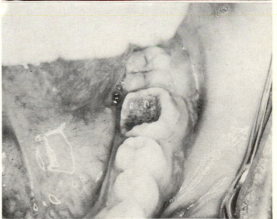

B

322. This solitary soft mass **(A)** on the alveolar mucosa in the mandibular molar region is *most* likely:

a. a papilloma.
b. a parulis.
c. a fibroma.
d. a lipoma.
e. a mucocele.

323. A painless swelling of the buccal aspect of the alveolar process in the right maxilla brought this 19-year-old man in for a consultation. All the maxillary teeth on that side of the arch were asymptomatic and tested vital. The *most* likely diagnosis is:

a. a globulomaxillary cyst.
b. a lateral radicular cyst.
c. a nasolabial (nasoalveolar) cyst.
d. a traumatic bone cyst.
e. an adenomatoid odontogenic tumor.

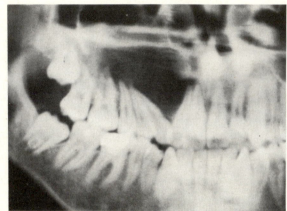

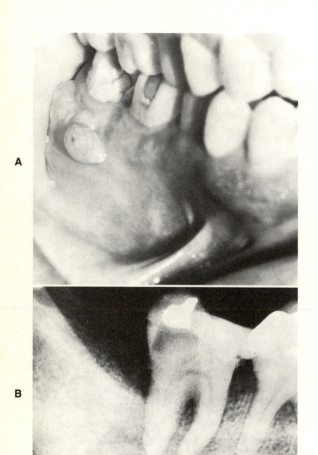

324. The asymptomatic radiolucency between the canine and lateral incisor teeth in this 14-year-old boy is *most* likely:
a. a globulomaxillary cyst.
b. a radicular cyst.
c. a primordial cyst.
d. an anatomic depression on the labial alveolar plate.
e. an anterior cleft.

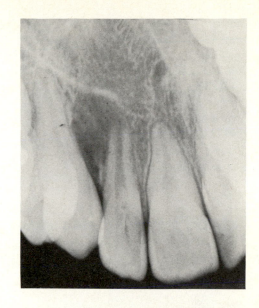

325. A concerned mother brought her 9-year-old child to the dentist for diagnosis and treatment of a tender swelling of the left mandible in the deciduous molar and first molar region. The swelling *(arrows)* at the inferior border of the mandible was bony hard. The deciduous second molar and the permanent first molar teeth were grossly carious and painful to percussion. The dentist extracted these teeth right away. This child *most* likely had:
a. Ewing's sarcoma.
b. osteogenic sarcoma.
c. proliferative periostitis (Garré's osteomyelitis).
d. fibrous dysplasia.
e. Caffey's disease (generalized cortical hyperostosis).

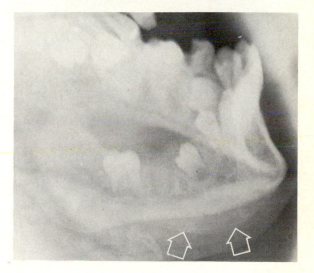

326. This 16-year-old boy presented for treatment of this painful swelling on the palate. He first noticed it 3 days previously and stated that it had increased in size very rapidly and had become more painful. The mass was soft to rubbery in consistency, painful to touch, and fluctuant. The mucosa over it was slightly redder than the remainder of the palate. This exophytic lesion is *most* likely:
a. an infected nasoalveolar cyst.
b. an infected globulomaxillary cyst.
c. an infected midline cyst of the palate.
d. a minor salivary gland tumor.
e. a palatal space abscess originating from a periapical abscess.

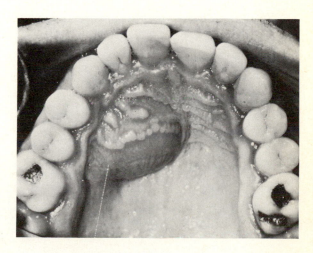

327. During examination of this 46-year-old woman, this asymptomatic palatal mass *(arrow)* was found. The solitary mass was firm, painless, and covered with mucosa of normal color. This exophytic lesion *most* likely is:

a. a palatal space abscess.
b. a minor salivary gland tumor.
c. fibrous dysplasia.
d. squamous cell carcinoma.
e. osteogenic sarcoma.

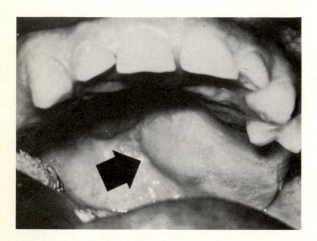

328. This 32-year-old woman presented for diagnosis and treatment of this painless mass on the anterior palate, which she stated had been present for about 2 months and had become significantly larger during that time. The mass was soft to rubbery in consistency, was fluctuant, and could not be emptied. The covering mucosa was a normal pink in color. The ten most anterior teeth tested vital.

A. The mass is *most* likely:
  a. a palatal space abscess.
  b. a cavernous hemangioma.
  c. a lipoma.
  d. a nasopalatine duct cyst or a midline palatal cyst.
  e. a mucocele.

B. The next step in the workup of the patient would be to:
  a. obtain specimen for culture and sensitivity testing.
  b. attempt to aspirate the lesion.
  c. obtain radiographs of the region.
  d. recheck the family history.
  e. take a blood specimen for serum chemistry test.

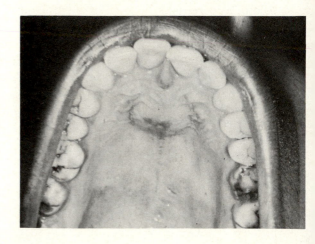

329. The mixed radiolucent-radiopaque condition in this radiograph is *most* likely produced by:
a. osteomyelitis.
b. fibrous dysplasia.
c. periapical cementomas.
d. lingual tori.
e. condensing and rarefying osteitis.

330. This asymptomatic mixed radiolucent-radiopaque lesion was observed during routine dental examination in a 45-year-old lady. The lesion is *most* likely:
a. a rarefying and condensing osteitis.
b. fibrous dysplasia.
c. a complex odontoma.
d. a lingual torus.
e. a periapical cementoma.

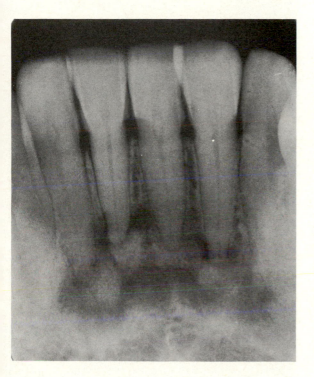

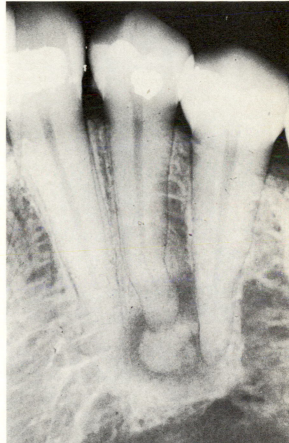

331. After this mixed radiolucent-radiopaque lesion was seen on the periapical film (**A**), a maxillary occlusal film (**B**) was taken of this 61-year-old man. The lesion in the periapical film is *most* likely:

a. cementoma.
b. a rarefying and condensing osteitis lesion.
c. exostosis.
d. hypercementosis.
e. a cotton-wool lesion of Paget's disease.

332. The radiopacity at the root end of the lateral incisor tooth is *most* likely:

a. a buckshot pellet.
b. an amalgam retrograde filling.
c. gutta-percha.
d. root canal sealer.
e. an artifact.

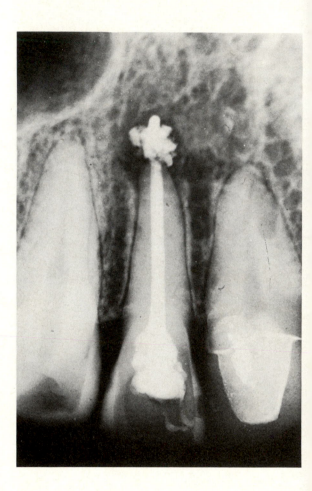

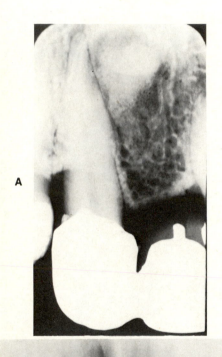

A

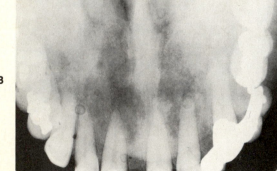

B

333. This large, asymptomatic periapical radiopacity found as a solitary lesion on full-mouth radiographs of a 39-year-old patient was *most* likely:

a. a lingual torus.
b. idiopathic osteosclerosis.
c. osteomyelitis.
d. cementoma.
e. condensing osteitis.

334. This asymptomatic radiopacity was discovered at the apex of the vital first premolar tooth during routine examination of a 22-year-old man. The first premolar tooth was completely asymptomatic. Shift shots were used, but the radiopacity could not be shifted from the apex of this tooth. The remaining findings were noncontributory. This radiopacity was *most* likely:

a. a condensing osteitis.
b. idiopathic osteosclerosis.
c. a cementoma.
d. an exostosis or torus.
e. pathognomonic for sickle cell anemia.

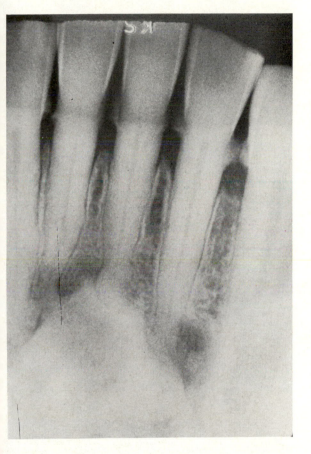

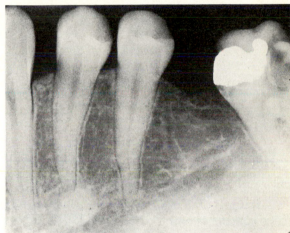

335. The radiopacity over the apex of the central incisor tooth is *most* likely:
   a. a retrograde amalgam filling.
   b. an amalgam tattoo.
   c. a small exostosis.
   d. a buckshot pellet.
   e. an artifact.

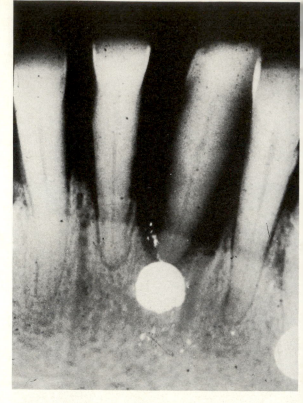

336. What is the *most* likely diagnosis of the radiopaque shadow that lies at the end of the first molar apices and was detected during routine oral examination of a 40-year-old woman? The first molar tested nonvital but was asymptomatic.
   a. a mucosal cyst of the sinus floor.
   b. periapical condensing osteitis.
   c. a projected image of a torus.
   d. periapical idiopathic osteosclerosis.
   e. a periapical cementoma.

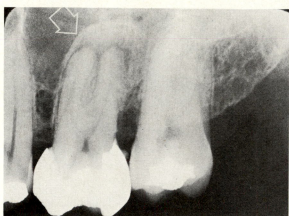

337. This radiopacity was detected on this radiograph, taken soon after a painful second premolar was extracted. The radiopacity is *most* likely:
   a. a residual radicular cyst.
   b. a mucosal cyst of the sinus floor.
   c. an antrolith.
   d. a projected image of a torus.
   e. hyperplasia of the sinus mucosa secondary to odontogenic infection.

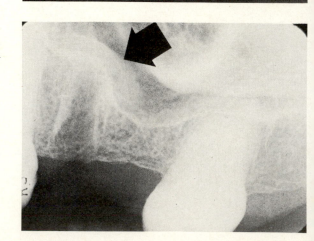

338. The asymptomatic radiopacity above the apices of the vital first molar tooth was found on routine radiographs of a 20-year-old woman. The radiopacity is *most* likely:
a. a condensing osteitis.
b. a mucosal cyst of the sinus floor.
c. hyperplasia of the mucosa of the sinus floor secondary to odontogenic infection.
d. the ala of the nose.
e. a benign tumor of the sinus.

339. The asymptomatic radiopacity over the apex of the second premolar tooth, which has just been root-canal filled, is *most* likely:
a. a condensing osteitis.
b. a mucosal cyst of the sinus floor.
c. hyperplasia of the mucosa of the sinus floor secondary to odontogenic inflammation or infection.
d. the ala of the nose.
e. a benign tumor of the sinus.

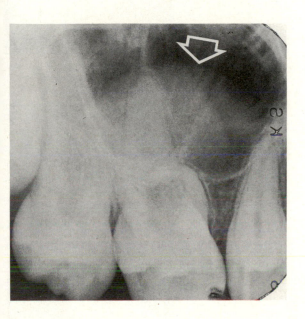

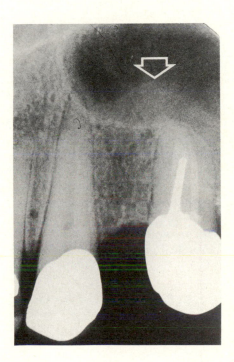

340. The moderately radiopaque shadow indicated by the arrow is *most* likely:
   a. a benign mucosal cyst of the sinus floor.
   b. a hyperplasia of the mucosa of the sinus floor secondary to dental infection.
   c. produced by fluid air level in the sinus.
   d. a palatal torus.

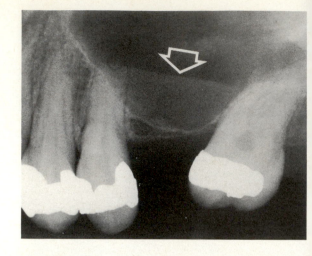

341. Which one of the following statements concerning the premolar tooth and its periapical radiolucency is *most* likely incorrect?
   a. The radiolucency is pulpal in origin.
   b. The root end and its associated pathology are in the sinus cavity.
   c. The root end and its associated pathology are within bone.
   d. The periapical radiolucency is probably a periapical granuloma or a radicular cyst.

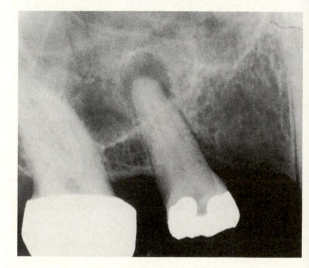

342. The arrow indicates:
   a. a large nutrient canal.
   b. the anterior palatine foramen.
   c. squamous cell carcinoma.
   d. a discontinuity in the bony floor of the sinus.

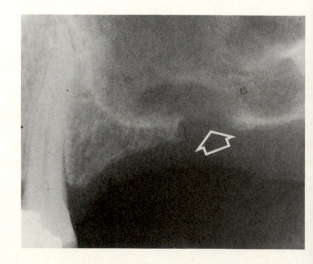

343. The arrows indicate:
   a. bilateral benign mucosal cysts of the sinuses.
   b. palatal tori.
   c. the dorsal surface of the tongue.
   d. the floor of the nasal cavity.

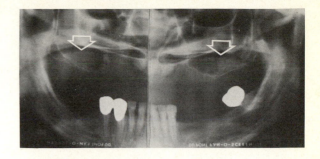

344. This radiopacity is *most* likely:
   a. a lingual torus.
   b. a cementoma.
   c. condensing osteitis from a nonvital second premolar.
   d. idiopathic osteosclerosis (enostosis).
   e. a condensation of bone caused by hyperocclusion.

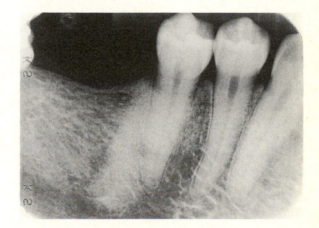

345. This radiopacity, which is surrounded by a faint radiolucent rim that in turn is surrounded by a thin radiopaque rim, is *most* likely:
   a. idiopathic osteoclerosis (enostosis).
   b. condensing osteitis.
   c. a sialolith.
   d. a lingual torus.
   e. a mass of calcified dental tissue in bone (for example, cementoma).

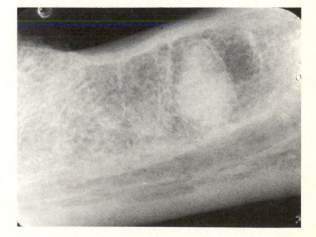

346. This dense radiopacity *(arrow)* is *most* likely:
a. a 38-caliber bullet.
b. an amalgam fragment.
c. a salivary stone.
d. a fragment of rubber base impression material.

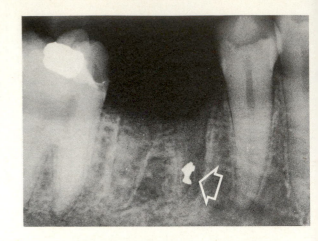

347. These radiopacities are *most* likely:
a. calcified blood vessels.
b. rubber base impression material.
c. calcified vegetable fiber.
d. retained root-canal filling material.

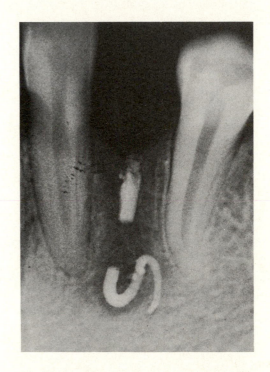

348. This solitary asymptomatic lesion was found on radiographic examination of the edentulous jaws of a 62-year-old patient. The diagnosis is *most* likely:
a. Paget's disease.
b. fibrous dysplasia.
c. cementoma.
d. odontoma.
e. lingual torus.

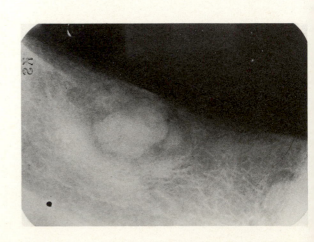

349. **A** shows the asymptomatic radiopacity in the periapical film, while **B** shows the location in an occlusal film. What is the *most* probable diagnosis?
a. salivary stone.
b. idiopathic osteosclerosis (enostosis).
c. lingual torus.
d. cementoma.

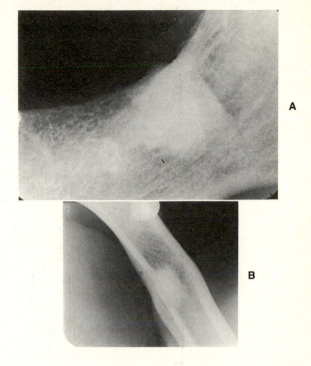

350. This periapical radiograph of the premolar-molar region of the mandible shows interesting shadows that are most compatible with:
a. Paget's disease.
b. sclerosed tooth sockets.
c. multiple retained roots.
d. osteogenic sarcoma.

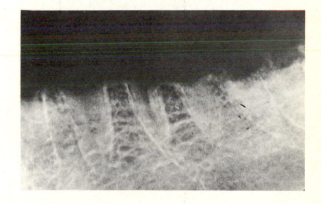

351. This radiographic appearance is best described as:
a. ground-glass pattern.
b. cotton-wool pattern.
c. worm-hole pattern.
d. tramcar-tracks pattern.

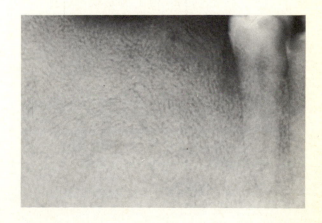

352. This 64-year-old man presented for full dentures. In addition to his obvious dental problems, he had a sore throat that had been bothering him for some years, particularly on the right side. This disappeared 2 years previously. This radiopacity *(arrow)* was found on the Orthopan radiograph, and this image was found to shift quite considerably on a Panorex film. The parotid examination was uneventful, and a satisfactory quantity of clear saliva could be readily milked from the right Stensen's duct. This radiopacity is *most* likely:

a. a foreign metal fragment.
b. a root fragment within the bone.
c. a condensing osteitis.
d. a sialolith.
e. a tonsillolith.

353. This asymptomatic radiopacity was found during routine examination of a 34-year-old woman. The remaining findings were totally noncontributory. This radiopacity is *most* likely:

a. idiopathic osteosclerosis or condensing osteitis.
b. a cementoma.
c. a torus.
d. a sialolith.
e. sclerosing osteomyelitis.

354. One week after having crowns placed in this region, a 25-year-old senior dental student complained of soreness of the gingiva just lingual to the molar tooth. A radiograph was taken and this radiopacity *(arrow)* was found. It is *most* likely:

a. a sialolith.
b. an exostosis.
c. condensing osteitis.
d. a foreign body (for example, a fragment of rubber base impression material).
e. a fragment of amalgam.

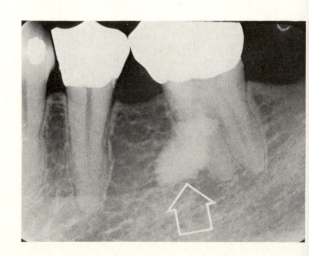

355. This radiopaque mass was detected on radiographs of a 64-year-old man that were taken to investigate the cause of chronic painful swelling he was experiencing on that side. This radiopacity is *most* likely:
a. shrapnel.
b. calcified lymph nodes.
c. a sialolith in the submaxillary salivary gland.
d. a phlebolith.
e. a calcified hematoma.

356. These several asymptomatic radiopacities found on radiographs of a 68-year-old man who had spent considerable time in a municipal tuberculosis sanitarium are *most* likely:
a. calcified hematomas.
b. phleboliths.
c. sialoliths.
d. shrapnel.
e. calcified lymph nodes.

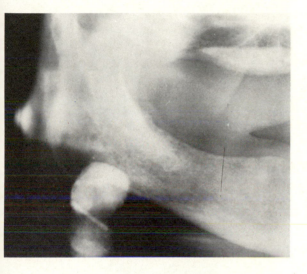

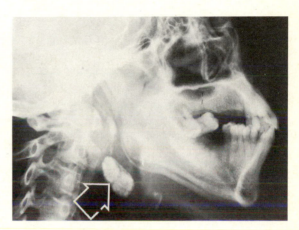

357. This painless radiopacity was detected on routine examination of a 25-year-old woman. It is *most* likely:
a. a cementoma.
b. idiopathic osteosclerosis.
c. a torus.
d. a sialolith.
e. a cotton-wool lesion of Paget's disease.

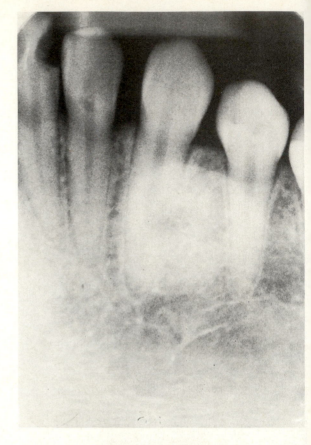

358. These asymptomatic radiopacities were discovered in a 54-year-old woman enjoying good health. They were *most* likely:
a. multiple cementomas.
b. multiple odontomas.
c. multiple areas of condensing osteitis.
d. root fragments.
e. cotton-wool lesions of Paget's disease.

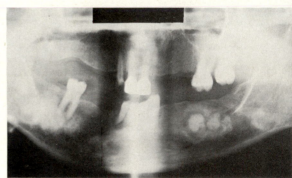

359. This 65-year-old man presented with pain and swelling in the posterior region of the left mandible. He stated that the problem started when his dentist treated the nerve of the second molar tooth with arsenic. The tooth became so painful within 2 or 3 days that it had to be extracted. Protracted pain and swelling had occurred after the extraction. This condition *most* likely is:
a. a cementoma.
b. a complex odontoma.
c. a fracture.
d. osteomyelitis.
e. chondrosarcoma.

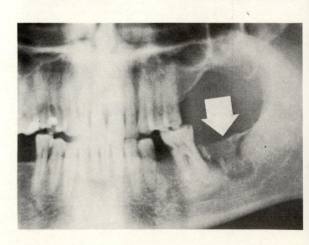

360. This radiopacity *(arrow)* is *most* likely:
   a. an evulsed tooth.
   b. the hyoid bone.
   c. a torus.
   d. a salivary stone.
   e. an osteogenic sarcoma.

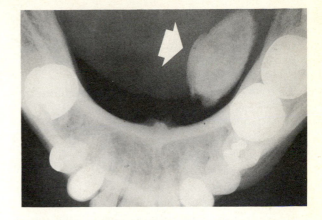

361. The radiopacity indicated by the arrow is *most* likely:
   a. an impacted tooth.
   b. an antrolith.
   c. a calcified node.
   d. a sialolith.

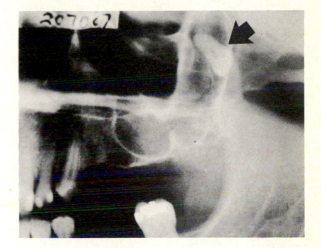

362. A panoramic radiograph of a very large 68-year-old black man who presented for new dentures. Aside from bouts with angina pectoris and essential hypertension, his medical history was unremarkable. The dense radiographic appearance of the jawbones indicates that he *most* likely has:
   a. Paget's disease.
   b. benign osteopetrosis.
   c. malignant osteopetrosis.
   d. sclerotic cemental masses (gigantiform cematomas, florid osseous dysplasia).
   e. a bony architecture that falls within the normal range.

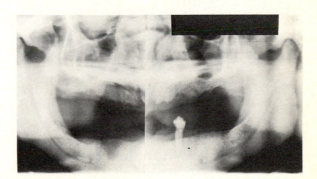

363. This 48-year-old black woman in apparently good health presented for new dentures. The panoramic radiograph revealed this radiopaque pattern. She *most* likely has:
a. Paget's disease.
b. sclerotic cemental masses (gigantiform cementomas, florid osseous dysplasia).
c. benign osteopetrosis.
d. malignant osteopetrosis.
e. Gardner's syndrome.

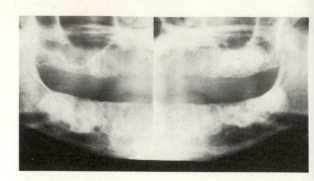

364. This 68-year-old man with various skeletal complaints had a serum alkaline phosphatase of 112 King-Armstrong units. What is the *most* likely diagnosis?
a. fibrous dysplasia.
b. hyperparathyroidism.
c. Paget's disease.
d. cleidocranial dysostosis.

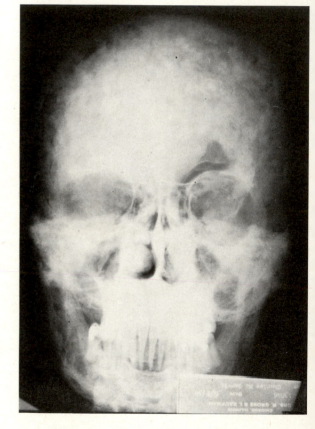

365. This 28-year-old man presented with a chief complaint of pain and swelling of the left mandible. Examination revealed a painful red swelling at the inferior border of the mandible in the region of the mixed radiolucent-radiopaque lesion. The lesion is *most* likely:
a. a cementoma.
b. osteogenic sarcoma.
c. fibrous dysplasia.
d. osteomyelitis.
e. condensing and rarefying osteitis.

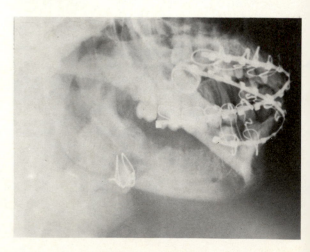

366. This 19-year-old woman was observed to have facial asymmetry because of an asymptomatic expansion of the jaw on one side. The remainder of the examination was negative. She *most* likely has:

a. Ewing's sarcoma.

b. proliferative periostitis (Garré's osteomyelitis).

c. osteogenic sarcoma.

d. fibrous dysplasia.

e. Paget's disease.

367. This 58-year-old man presented for treatment of pain and swelling of the left mandible. He had received radiation treatments 6 years previously for a malignancy of the left submandibular salivary gland. The swollen tissue was tender to palpate and there was a sinus on the skin at the inferior border of the mandible. The current lesion *most* likely is:

a. fibrous dysplasia.

b. chronic osteomyelitis (osteoradionecrosis).

c. radiation sarcoma.

d. Paget's disease (intermediate stage).

e. metastatic carcinoma.

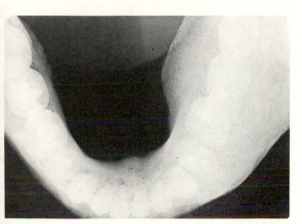

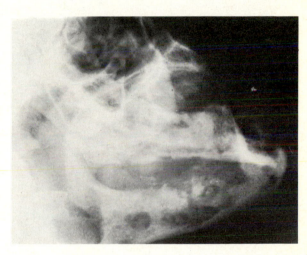

368. A concerned mother brought her 14-year-old son for a consultation concerning the delayed eruption of the right maxillary canine and also the moderate-sized painless expansion of the buccal plate in Figure **A. B** shows the histopathology of the lesion. The final diagnosis is:

a. a dentigerous cyst.

b. ameloblastoma.

c. early odontoma.

d. an adenomatoid odontogenic tumor.

e. osteogenic sarcoma.

369. This salt-and-pepper appearance was observed in a 46-year-old woman who had a painless swelling of the jaw in the molar and ramus region. Although she had no pain, she was unable to open her jaw more than 1.5 cm. She had a mastectomy 2 years previously. This condition in the mandible is *most* likely:

a. osteomyelitis.

b. fibrous dysplasia.

c. metastatic tumor.

d. osteopetrosis.

e. not a pathologic condition, since the appearance is within the normal range.

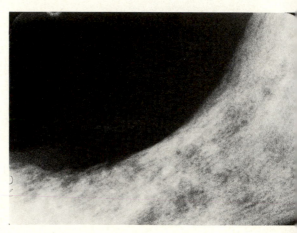

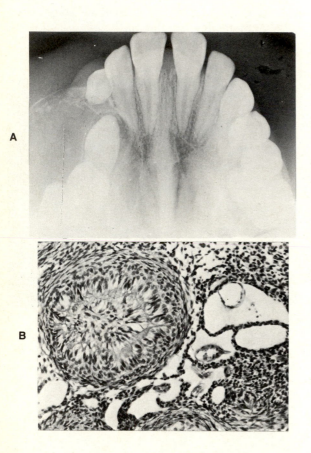

A

B

370. This 11-year-old boy was troubled with an expanding swelling of the left side of the jaw, which he first noticed about 6 weeks previously. He now complains of numbness of the lower lip on the left side. He *most* likely has:
a. fibrous dysplasia.
b. chondrosarcoma.
c. squamous cell carcinoma.
d. acute osteomyelitis.
e. osteogenic sarcoma.

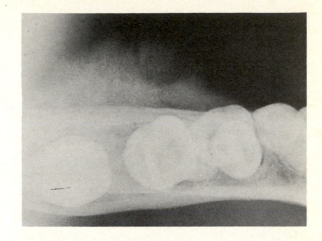

371. This 30-year-old man has had pain and looseness of the anterior teeth for the last 4 months. There is now expansion of the mandible in this region. Notice the peculiar widening of the periodontal ligament shadows. The diagnosis is *most* likely:
a. fibrous dysplasia.
b. Paget's disease.
c. osteosarcoma.
d. squamous cell carcinoma.

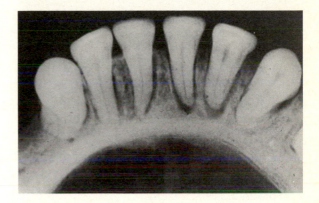

372. The asymmetric, bandlike widening of the periodontal ligament on the mesial aspect of the lateral incisor in this 15-year-old youth is *most* likely caused by:
a. calculus.
b. an osteolytic sarcoma.
c. Ewing's sarcoma.
d. chondrosarcoma.
e. orthodontic movement.

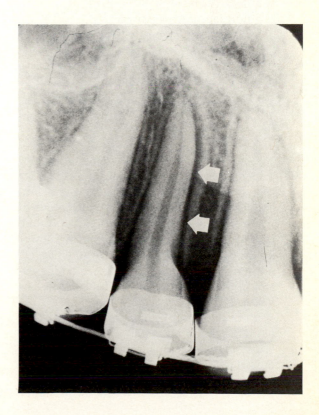

373. The asymmetric, bandlike widening of the periodontal ligament on the mesial of the canine in this 45-year-old woman is *most* likely caused by:
a. occlusal trauma.
b. calculus.
c. squamous cell carcinoma.
d. metastatic carcinoma.
e. chondrosarcoma.

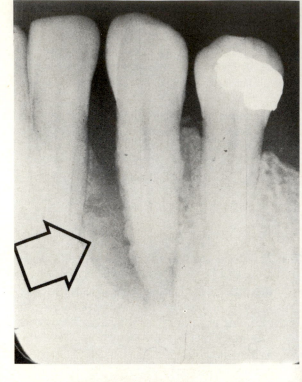

374. This painless, ragged, ill-defined radiolucency in the anterior border of the ramus, covered with normal mucosa, in a 24-year-old man is *most* likely:
a. a dentigerous cyst.
b. a normal marrow pattern.
c. an infection or malignancy.
d. a lingual salivary gland depression.

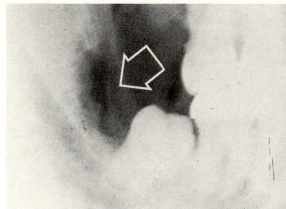

375. This radiolucent lesion in the left retromolar region of this 61-year-old man was a firm exophytic mass with an ulcerated, reddish-white surface. He complained of pain in the jaw and of a tingling sensation of the lower lip on that side. There was a firm, enlarged, nontender mass fixed to the surrounding tissue in the left submaxillary space. This jaw lesion is *most* likely:
a. chronic osteomyelitis.
b. metastatic carcinoma.
c. osteolytic sarcoma.
d. fibrous dysplasia.
e. squamous cell carcinoma.

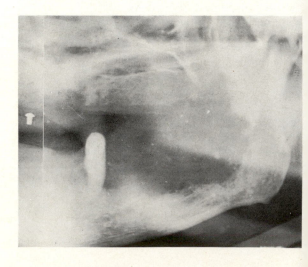

76. This radiolucency *(arrow)* was discovered when a 54-year-old woman presented for diagnosis of pain in the jaw and a tingling sensation of the lip on that side. She gave a history of treatment for carcinoma of the cervix 2 years previously. This radiolucency is *most* likely:
a. chondrosarcoma.
b. a metastatic tumor.
c. a lingual salivary gland invagination.
d. a residual cyst.
e. a traumatic bone cyst.

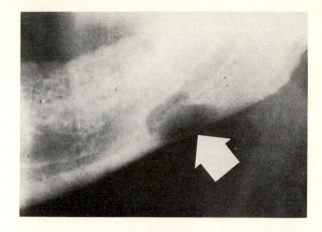

77. This is a panoramic radiograph of a 56-year-old woman who has spent much of the last 20 years in and out of hospitals for a chronic kidney ailment. It is *most* likely that she has:
a. postmenopausal osteoporosis.
b. primary hyperparathyroidism.
c. secondary hyperparathyroidism.
d. thalassemia.
e. Paget's disease (stage of osteoporosis circumscripta).

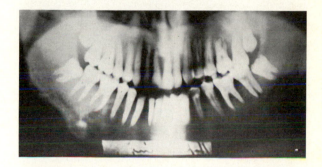

78. This radiolucency *(arrow)* was found on routine examination of a 15-year-old boy. The diagnosis is *most* likely:
a. a lateral periodontal cyst.
b. a primordial cyst.
c. a traumatic bone cyst.
d. lingual salivary bone invagination.
e. ameloblastoma.

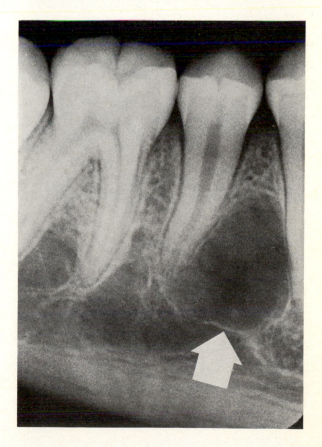

379. This radiolucency *(arrow)* was detected during routine dental examination of a 61-year-old man. There was a slight but definite expansion of the buccal plate over the region of the radiolucency. The remainder of the examination was essentially noncontributory. The radiolucency is *most* likely:

a. an ameloblastoma.
b. a residual cyst.
c. a traumatic bone cyst.
d. a cystlike marrow pattern.
e. a lingual salivary gland invagination.

380. These three bony lesions were found in association with the three impacted third molar teeth during routine dental examination of a 38-year-old man. A chest radiograph revealed two bifid ribs. This patient *most* likely has:

a. conventional cysts (no syndrome).
b. the basal cell nevus syndrome.
c. multiple giant cell lesions of hyperparathyroidism.
d. multiple ameloblastomas.
e. multiple myeloma.

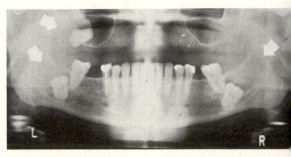

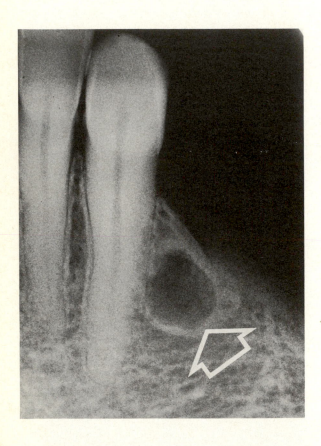

381. If these two teeth are vital, the *most* likely diagnosis of this radiolucency in a 46-year-old man is:

a. a primordial cyst.
b. a residual cyst.
c. a lateral periodontal cyst.
d. a traumatic bone cyst.
e. a globulomaxillary cyst.

382. This radiolucency was found in a 25-year-old man **(A)**. There was a similar lesion on the opposite side where the third molar had been extracted 5 years previously. **B** is a photomicrograph that was similar for both lesions. The final diagnosis is:

a. ameloblastoma.
b. odontogenic keratocyst.
c. cherubism.
d. squamous cell carcinoma.

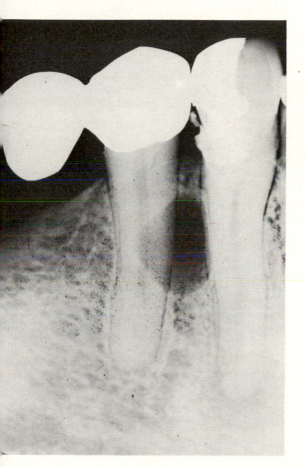

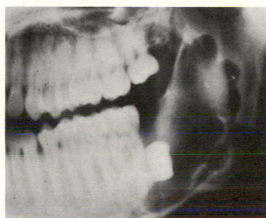

A

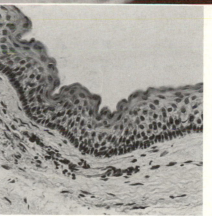

B

383. This large, multilocular radiolucent lesion in a 62-year-old man is *most* likely:
   a. an ameloblastoma.
   b. a central giant cell granuloma.
   c. an odontogenic myxoma.
   d. a giant cell lesion of hyperparathyroidism.
   e. a central hemangioma.

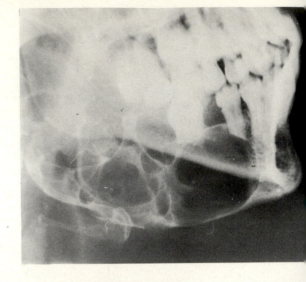

384. This asymptomatic radiolucency associated with the crown of the impacted third molar tooth in a 42-year-old man is *most* likely:
   a. a dentigerous cyst.
   b. a mural ameloblastoma.
   c. an ameloblastoma.
   d. an enlarged follicle but within normal limits.
   e. an adenomatoid odontogenic tumor.

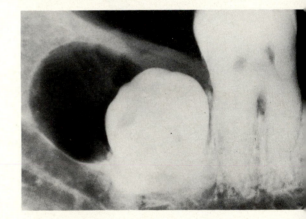

385. This patient presented with the chief complaint of a swelling of the right jaw. Attempts to aspirate this radiolucency (**A**) yielded a straw-colored fluid. At surgery, a mass was seen projecting into the lumen. The microscopy of this mass is shown in **B.** The final diagnosis is:
   a. a dentigerous cyst.
   b. a dentigerous cyst with a mural nodule of granulation tissue.
   c. an odontogenic keratocyst.
   d. a dentigerous cyst with a mural ameloblastoma.
   e. a dentigerous cyst with a mural adenomatoid odontogenic tumor.

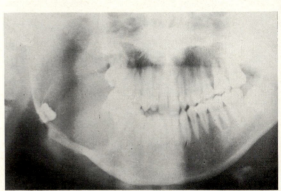

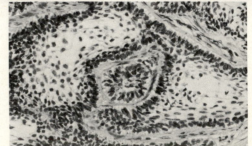

B

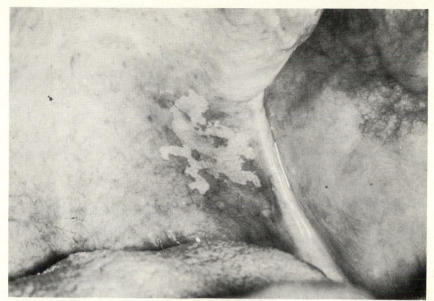

A

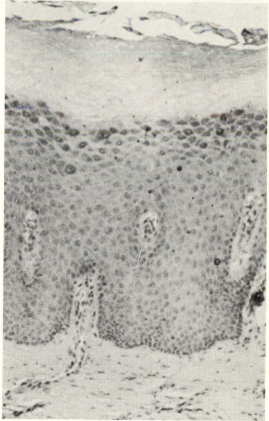

B

386. This solitary white lesion (**A**) was found during routine examination of a 52-year-old man who has smoked 1½ packs of cigarettes a day for the last 35 years. The white lesion cannot be scraped off. If **B** shows the microscopic picture of this lesion:

A. What is the final diagnosis?
    a. epithelial hyperplasia with hyperkeratosis and acanthosis (leukoplakia).
    b. squamous cell carcinoma.
    c. verrucous carcinoma.
    d. lichen planus.
    e. candidiasis.

B. What is the best initial management approach to this lesion?
    a. exfoliative cytology.
    b. incisional biopsy.
    c. excisional biopsy.
    d. toluidine staining.
    e. have the patient discontinue smoking immediately and reevaluate the lesion in 2 weeks.

387. This white condition involves several of the oral mucosal surfaces of a 45-year-old woman who has been using tetracycline mouth rinses for the last week as treatment for recurrent aphthous stomatitis. The white curds may be readily scraped off with a tongue blade. When this is done, a raw bleeding surface is found underneath.

A. The diagnosis *most* likely is:
   a. leukoplakia.
   b. gangrenous stomatitis.
   c. pemphigus.
   d. candidiasis.
   e. aspirin burn.

B. Correct management of this patient should include:
   a. an incisional biopsy.
   b. administration of penicillin.
   c. administration of nystatin.
   d. continuance of the tetracycline mouth rinse.
   e. immediate hospitalization for extensive tests to rule out diseases such as leukemia.

388. This linear white condition was seen on the buccal mucosa of a 56-year-old woman during a periodic dental examination. The remainder of the findings were noncontributory. The white condition is *most* likely:
a. a variation of linea alba.
b. lichen planus.
c. leukoplakia.
d. leukoedema.
e. hypertrophic candidiasis.

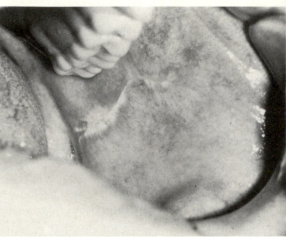

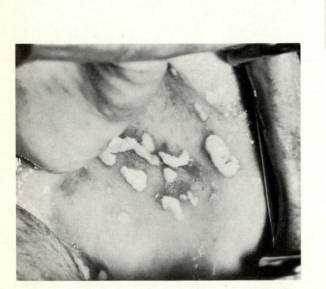

389. This 65-year-old man presented with the solitary asymptomatic white lesion shown in **A.** The white material could not be scraped off. **B** shows the patient 2 weeks later when the white condition had been successfully eliminated through conservative management. What was the *most* likely diagnosis of the white lesion?

a. squamous cell carcinoma.
b. snuff dipper's leukoplakia (reversible in this case).
c. candidiasis.
d. lichen planus.
e. white sponge nevus.

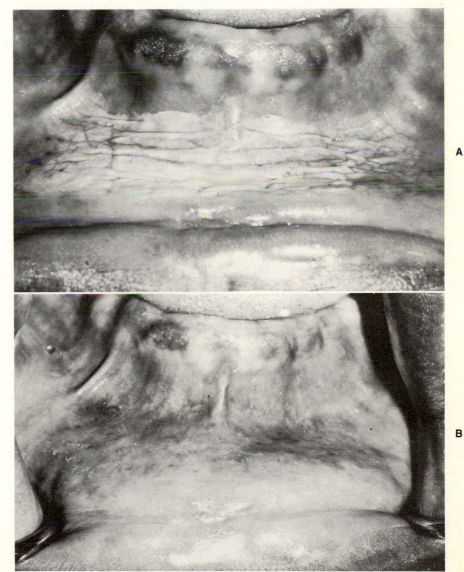

A

B

390. This 45-year-old black man has this white condition on the mucosa of both cheeks. When the cheek is stretched, the white appearance disappears. The patient was not aware of a problem. The correct diagnosis is:

   a. leukoedema.
   b. leukoplakia.
   c. candidiasis.
   d. lichen planus.
   e. white sponge nevus.

391. When this nervous, 46-year-old woman presented for a periodic dental examination, this asymptomatic white condition was found on both buccal mucosas and also on the lateral borders of the tongue. The white material could not be scraped off. The patient was unaware of the condition. She denied taking drugs or medication of any kind but admitted to smoking 1 pack of cigarettes a day and also to considerable alcohol consumption.

A. The *most* likely diagnosis is:
   a. leukoplakia.
   b. lichen planus.
   c. leukoedema.
   d. ectopic geographic tongue.
   e. hypertrophic candidiasis.

B. The correct approach to the management of this case is to:
   a. perform exfoliative cytology.
   b. do toluidine blue staining.
   c. prescribe systemic corticosteroids immediately.
   d. inform the patient about the condition and reexamine her periodically.

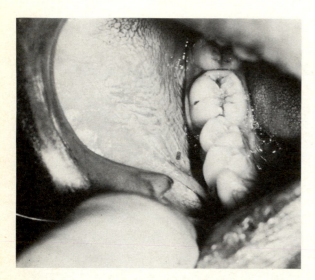

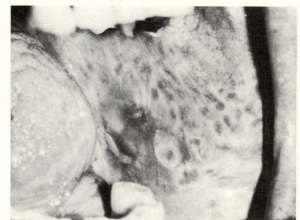

392. A. During examination of a 60-year-old man who presented only sporadically for dental treatment, you noticed this asymptomatic whitish condition on the palate. The condition is *most* likely:
  a. squamous cell carcinoma.
  b. papillary hyperplasia (multiple papillomatosis).
  c. hypertrophic candidiasis.
  d. nicotine stomatitis.
  e. lichen planus.
B. Which *one* of the following is the indicated management?
  a. Strip the palate and send for microscopic study.
  b. Prescribe topical cortisone applications.
  c. Tell the patient to discontinue pipe smoking and reexamine in 2 weeks.
  d. Prescribe nystatin ointment.

393. This asymptomatic white-and-red lesion was found during periodic examination of a 58-year-old man. He was unaware of the lesion. He admitted to smoking 1½ packs of cigarettes a day for the previous 40 years and to heavy consumption of alcohol. The white material could not be scraped off. The remainder of the examination was unremarkable.
A. This lesion is *most* likely:
  a. hypertrophic candidiasis.
  b. white sponge nevus.
  c. a papilloma.
  d. lichen planus.
  e. speckled leukoplakia.
B. The correct management of this lesion is:
  a. having the patient discontinue smoking and drinking entirely, and reevaluating the lesion in 2 months.
  b. painting the lesion with toluidine blue.
  c. performing an exfoliative cytologic test.
  d. performing an incisional biopsy as soon as possible.
  e. performing an excisional biopsy as soon as possible.

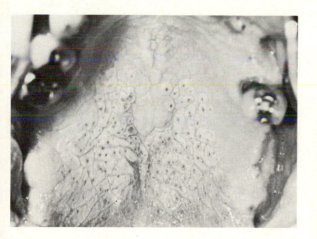

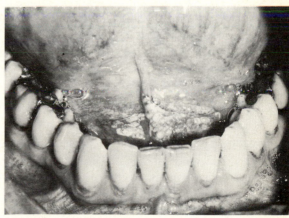

394. This white condition was found on several of this 45-year-old man's oral mucosal surfaces when he presented for extraction of a painful tooth. The white condition was not painful but could not be scraped off, and stretching the cheek did not eliminate it. The man denied ever having used alcohol or tobacco. He said he had had this white condition all his life. The correct diagnosis is *most* likely:

a. extensive leukoplakia.
b. white sponge nevus.
c. hypertrophic candidiasis.
d. leukoedema.
e. lichen planus.

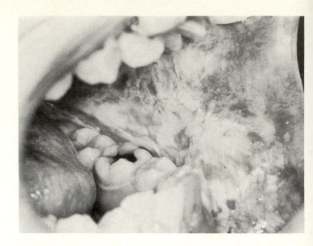

395. A. What question concerning etiology should you ask this 38-year-old man who presents with these changes *(arrows)*?

a. Do you smoke a pipe?
b. Do you use a toothbrush with stiff bristles?
c. Do you use lemon drops excessively?
d. Do you use smokeless tobacco?

B. If the patient uses snuff, which *one* is the correct approach in this case?

a. Have the patient discontinue its use.
b. Have the patient discontinue its use and reexamine him in 2 weeks.
c. Perform an excisional biopsy and send for a microscopic study.
d. Refer the patient for irradiation.

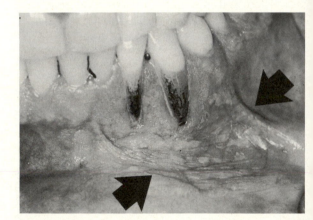

396. A. This solitary, white, asymptomatic lesion was found in a 52-year-old man who smokes a pack of cigarettes a day. The *most* likely diagnosis is:

a. candidiasis.
b. leukoplakia.
c. lichen planus.
d. verrucous carcinoma.

B. What is the approximate risk of this lesion being malignant now or becoming malignant during the life of this patient?

a. almost none.
b. 5% to 10%.
c. 20% to 40%.
d. 80% to 90%.

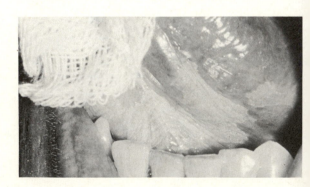

397. This red-and-white pattern was observed bilaterally on the anterior buccal mucosa during routine examination of an apprehensive 18-year-old man. Close examination revealed that the white component was composed of ragged tags. This condition is *most* likely:
a. lichen planus.
b. candidiasis.
c. bilateral speckled leukoplakia.
d. the result of chronic cheek biting.

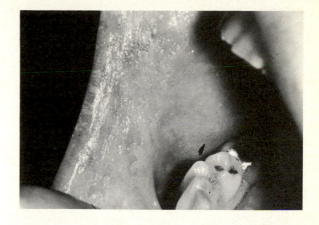

398. What is the most likely cause of this leukoplakia?
a. smoking.
b. an ill-fitting denture.
c. smokeless tobacco.
d. frequent drinking of hot coffee.

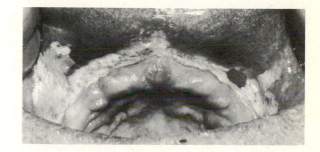

399. This firm, broad-based, moderately elevated, painless white lesion has been slowly increasing in size for the last 5½ years in this 65-year-old man. What is the *most* likely diagnosis?
a. leukoplakia.
b. squamous cell carcinoma.
c. condyloma acuminatum.
d. verrucous carcinoma.

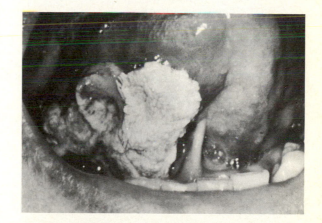

400. This firm, white, painless lesion was first noticed 4 months ago by this 54-year-old man. The *most* likely diagnosis is:
a. squamous cell carcinoma.
b. verrucous carcinoma.
c. rhabdomyosarcoma.
d. pyogenic granuloma.

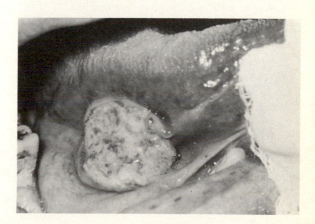

401. This 22-year-old man has enjoyed good health up until a year ago when he contracted this painful condition of the mouth and angles of the lips (**A** and **B**). Nystatin administration clears the condition up for short periods, but it soon returns. Serious consideration should be given to the possibility that the patient has:

a. an allergy to his toothpaste.
b. a severe herpes infection of the oral cavity.
c. an inherited immunodeficiency disease.
d. acquired immunodeficiency syndrome (AIDS).

402. This tender white condition was observed on the soft palate, fauces, and pharynx of a chronic adult asthmatic. The white material could be readily scraped off, and pseudohyphae could be seen on microscopic study of the smears. What *most* likely predisposed this patient to the candidal infection?

a. tetracycline use.
b. concomitant uncontrolled diabetes.
c. theophylline use.
d. oral cortisone inhaler use.

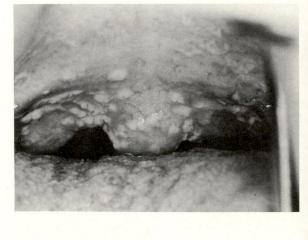

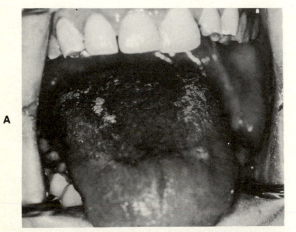

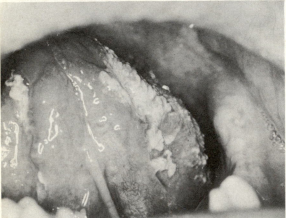

403. A. This asymptomatic condition found bilaterally on the buccal mucosa of a 43-year-
old woman is *most* likely:
   a. candidiasis.
   b. speckled leukoplakia.
   c. leukoedema.
   d. lichen planus.
B. Proper management in this case is to:
   a. prescribe systemic cortisone.
   b. prescribe topical cortisone ointment.
   c. perform several incisional biopsies to
   check for malignant change.
   d. inform the patient of the condition and
   reexamine periodically.

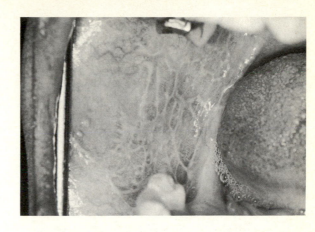

404. This tender red-and-white lesion occurred
after this temporary filling was placed in the
molar tooth. The diagnosis is *most* likely:
   a. aspirin burn.
   b. allergy to the filling material.
   c. candidiasis.
   d. speckled leukoplakia.

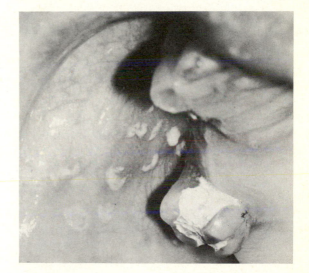

405. This 65-year-old man gives a history of extensive local surgery of the floor of the mouth
for cancer about 10 years previously. The
asymptomatic solitary white condition indicated by an arrow in the floor of the mouth
is *most* likely:
   a. leukoplakia.
   b. white sponge nevus.
   c. hypertrophic candidiasis.
   d. scar tissue.
   e. a skin graft.

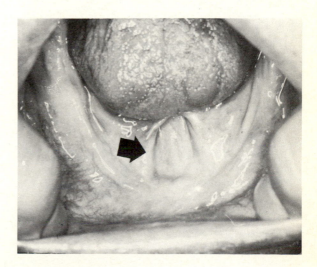

406. This white lesion on the posterolateral region in a 42-year-old woman has been present for about 6 months. It is not painful and does not appear to be enlarging. The patient denies the use of tobacco products or alcohol. The lesion is quite pedunculated.

A. The diagnosis is *most* likely:
    a. squamous cell carcinoma.
    b. a papilloma.
    c. a fibroma.
    d. verrucous carcinoma.
    e. a minor salivary gland tumor.

B. Ideal management would be to:
    a. evaluate the lesion again in 6 months.
    b. perform an incisional biopsy.
    c. perform an excisional biopsy.
    d. perform exfoliative cytology.
    e. make an intralesional injection of cortisone.

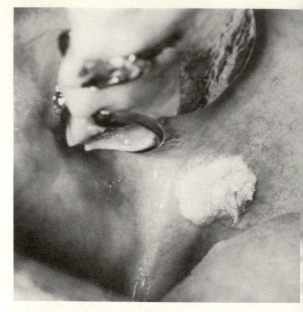

407. This solitary, asymptomatic white lesion at the junction of the ventral surface of the tongue and the floor of the mouth was found in this 62-year-old man during an extraction appointment. He was examined 12 months previously and the lesion was not present at that time. The lesion was firm and painless and the underlying tissue was indurated. There were enlarged, fixed submaxillary nodes on the left side. He admitted to smoking 2 packs of cigarettes per day and to heavy consumption of alcohol. The lesion is *most* likely:

a. squamous cell carcinoma.
b. verrucous carcinoma.
c. a sloughing type of traumatic lesion.
d. a malignant salivary gland tumor.
e. reversible leukoplakia.

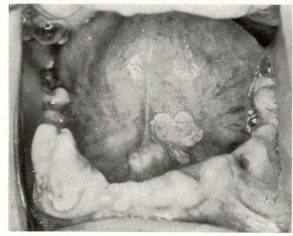

408. This 48-year-old man came for diagnosis and treatment of this painful ulcer, which had been present for 2 weeks. Dark-field examination was negative. The diagnosis is *most* likely:

a. squamous cell carcinoma.
b. recurrent herpetic ulcer.
c. chancre.
d. traumatic ulcer.

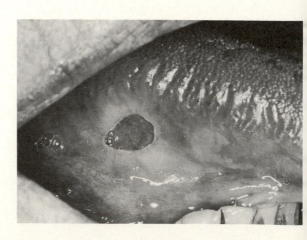

409. This ulcer had been present for about 5 days. When it first appeared, it was very painful. Now pictured in its healing phase, the discomfort was almost all gone. This lesion *most* likely is:

a. a recurrent aphthous ulcer.

b. an odontogenic ulcer.

c. a recurrent herpetic ulcer.

d. a traumatic ulcer.

e. a chancre.

410. This 25-year-old man presented with a chief complaint of a painful ulcer on the lingual frenum that had been bothering him on and off for about a year. The white material could not be scraped off. Except for the presence of a partial ankyloglossia, the remainder of the examination was nonsignificant. This lesion is *most* likely:

a. squamous cell carcinoma.

b. a traumatic lesion possibly related to oral sex.

c. a recurrent aphthous ulcer.

d. candidiasis.

e. a lesion of erosive lichen planus.

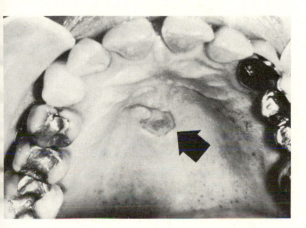

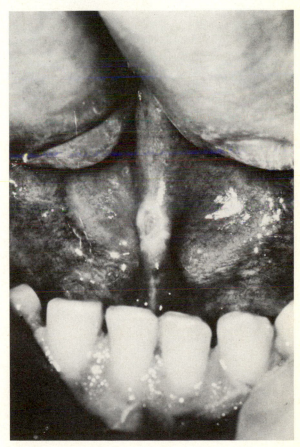

411. This tender, solitary ulcer was found when a 65-year-old man presented for new dentures. He had worn the present denture for some 20 years. The remainder of the oral examination was unremarkable. The ulcer is *most* likely:

a. a recurrent aphthous ulcer.
b. a recurrent herpetic ulcer.
c. squamous cell carcinoma.
d. caused by a retained root fragment.
e. osteogenic sarcoma.

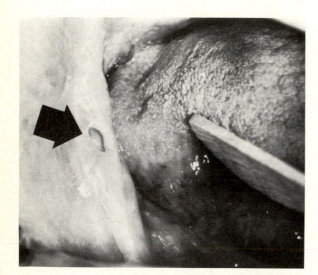

412. This 45-year-old woman presented for diagnosis and treatment of this solitary, painful ulcer *(arrow)*. She said it had been present for about 6 weeks and she thought it had started when she bit her tongue. The borders of the ulcer were slightly indurated. There were several enlarged and slightly tender neck "nodes" on that side. A careful intraoral examination failed to reveal any sharp teeth or appliances. No white lesions are present.

A. The correct approach to this lesion is to:
   a. stain with toluidine blue.
   b. perform an excisional biopsy.
   c. perform an incisional biopsy.
   d. prescribe cortisone in an emollient base and reexamine in 1 month.
   e. take a smear for exfoliative cytology.

B. The *most* likely diagnosis is:
   a. persistent traumatic ulcer or squamous cell carcinoma.
   b. recurrent aphthous ulcer.
   c. recurrent herpetic ulcer.
   d. histoplasmosis.
   e. erosive lichen planus.

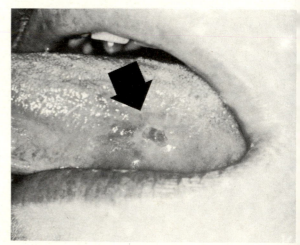

413. This 14-year-old boy suffers from recurrent episodes of this painful ulcerative condition of the hard palate just in this region. The lesions last for approximately 7 to 10 days. This condition is *most* likely:

a. recurrent aphthous ulcers.
b. erythema multiforme.
c. pemphigus.
d. recurrent herpetic lesions.

414. This 35-year-old patient presented for diagnosis and treatment of this solitary, painful palatal ulcer of 4 days' duration (**A**). **B** shows the lesions that involved the palms. The oral ulcer is *most* likely:

a. a major aphthous ulcer.
b. a recurrent herpetic ulcer.
c. a traumatic ulcer.
d. a lesion of erosive lichen planus.
e. a lesion of erythema multiforme.

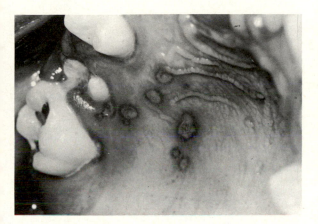

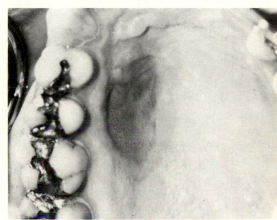

A

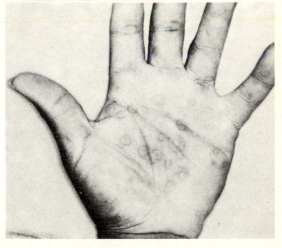

B

415. This ulcerative lesion was examined when a 59-year-old man presented for treatment. The diagnosis is *most* likely:
a. a minor salivary gland tumor.
b. a persistent traumatic ulcer.
c. gumma.
d. osteogenic sarcoma.
e. squamous cell carcinoma.

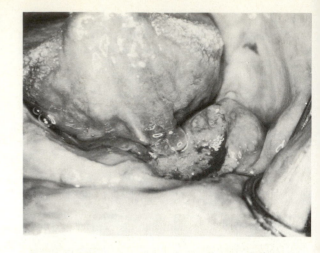

416. This solitary, firm, painless, ulcerated red lesion *(arrow)* on the ventral surface of the tongue just to the right side of the lingual frenum was found in a 58-year-old man who had smoked heavily all his life. The lesion is *most* likely:
a. a traumatic erythema.
b. an erythematous patch caused by a burn.
c. squamous cell carcinoma.
d. fissured tongue.
e. actinomycosis.

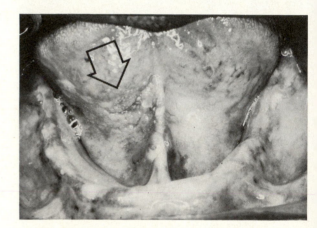

417. The reddish condition of the gingiva was observed in a 34-year-old Asian patient who was 6 months' pregnant. The basic pathologic response is related to:
a. leukemia.
b. medication.
c. folic acid deficiency.
d. ANUG.
e. the presence of local irritants (probably calculus).

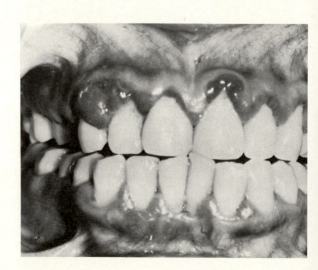

418. This firm nodular mass *(arrow)* was found during routine examination of a 43-year-old man.
   A. This exophytic lesion is *most* likely:
      a. a pyogenic granuloma.
      b. a fibroma.
      c. a myoma.
      d. a myosarcoma.
      e. a papilloma.
   B. This lesion originally was *most* likely:
      a. a papilloma.
      b. a myoma.
      c. a lipoma.
      d. a neuroma.
      e. a pyogenic granuloma.

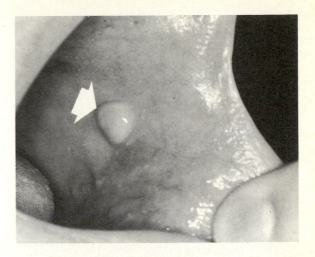

419. This solitary, firm, painless mass is *most* likely:
      a. an epulis fissurata.
      b. a papilloma.
      c. verrucous carcinoma.
      d. squamous cell carcinoma.
      e. condyloma latum.

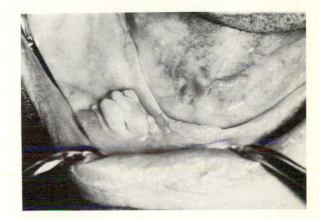

420. This solitary painless lesion was discovered by a 41-year-old patient about 4 months previously. She thought it had begun after she had bitten her cheek one day. She then seemed to bite the mass repeatedly and it continued to grow. The lesion was moderately soft to palpation and bled readily. The whitish material could be scraped off. She smoked 1½ packs of cigarettes per day. The lesion is *most* likely:
      a. a fibroma.
      b. squamous cell carcinoma.
      c. a papilloma.
      d. a pyogenic granuloma.
      e. a lipoma.

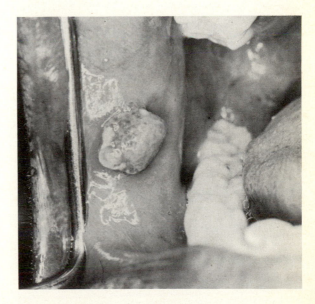

421. Ten days after the right central incisor was extracted, this 52-year-old patient returned because of this soft tissue growth *(arrow)* from the socket. New radiographs yielded no significant findings. The diagnosis *most* likely is:

a. epulis granulomatosa.
b. pulp polyp.
c. osteogenic sarcoma.
d. squamous cell carcinoma.

422. A 68-year-old man presented with this solitary, firm, expanding mass **(A)**. **B** shows the representative histopathology. The *final* diagnosis is:

a. fibroma.
b. pyogenic granuloma.
c. papilloma.
d. squamous cell carcinoma.
e. lipoma.

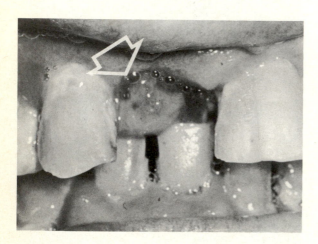

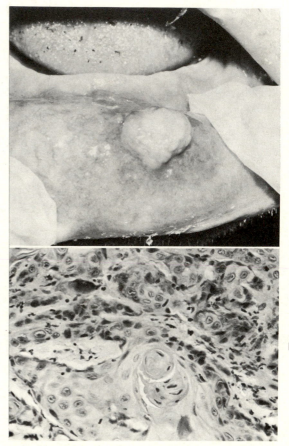

423. An 18-year-old man presented for diagnosis and treatment of this large, bluish, painless mass, which he first noticed about 1 month previously. The mass was soft to rubbery in consistency and fluctuant and could not be emptied with digital pressure. This mass is *most* likely:
a. a ranula.
b. a dermoid cyst.
c. a hemangioma.
d. a melanoma.
e. a lymphangioma.

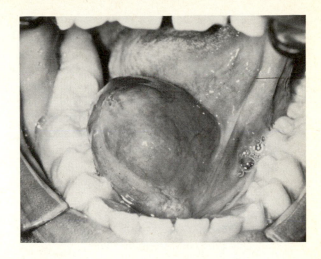

424. An 18-year-old man presented with this sublingual mass, which he noticed for the first time a couple of years previously. He stated that it was painless, had grown slowly, and had become so bulky that it interfered with mastication. The covering mucosa was a normal pink in color. The mass was fluctuant and firmly doughy and moved quite freely in the tissues. Particularly, the mucosa could be moved freely over the mass. The lesion is *most* likely:
a. a ranula.
b. a dermoid cyst.
c. a cavernous hemangioma.
d. a lipoma.
e. a sublingual abscess.

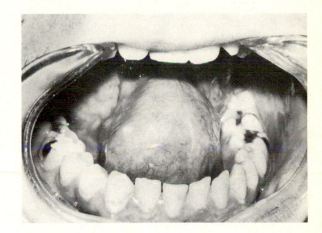

425. This firm, painless, slow-growing mass *(arrow),* which this 53-year-old woman first noticed 3½ years previously is *most* likely:
a. a palatal space abscess.
b. a malignant tumor of the maxillary sinus.
c. an exostosis.
d. a tumor of minor salivary glands.

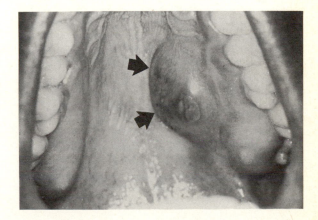

426. This very firm, painless mass occurred in a 25-year-old man. He watched it enlarge for several months before seeking professional help. The teeth in the region registered vital by the various pulp-testing procedures and had no restorations or caries. Occlusal radiographs revealed thin spicules of bone protruding from the buccal aspect of the outer cortical plate. This lesion is *most* likely:
a. an exostosis.
b. a peripheral fibroma with ossification (peripheral odontogenic fibroma).
c. osteogenic sarcoma.
d. chondrosarcoma.
e. a calcifying odontogenic cyst.

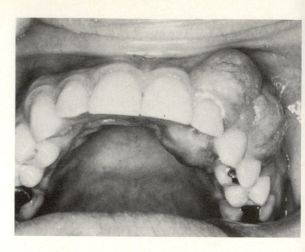

427. This solitary elevated mass in an infant was rubbery, painless, and fluctuant. It is *most* likely:
a. an eruption cyst.
b. a congenital epulis of the newborn.
c. a hemangioma.
d. a mucocele.
e. an Epstein's pearl.

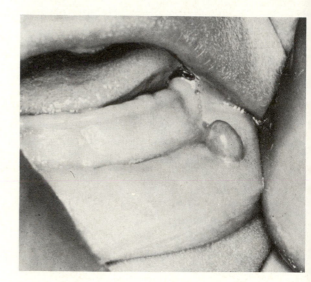

428. A pediatrician requested a dental consultation because of the mass in this newborn's mouth. The firm and nontender mass was polypoid in shape and was attached to the anterior portion of the mandibular ridge. It is *most* likely:
a. a congenital epulis of the newborn.
b. an eruption cyst.
c. a hemangioma.
d. an Epstein's pearl.
e. a metastatic tumor.

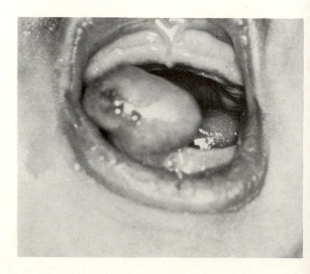

429. A mother brought her 6-month-old daughter to an oral surgeon with the chief complaint of this solitary, painless, bluish mass. It was soft to rubbery, fluctuant, and painless and could not be emptied with digital pressure. This lesion *most* likely is:

a. a congenital epulis of the newborn.
b. an Epstein's pearl.
c. a hemangioma.
d. a mucocele.
e. an eruption cyst.

430. This painless bluish mass (**A**, *arrow*), which was soft and fluctuant in one spot and firm in other areas, was found on routine dental examination. The histopathology of the lesion is illustrated in **B**. The final diagnosis is:

a. a mucocele.
b. a hemangioma.
c. a mucoepidermoid tumor.
d. lymphangioma.
e. giant cell granuloma.

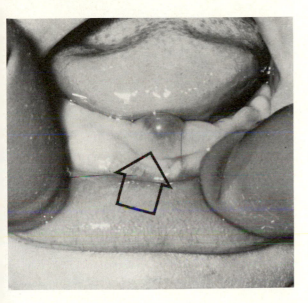

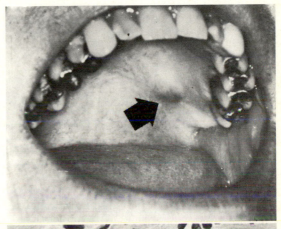

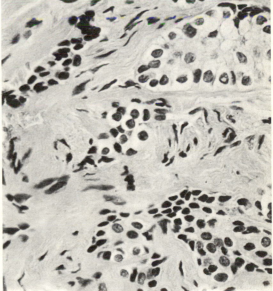

431. This 45-year-old man experienced a tremendous expansion of the posterior ridge on this side only during the previous 6 months. He is now biting on the tuberosity with the lower molars. The expansion is very firm and nontender. Serum studies and blood cell counts are within normal limits. A Waters' radiograph reveals an opacity of the sinus and also some loss of bony walls. The patient *most* likely has:

a. squamous cell carcinoma of the soft tissue covering the tuberosity.
b. an exostosis.
c. Paget's disease.
d. a malignant tumor of the maxillary sinus.

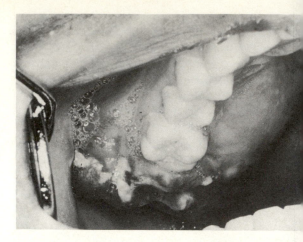

432. This 34-year-old woman stated that these two soft masses had been present for many years. She also had many soft nodules distributed over many skin surfaces as well as several tan macules of varying sizes. The intraoral nodules are *most* likely:

a. multiple lipomas.
b. basal cell nevi.
c. multiple metastatic carcinomas.
d. multiple neurofibromatosis.
e. multiple papillomas.

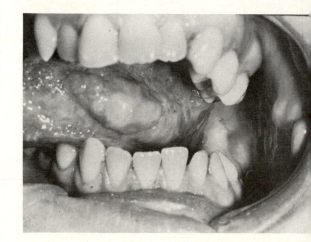

433. A 21-year-old man presented for diagnosis and treatment of this solitary bluish mass *(arrow)* on the lower lip. He said he first became aware of it about 6 months previously, and that it was never painful and sometimes disappeared completely only to return again. The mass was soft to rubbery in consistency, was fluctuant, and could not be emptied by digital pressure. It *most* likely is:

a. a hemangioma.
b. a hematoma.
c. a mucocele.
d. a mucus-producing salivary tumor.
e. a pyogenic granuloma.

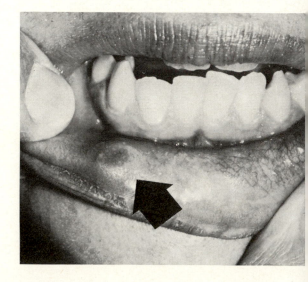

434. This solitary bluish mass was discovered during a periodic dental examination of a 42-year-old woman. The mass was soft and fluctuant and could be slowly reduced in size by slow, judicial digital pressure. The patient admitted to having known of its presence for several years but said it had not increased in size during all that time. The mass is *most* likely:

a. a mucocele.
b. a lymphangioma.
c. a hematoma.
d. a mucus-producing salivary tumor.
e. a hemangioma.

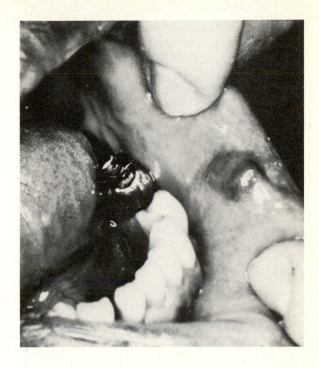

435. This soft-to-rubbery bluish mass was found during routine examination of a 56-year-old man who enjoyed good health. Digital pressure did not produce emptying of the mass. The mass does not vary much in size. The diagnosis is *most* likely:

a. a hemangioma.
b. a hematoma.
c. a varicosity.
d. a ranula.

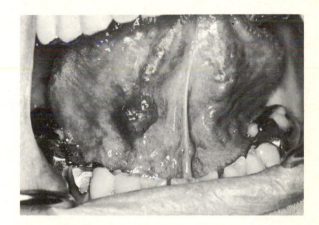

436. The attending dentist had kept this pigmented macule *(arrow)* under surveillance for several months, but it had not changed in appearance. He was unable to blanch it with digital pressure. The lesion in this 44-year-old blonde patient is *most* likely:

a. melanoplakia.
b. an amalgam tattoo.
c. a hemangioma.
d. a junctional nevus.
e. a hematoma.

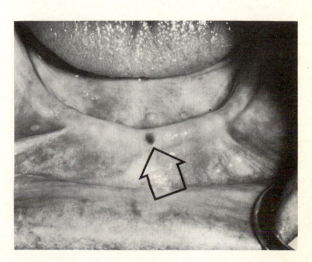

437. During examination of a 65-year-old man a day after he was involved in an automobile accident, a dentist found this dark bluish lesion. The lesion was moderately soft to palpation and basically painless except that digital pressure on the lesion produced a stinging sensation at its periphery. This condition is *most* likely:

a. a melanoma.

b. a hematoma.

c. a hemangioma.

d. a ranula.

e. melanoplakia.

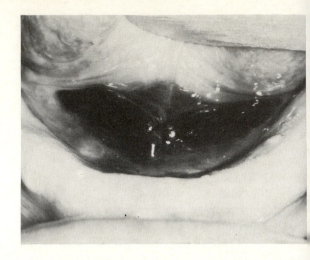

438. This rapidly growing, firm, bluish-black mass occurred in a 55-year-old black woman. She had watched a black patch in her mouth grow slowly over the years and had noticed a nodule develop in the macule 6 months previously. This nodule proceeded to increase in size very rapidly. The mass is *most* likely:

a. squamous cell carcinoma.

b. giant cell granuloma.

c. hemangiosarcoma.

d. a metastatic tumor.

e. a melanoma.

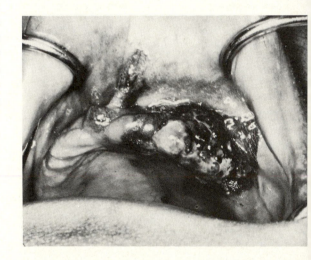

439. These bluish-black ribbons seen in this 28-year-old woman are probably examples of:

a. Addisonian pigmentation.

b. melanoplakia.

c. heavy metal line.

d. argyria.

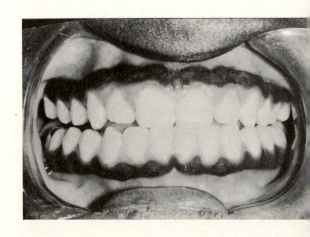

440. This asymptomatic red lesion did not regress when this 55-year-old tobacco smoker left his dentures out for 3 weeks, but rather showed growth. It is *most* likely:
a. an erythroplakia.
b. a hemangioma.
c. traumatic erythema.
d. early-stage epulis fissurata.

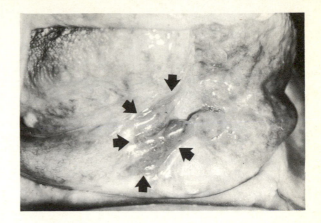

441. This reddish condition was noted under a U-shaped acrylic partial denture. It is *most* likely:
a. atrophic candidiasis.
b. nicotine stomatitis.
c. a denture base allergy.
d. related to a xerostomia.
e. papillary hyperplasia.

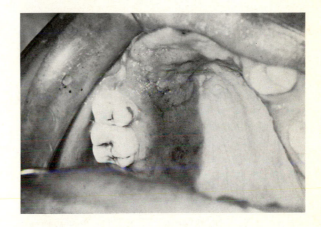

442. This 64-year-old patient experienced surgical removal of a squamous cell carcinoma of the left side of the floor of the mouth 2 years previously. The present solitary, painless, red, firm lesion on the right side of the floor of the mouth had been present for at least 6 weeks and was slowly enlarging. The present lesion is *most* likely:
a. a new squamous cell carcinoma.
b. a secondary carcinoma.
c. a papilloma.
d. an early inflammatory hyperplasia lesion (epulis fissurata).
e. traumatic erythema.

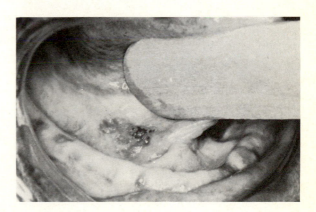

443. This otherwise healthy 32-year-old patient complained of this painful bleb on her palate. She said she noticed it immediately after eating dinner the previous night. She had not experienced a similar lesion before. The painful condition is *most* likely:

a. related to a burn.
b. a friction blister.
c. a herald lesion of benign mucous membrane pemphigoid.
d. a recurrent herpetic lesion.
e. a herpangina lesion.

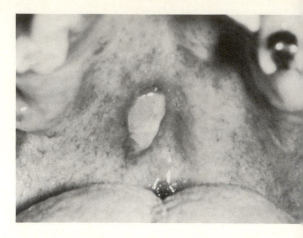

444. This 26-year-old man presented for treatment of a very sore mouth. The oral lesions as shown here were composed of blebs and ulcers. The salivary pool was found to be generous, and except for the presence of "bull's eye" lesions on the palms, the remainder of the examination was unremarkable. This patient *most* likely has:

a. primary herpetic gingivostomatitis.
b. erythema multiforme.
c. recurrent aphthous stomatitis.
d. pemphigus.
e. sicca syndrome.

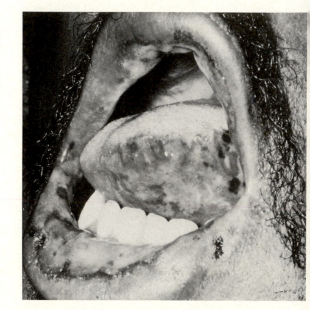

445. While a periodic dental examination was being performed in this 18-year-old man, these asymptomatic reddish macules were found on several oral surfaces. He *most* likely has:

a. Reiter's syndrome.
b. primary herpetic gingivostomatitis.
c. atrophic candidiasis.
d. ectopic geographic tongue.
e. an early stage of erythema multiforme.

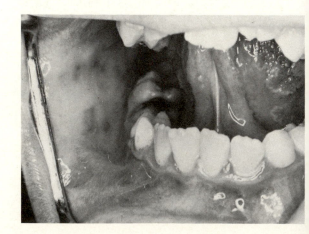

446. A. This 67-year-old man complained of a tender mouth, dysphasia, and itching conjunctivae. **A** shows the lesions on the soft palate and **B** shows the conjunctival involvement. The salivary pool was found to be quite copious. This man *most* likely is suffering from:

a. erythema multiforme.
b. recurrent aphthous stomatitis.
c. primary herpetic stomatitis.
d. benign mucous membrane pemphigoid.
e. Sjögren's syndrome.

B. In differentiating between pemphigus and benign mucous membrane pemphigoid, the following test is helpful:

a. Fluorescent treponema antibody.
b. differential white count.
c. Paul-Bunnell heterophil.
d. immunofluorescent tissue test.

447. This 25-year-old woman presented to her dentist for treatment of a sore mouth. Oral examination revealed several painful reddish macules on various mucosal surfaces similar to those shown here. She also complained of a smarting of the eyes, pain in the joints, and burning on urination. While examining her intraorally, the dentist noted the lack of formation of a salivary pool in the floor of the mouth. This patient *most* likely has:

a. erosive lichen planus.
b. Sjögren's syndrome.
c. Reiter's syndrome.
d. erythema multiforme.
c. pemphigus.

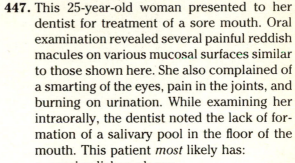

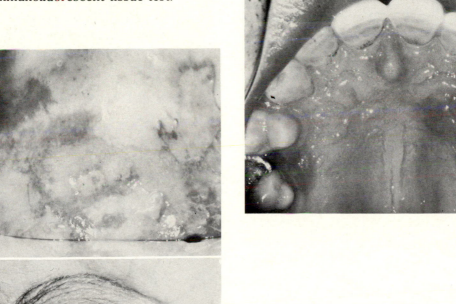

A

B

448. The palatal lesion illustrated here is most likely:
- a. probably squamous cell carcinoma.
- b. a minor salivary gland tumor.
- c. a gumma.
- d. a papillary hyperplasia type of condition.
- e. a traumatic lesion caused by a suction cup on a denture.

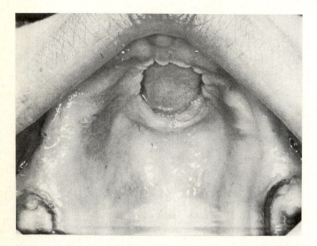

Dr. Danny Sawyer authored questions 449 through 462.

449. A. The examiner is palpating a hard, movable, painless mass in the floor of the mouth *(arrow),* which is tender when the denture flange impinges on the area during mastication. The working diagnosis is *most* likely:
- a. squamous cell carinoma.
- b. dermoid cyst.
- c. sialolithiasis.
- d. hyperplasia of the genial tubercle.
- c. mucous retention phenomenon (ranula).

B. The *most* useful clinical or laboratory aid in diagnosis of this lesion is:
- a. determination of salivary IgA levels.
- b. determination of seromucoid levels.
- c. an occlusal x-ray.
- d. a cytologic smear.
- e. aspiration of the mass.

C. Treatment of the condition may include:
- a. expression, by manipulation, of the stone if it is near the orifice.
- b. no treatment.
- c. radical surgical excision.
- d. antibiotic therapy.
- e. surgical drainage of the lesion.

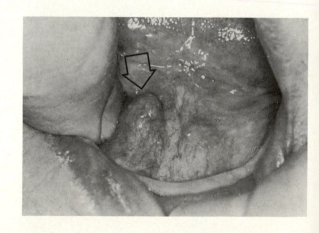

450. A. This 22-year-old man complained of sore throat, fever, and headache. In addition to the multiple petechiae, he manifested a tonsillitis and bilateral cervical lymphadenitis. Clinical differential diagnosis should include all the following *except:*
   a. mucocele.
   b. blood dyscrasia.
   c. hereditary hemorrhagic telangiectasia.
   d. infectious mononucleosis.
   e. trauma.
   B. The most helpful laboratory or clinical aid is:
   a. a Mantoux test.
   b. a Paul-Bunnell test.
   c. an excisional biopsy.
   d. radiographs.
   e. an FTA-ABS test.
   C. Blood analysis demonstrated a relative lymphocytosis with atypical lymphocytes. The *most* likely diagnosis in this case is:
   a. trauma.
   b. hereditary hemorrhagic telangiectasia.
   c. melanoma.
   d. infectious mononucleosis.
   e. herpangina.
   D. The disease is *probably* caused by:
   a. trauma.
   b. a rickettsial organism.
   c. a fungus.
   d. a bacteria.
   e. a virus.

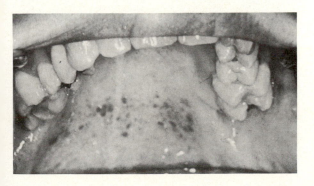

451. A. This denture patient had worn the same dentures 24 hours per day for the past 20 years. The red lesions were slightly tender and the patient complained of a "burning" sensation. Differential diagnosis should include all the following *except:*
   a. candidiasis.
   b. denture allergy.
   c. leukoplakia.
   d. inflammatory papillary hyperplasia.
   e. denture stomatitis (denture-sore mouth).
   B. The *most* likely final diagnosis of the lesion is:
   a. candidiasis.
   b. denture allergy.
   c. leukoplakia.
   d. inflammatory papillary hyperplasia.
   e. denture stomatitis (denture-sore mouth).
   C. As in this case, when the lesions are red (in the early inflammatory stages), papillary hyperplasia of the palate may frequently be treated successfully by:
   a. removal of the denture at night and the use of a tissue conditioner.
   b. antibiotic therapy.
   c. surgical excision.
   d. antiviral agents.
   e. cryosurgery.
   D. Inflammatory papillary hyperplasia:
   a. is a premalignant condition.
   b. is also known as nicotine stomatitis.
   c. is a condition in which the inflammatory lesions (red) may persist and become fibrotic.
   d. requires no treatment.

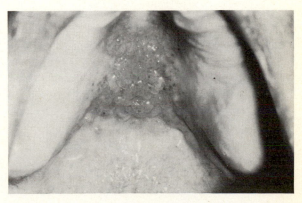

452. A. The white lesion in this case was tender and the material itself could be easily removed. The lesion was opposite a carious molar tooth. In this case, differential diagnosis should include all the following *except:*
   a. aspirin burn.
   b. leukoedema and cheek biting.
   c. candidiasis.
   d. leukoplakia.
   B. The *best* diagnostic aid in this case is:
   a. a cytologic smear.
   b. radiographs.
   c. palpation.
   d. a biopsy.
   e. careful questioning of the patient regarding topical aspirin usage.

453. A. This 30-year-old man presented with hyperplastic and bleeding gingivae. He complained of dizziness and fever. He was pale in appearance, and clinical examination revealed bilateral cervical lymphadenopathy. The working diagnosis in this case is *most* likely:
   a. hyperplastic gingivitis.
   b. blood dyscrasia: acute leukemia.
   c. ANUG.
   d. erythema multiforme.
   B. The *most* definitive laboratory/clinical aid in establishing a correct diagnosis would be:
   a. a biopsy.
   b. a radiographic examination.
   c. a cytology/smear.
   d. aspiration.
   e. a hemogram and bone marrow examination.

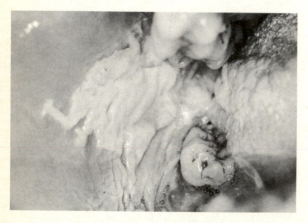

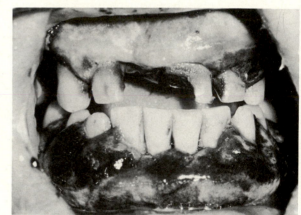

454. A. This elderly outdoor worker noticed this ulcerated lesion with a smooth rolled border on her cheek several months ago. It has progressively enlarged despite reported attempts at healing. The *most* likely final diagnosis is:

    a. basal cell carcinoma.
    b. melanocarcinoma.
    c. sebaceous cyst.
    d. keratoacanthoma.
    e. squamous cell carcinoma.

  B. Basal cell carcinomas may be treated by:

    a. surgery.
    b. electrocauterization.
    c. cryosurgery.
    d. all the methods above.
    e. none of the methods above.

455. A. This adult patient presented with these multiple asymptomatic, bilateral, firm swellings, which had been present several years on the lingual aspect of the mandible adjacent to the premolar teeth. The *most* likely diagnosis is:

    a. chondromas.
    b. osteomas.
    c. osteochondromas.
    d. tori mandibularis.
    e. odontomas.

  B. The treatment indicated for this case, which requires a partial denture, is:

    a. none.
    b. surgical removal.
    c. a full workup for Paget's disease.
    d. removal by use of laser techniques.

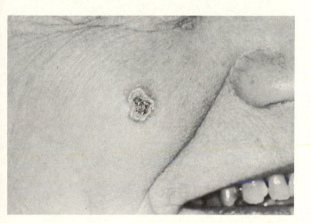

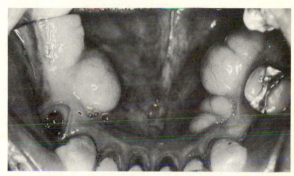

456. A. This patient had a large, soft, smooth, reddish-yellow mass in the region of the palatoglossal and palatopharyngeal arches. This painless mass was not attached to the uvula. The *most* likely diagnosis is:
   a. lipoma.
   b. fibroma.
   c. enlarged palatine tonsil (benign).
   d. papilloma.
   e. lymphoma.

   B. The correct management for this lesion is:
   a. to inform the patient of its presence and reexamine in 6 months.
   b. to tell the patient that it is within normal limits.
   c. surgical excision and microscopic study.
   d. irradiation.

457. A. This painless lesion on the palate of a 38-year-old woman is *most* likely:
   a. papilloma.
   b. condyloma acuminatum.
   c. fibroma.
   d. pyogenic granuloma.
   e. verrucous carcinoma.

   B. The *most* correct management of the lesion should consist of:
   a. radiation therapy.
   b. chemotherapy.
   c. surgical excision through the stalk.
   d. surgical excision including some adjacent normal tissue.
   e. periodic observation.

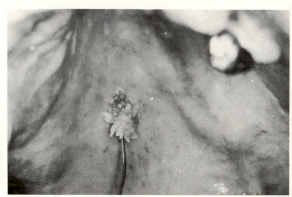

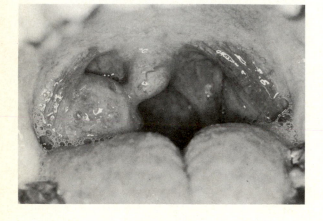

458. A. This male patient presented with patchy, circinate, and irregular areas of surface erosion. The lesions are sharply demarcated by whitish raised lines at the periphery of the lesions. The *most* likely diagnosis is:
   a. geographic tongue.
   b. erosive lichen planus.
   c. oral psoriasis.
   d. Reiter's syndrome.
   e. median rhomboid glossitis.
 B. The lesions in this case might include all the following characteristics *except:*
   a. they are usually multiple.
   b. they may spontaneously disappear.
   c. they often undergo malignant change.
   d. they may be quite painful.
   e. they are usually migratory.
 C. Geographic tongue:
   a. is relatively common (1% to 2% of population).
   b. is more commonly seen in male patients.
   c. is known to be caused by stress in all cases.
   d. is also known as median rhomboid glossitis.

459. A. This elderly man in congestive heart failure first noticed this lesion *(arrow)* some 20 years previously. The lesion was bluish-black in color, compressible, and asymptomatic. The diagnosis is *most* likely:
   a. a mucocele.
   b. a hemangioma.
   c. a hematoma.
   d. a melanoma.
 B. Indicated management of the lesion is to:
   a. remove with surgical excision.
   b. treat with topical cortisone.
   c. reexamine the lesion periodically.
   d. remove the lesion with cryotherapy.

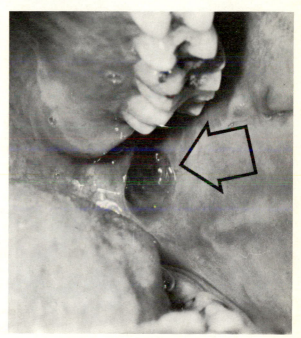

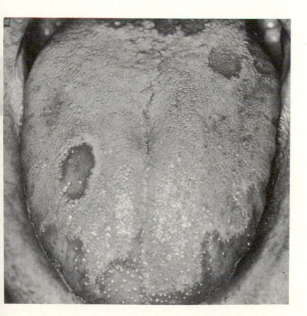

460. A. During routine examination of this 55-year-old woman you find this bony-hard palatal lesion. The patient indicates that it had been present for many years. The *most* likely diagnosis of the lesion is:

a. osteogenic sarcoma.

b. torus palatinus.

c. pleomorphic adenoma of minor salivary glands.

d. adenoid cystic carcinoma of minor salivary glands.

B. Surgical excision of tori may be required for all the following reasons *except:*

a. psychologic reasons.

b. if they are continually traumatized.

c. if they interfere with speech or mastication.

d. if they interfere with prosthesis fabrication.

e. because they frequently undergo malignant change.

461. A. This ulcerative lesion occurred on the palate of a 55-year-old white man. He had noticed a swelling of the area a "few" weeks previously. Differential diagnosis includes all the following. The *most* likely diagnosis is:

a. squamous cell carinoma or necrotizing sialometaplasia.

b. infected median palatal cyst or necrotizing sialometaplasia.

c. recurrent aphthous ulcer or squamous cell carcinoma.

d. necrotizing sialometaplasia or malignant minor salivary gland tumor.

e. necrotizing sialometaplasia or recurrent aphthous ulcer.

B. The *most* valuable diagnostic aid in this case would be:

a. biopsy.

b. radiographs.

c. aspiration.

d. cytology.

e. determination of salivary IgA levels.

C. The lesions of necrotizing sialometaplasia are:

a. self-limiting and heal spontaneously.

b. best treated by radiation therapy.

c. best treated by chemotherapy.

d. best treated by radical surgical excision.

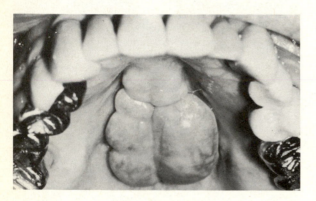

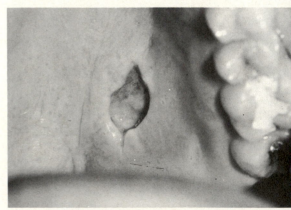

462. This adult male presented with this extensive destruction and necrosis of the hard palate, which he noticed for the first time 6 weeks previously. The *most* likely diagnosis is:
a. squamous cell carcinoma.
b. recurrent herpes lesion.
c. midline malignant reticulosis.
d. chancre.

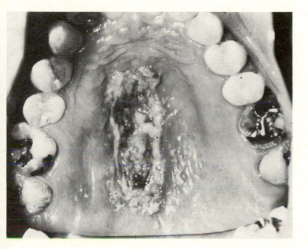

463. This 25-year-old woman presented for treatment of this painful ulcer, which had been present for about 2 days. She stated that she frequently gets these ulcers when under stress and that they usually last for about 7 days. The submandibular nodes are tender on that side.
A. The lesion is *most* likely:
    a. a traumatic ulcer.
    b. a recurrent aphthous ulcer.
    c. a recurrent herpetic ulcer.
    d. squamous cell carcinoma.
    e. a chancre.
B. The proper approach to this lesion should include:
    a. exfoliative cytology.
    b. excisional biopsy.
    c. systemic penicillin.
    d. toluidine staining.
    e. topical applications of corticosteroid in an emollient base.

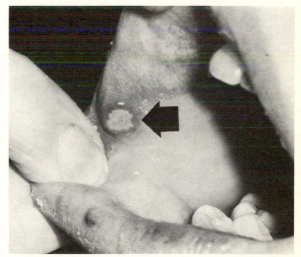

464. A. This 40-year-old woman had developed these lip lesions over the previous 3 months. She had reddish lesions on the skin of her face and forearms. The whitish plaques on the lips were painless. She had arthritis and complained of tiredness and photosensitivity. All the following are included in the differential diagnosis of these lesions *except:*
a. lichenoid drug reaction.
b. lichen planus.
c. basal cell carcinoma.
d. lupus erythematosus.

B. The *most* likely diagnosis based on the history is:
a. lichenoid drug reaction.
b. lichen planus.
c. squamous cell carcinoma.
d. lupus erythematosus.

465. This illustration shows the buccal mucosa, buccal sulcus, and gingivae of an adult patient 2 days after dental treatment of a carious first mandibular molar. The lesion was white, well demarcated, and painful. The superficial epithelial cells were necrotic and sloughing. Differential diagnosis of this lesion includes all the following *except:*
a. recurrent herpes.
b. chemical burn.
c. leukoplakia.
d. candidiasis.

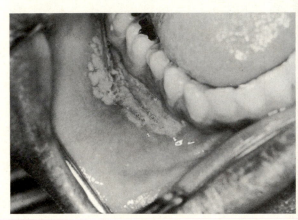

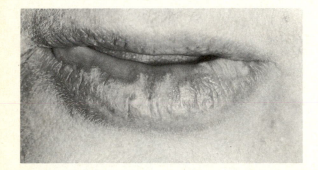

466. A. This adult patient presented with a solitary white lesion that could not be stripped off on the lateral border of the tongue. The lesion was opposite a mandibular premolar tooth with sharp jagged edges. Differential diagnosis might include all the following *except:*
   a. leukoplakia.
   b. lichen planus.
   c. nicotine stomatitis.
   d. verrucous carcinoma.

B. What is the *most* likely diagnosis?
   a. leukoplakia (benign microscopic changes).
   b. speckled leukoplakia.
   c. squamous cell carcinoma.
   d. verrucous carcinoma.

C. The indicated management of this lesion is to:
   a. excise immediately with a wide border of normal tissue.
   b. irradiate.
   c. tell the patient that nothing need be done.
   d. eliminate the sharp edges on the premolar tooth and reexamine in 2 weeks.

D. The overall malignant transformation rate of all oral leukoplakic lesions in the United States is approximately:
   a. less than 1%.
   b. 1% to 3%.
   c. 10% to 15%.
   d. 3% to 6%.
   e. over 20%.

467. A. This photograph shows a granular, red, and erosive gingival surface. This 50-year-old white woman had two or three areas like this on the gingiva. Differential diagnosis includes all the following *except:*
   a. erosive lichen planus.
   b. desquamative gingivitis.
   c. benign mucous membrane pemphigoid.
   d. pemphigus vulgaris.
   e. recurrent aphthous ulcer.

B. If a region showing a white lattice pattern is found on the oral mucosa, this would prompt a working diagnosis for the gingival condition of:
   a. erosive lichen planus.
   b. desquamative gingivitis.
   c. benign mucous membrane pemphigoid.
   d. pemphigus vulgaris.

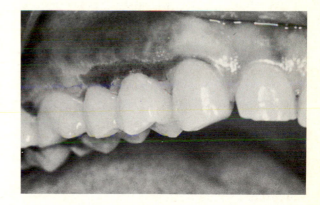

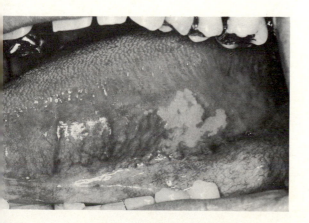

468. This young patient's chief complaint was the appearance of her teeth. The teeth affected are the central incisors, canines, and first permanent molars. The *most* likely diagnosis is:

a. hypocalcification.

b. syphilitic teeth.

c. Turner's teeth.

d. hypoplasia as a result of systemic infection or fever.

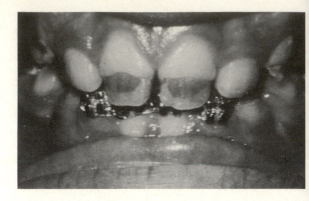

469. This radiograph is of a 9-year-old girl whose grandparents were from Greece. She had experienced a sickly childhood and was continually under a physician's care. Both the jaws and skull showed a generalized radiolucency. This photograph has been underprinted (processed to make a less dark image) in order to retain the detail that was present. This patient *most* likely has:

a. sickle cell anemia.

b. hyperparathyroidism.

c. osteoporosis (drug induced).

d. Paget's disease (early stage).

e. thalassemia.

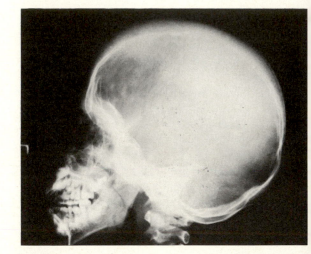

470. Several of these pigmented macules were found on various skin surfaces of this young girl who had experienced precocious development of puberty. She *most* likely has:

a. Addison's disease.

b. von Recklinghausen's disease.

c. Albright's syndrome.

d. Peutz-Jeghers syndrome.

e. Cushing's syndrome.

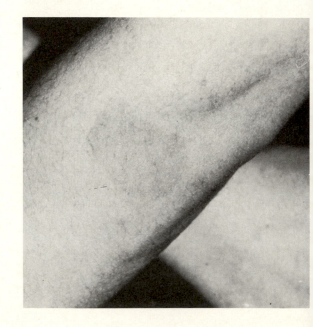

471. The two black areas seen here could be removed with a tongue blade, which revealed small discrepancies in the mucosa underneath. In addition there were some ecchymotic patches and some petechiae on the oral mucosa. This patient *most* likely:
a. has necrotic metastatic melanomas.
b. has thrombocytopenic purpura.
c. is suffering only from a recent traumatic incident.
d. has multiple giant cell granulomas.
e. has multiple pyogenic granulomas.

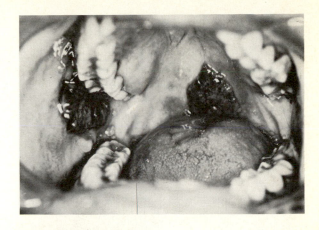

472. This 38-year-old man who has petechiae scattered over the skin and oral mucous membranes presented with a chief complaint of tender gums and bleeding gingiva. He *most* likely has:
a. ANUG.
b. mouth-breathing gingivitis.
c. leukemia.
d. phenytoin (Dilantin) gingivitis.
e. vitamin B deficiency.

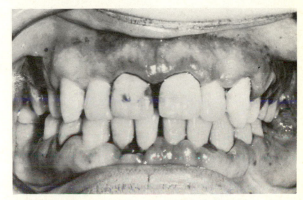

473. The entire skin of this 42-year-old person is covered with these tender reddish macules and papules. The rapid plasmin reagin card test is positive. The patient *most* likely has:
a. von Recklinghausen's disease.
b. basal cell nevus syndrome.
c. pityriasis rosea.
d. secondary syphilis.
e. lupus erythematosus.

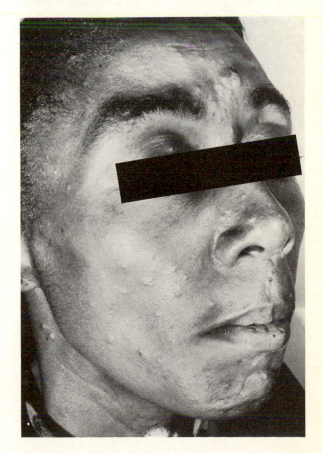

474. This patient, who has a few large brown macules on his back, *most* likely has:
   a. basal cell nevus syndrome.
   b. multiple keloids.
   c. multiple metastatic carcinoma.
   d. multiple melanomas.
   e. von Recklinghausen's disease.

475. It is a problem completing the dental procedure for this woman because her perioral tissues are so stiff that they greatly limit intraoral access. Full-mouth radiographs reveal a generalized widening of the periodontal ligament spaces. This patient *most* likely has:
   a. discoid lupus erythematosus.
   b. scleroderma.
   c. amyloidosis.
   d. submucous fibrosis.
   e. uncontrolled diabetes.

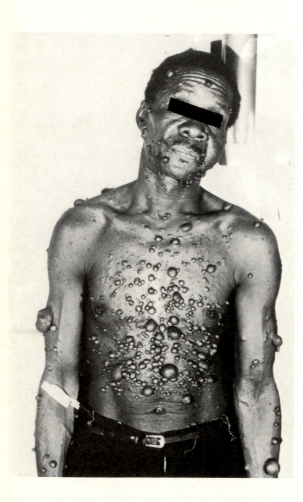

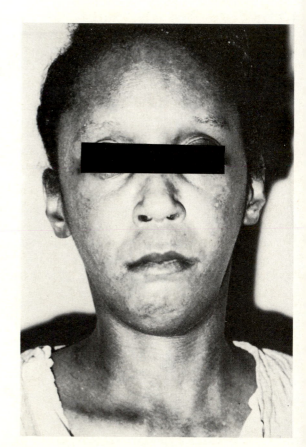

476. From the clinical and radiographic findings (**A** and **B**) in this man, the following diagnosis can be made:

a. basal cell nevus syndrome.
b. Albright's syndrome.
c. Addison's disease.
d. Sturge-Weber syndrome.
e. von Recklinghausen's disease.

477. This 65-year-old black man presented for a tooth extraction. The two lesions shown in **A** and **B** are painful. He *most* likely has:

a. leukemia.
b. sickle cell anemia.
c. uncontrolled diabetes.
d. syphilis.
e. congestive heart failure.

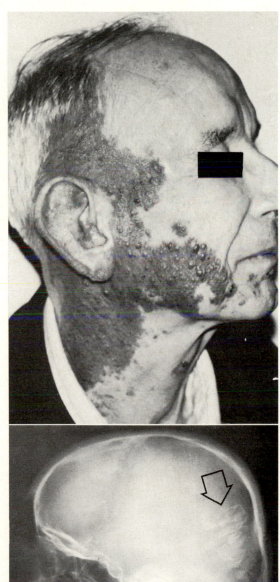

A

B

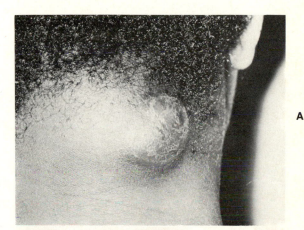

A

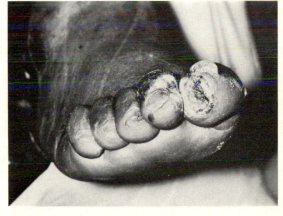

B

478. These painless, reddish lesions on the skin of the upper abdomen of this 48-year-old man blanch readily on digital pressure. They are usually an indication of:
a. alcoholic liver disease.
b. congestive heart failure.
c. hereditary telangiectasia.
d. leukemia.
e. essential hypertension.

479. A generalized bluish tint was seen on the oral mucosa and face of this 65-year-old man. He appeared to be in reasonably good heath except for some difficulties with hearing, sight, and smell. He *most* likely has:
a. cyanosis.
b. Addison's disease.
c. hemochromatosis.
d. argyria.
e. anemia.

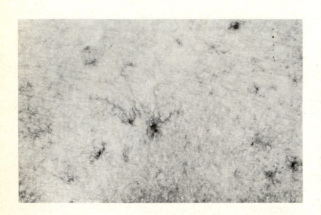

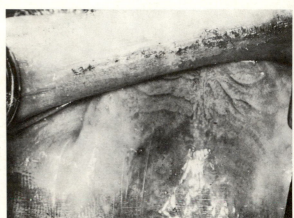

480. This 60-year-old woman (**A** and **B**) was under treatment for bone pain. Laboratory tests revealed a decreased albumin/globulin ratio and Bence Jones protein in the urine. This patient *most* likely has:

a. thalassemia.
b. multiple metastatic carcinoma.
c. multiple myeloma.
d. histiocytosis X.
e. disseminated tuberculosis.

481. This 21-year-old woman presented with the chief complaint of a sore mouth (**A**). Several of the mucosal surfaces were diffusely red (**B**). No ulcers were present at this time, but the lips were dry and the salivary pool was absent. Copious carious lesions were present, particularly in the lingual aspects of the lower anterior teeth. The patient had tender swellings of both parotid glands and tenderness of the conjunctivae. She was taking aspirin every 4 hours to minimize the arthritic discomfort. She *most* likely has:

a. erythema multiforme.
b. erosive lichen planus.
c. Sjögren's syndrome.
d. benign mucous membrane pemphigoid.
e. candidiasis.

A
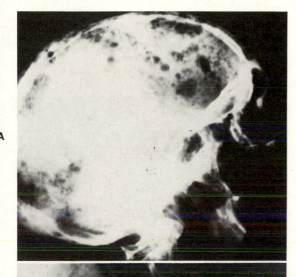
B
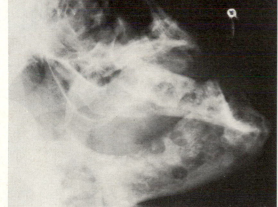

A
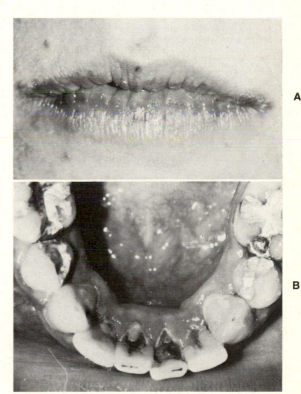
B

482. This swollen joint is characteristic of:
   a. osteoarthritis.
   b. gouty arthritis.
   c. rheumatoid arthritis.
   d. rheumatic heart disease.
   e. clubbing of the fingers.

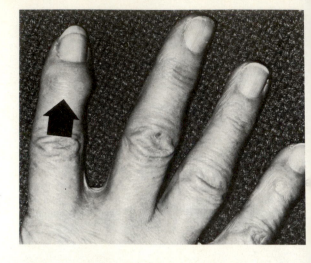

483. This swollen joint *(arrow)* is characteristic of:
   a. degenerative joint disease (osteoarthritis).
   b. gouty arthritis.
   c. rheumatoid arthritis.
   d. rheumatic heart disease.
   e. clubbing of the fingers.

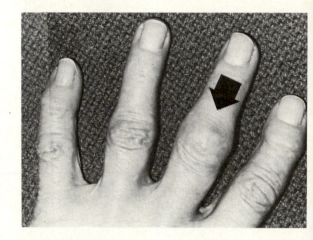

484. A. This 52-year-old man had been bothered for some weeks with a sore mouth. The small vesicles and ulcerations illustrated were seen on all the oral mucosal surfaces, and a few on the skin. The eyes were not involved and the salivary pool was quite generous. This patient *most* likely has:
   a. primary herpetic gingivostomatitis.
   b. pemphigus.
   c. Sjögren's syndrome.
   d. benign mucous membrane pemphigoid.
   e. erosive lichen planus.

B. Which of the following tests would be *most* helpful in making the diagnosis?
   a. immunofluorescent studies.
   b. Bence Jones test.
   c. FTS—ABS.
   d. differential white cell count.

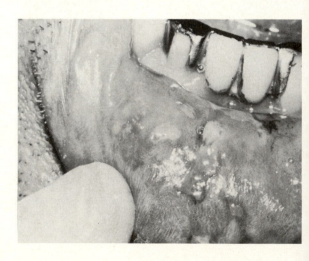

485. Both sides of the mandible had this appearance, but the maxilla appeared to be within normal limits in this 11-year-old girl who was continually tired and suffered from bleeding of the gingiva and epistaxis. She *most* likely has:
a. uncontrolled diabetes.
b. sickle cell anemia.
c. hyperparathyroidism.
d. leukemia.

486. This very painful lesion on the thumb of a 33-year-old dentist has recurred several times over the last 12 months. The dentist relates that it first occurred 2 days after treating a patient who had a painful lesion on the upper lip. This lesion is most likely:
a. a staphylococcal infection.
b. a herpetic whitlow.
c. a streptococcal infection.
d. a local hepatitis B infection.

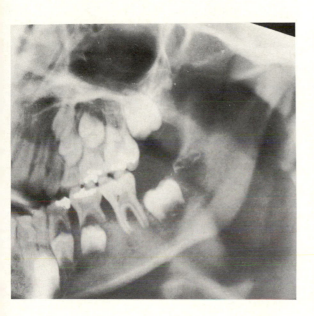

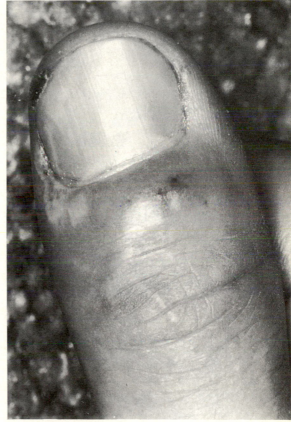

487. A. This 32-year-old man has enjoyed excellent health for years but now complains of malaise and fever for the previous 6 weeks. During the previous 6 months he has experienced recurrent bouts with oral candidiasis. During this periodic oral examination you notice these bluish-black painless lesions on the palate, which the patient says have been present for about 6 weeks. Serious consideration has to be given to the possibility that he may have:

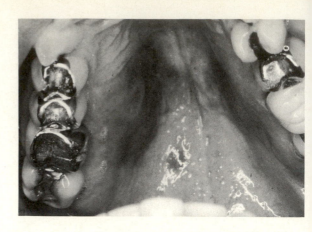

   a. an inherited immunoincompetence.
   b. thrombocytopenic purpura.
   c. melanoma.
   d. AIDS.

   B. AIDS is caused by:
   a. herpes virus.
   b. Epstein-Barr virus.
   c. human immunodeficiency virus (HTLV-III) virus.
   d. Coxsackievirus.

   C. The best preventive measure for dentists to follow in order to protect themselves against contracting AIDS is to:
   a. be immunized against the virus.
   b. use the barrier technique and other infection control measures.
   c. use protective eye covering.
   d. eliminate all patients from their practice who have a history of recurrent herpes infections.

   D. Which of the following items in patient history would *most* likely lead us to consider a possible diagnosis of AIDS?
   1. pneumonia due to *Pneumocystis carinii.*
   2. polycythemia.
   3. hairy leukoplakia.
   4. Kaposi's sarcoma of skin and mucous membranes.
      a. 1, 2, and 3 only.
      b. 1 and 4 only.
      c. 2 and 3 only.
      d. 1, 3, and 4 only.

488. This 15-year-old girl presented with this sore throat and soft palate in August. She suffered from fever, malaise, and these vesicles in the posterior aspect of the mouth. The attack lasted for about 2 weeks and there has been no recurrence. The rest of the oral cavity, lips, and skin are unaffected. The Paul-Bunnell test remained negative. The diagnosis is *most* likely:

a. herpangina (Coxsackievirus).
b. recurrent herpetic infection.
c. mononucleosis.
d. chickenpox.

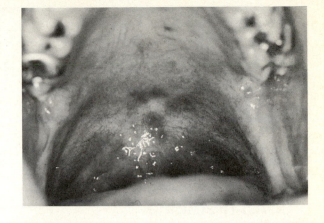

489. This 21-year-old woman presented 1 week before this picture was taken. The lesions at that time were a cluster of burning, itching vesicles. They soon ruptured and crusted over. The lesions disappeared in 10 days, but there have been three recurrences during the past year. The patient is otherwise in good health. The diagnosis *most* likely is:

a. recurrent herpes simplex lesion.
b. herpes zoster (shingles).
c. erysipelas.
d. candidiasis of the skin.

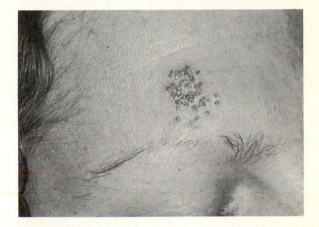

490. This 10-year-old girl has been suffering from fever and malaise for 4 days. These lesions were present on all the skin surfaces. Several small, tender vesicles could be seen in the oral cavity. This patient *most* likely has:

a. chickenpox.
b. primary herpes simplex infection.
c. measles.
d. herpangina.

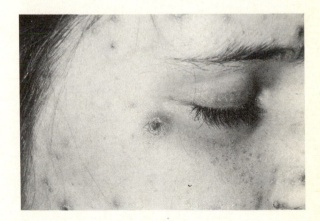

PART 2

Comprehensive treatment planning

Oral medicine

1. You have just administered a mandibular block injection to this patient, who appeared normal prior to the injection. You should advise her that:
   a. this is an entirely normal phenomenon.
   b. the sensation to the lower lip will return for certain within 6 months.
   c. it is anticipated that everything will return to normal within 3 to 4 hours.
   d. the asymmetry is attributable to the bulk of the anesthetic solution in the tissues.
   e. if she will just relax sufficiently, you will be able to reduce the dislocation of the right condyle.

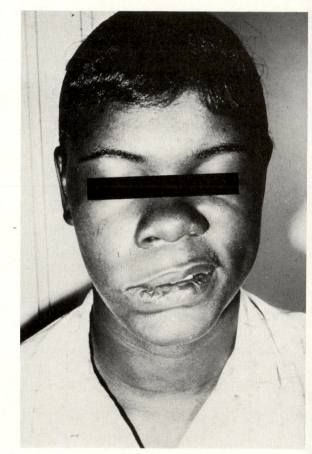

2. This lesion on the side of the nose is *best* treated by:
a. incisional biopsy.
b. excisional biopsy.
c. radiation.
d. cortisone ointment.
e. sclerosing solutions.

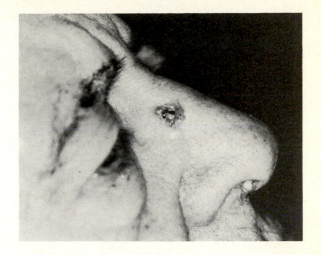

3. The remainder of the oral mucosal surfaces look just as pale as the dorsal surface of the tongue in this 9-year-old boy. Which one of the following tests would be *most* appropriate to order?
a. Exfoliative cytology.
b. Culture and sensitivity tests of the tongue.
c. Incisional biopsy of the tongue.
d. Total RBC, WBC, and hemoglobin.
e. 2-hour postprandial blood glucose.

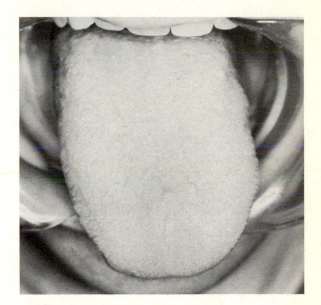

4. Which is the correct management of the radiopacity indicated by the arrow?
a. Take periodic radiographs and observe after informing the patient of its presence.
b. Take skeletal radiographs.
c. Remove the radiopacity surgically from a lingual approach and submit for microscopic study.
d. Remove the radiopaque lesion using a Caldwell-Luc procedure.
e. Continue to observe the lesion periodically but order a serum alkaline phosphatase test.

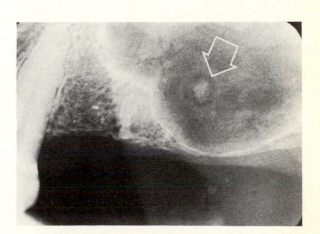

5. After evaluating these two periapical radiographs (**A** and **B**), which were taken in the patient during the same appointment, what treatment approach should you recommend for the radiolucency indicated by the arrow in **B**?
   a. No treatment.
   b. Perform surgical exploration and submit a specimen for microscopic study.
   c. Order skull radiographs.
   d. Perform a root canal filling on the second molar.
   e. Attempt to aspirate the area.

6. The premolar tooth requires:
   a. only a DO restoration.
   b. a DO restoration in addition to a pulpotomy.
   c. a DO restoration in addition to a root canal filling.
   d. a DO restoration and periodontal surgery.
   e. periodontal surgery and splinting to the canine tooth.

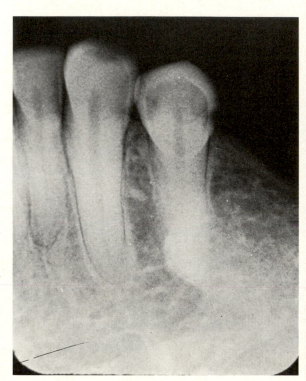

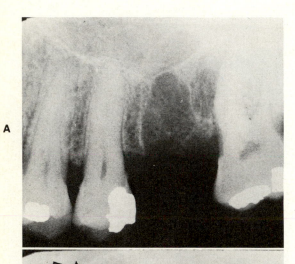

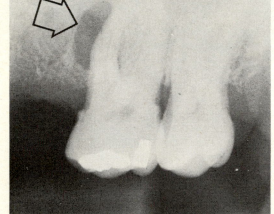

7. This situation is discovered during periodic dental examination of a 50-year-old woman. The remainder of the findings are basically nonsignificant. The correct advice to the patient would be:

a. to have lateral skull radiographs taken.

b. to have the root canals of these four incisors filled.

c. that this is an innocuous condition that will not need to be examined again.

d. that this area should be observed periodically.

e. that you would have expected to see purulent drainage from the alveolus in this region.

8. This radiopacity *(arrow)* is discovered on routine radiographs of a completely asymptomatic patient. The *most* correct approach would be to:

a. advise the patient of its presence and its identification and that treatment is required only if symptoms of sinus problems develop on that side.

b. advise the patient that it is the image of the palatal torus.

c. advise the patient that it is a hyperplasia of the mucosa of the sinus floor because of the diseased molar tooth that was removed 3 weeks previously.

d. advise the patient that it represents a serious antral pathologic condition that should be excised through a Caldwell-Luc approach.

e. advise the patient that it is an antrolith.

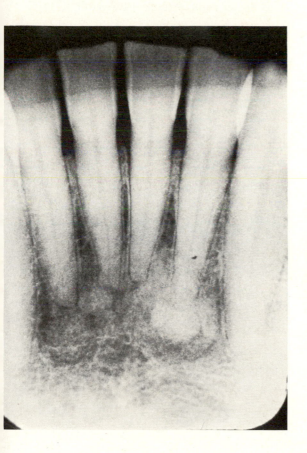

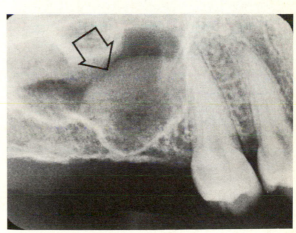

9. You find this radiopacity in a patient who had a myocardial infarction 3 months ago. He is currently experiencing comfortable function with his upper and lower dentures. The *most* correct approach would be to:

   a. remove it surgically right away so he won't have an opportunity to worry about it.

   b. remove it surgically after you obtain a verbal clearance from his physician.

   c. grind the inside of the lower denture over the lesion in question.

   d. inform your friend of the presence of the radiopacity and its diagnosis. Advise him that nothing should be done at the present time, but that you will reexamine it periodically.

   e. refer him to an oral surgeon for its removal.

10. An edentulous 70-year-old man with minimal ridges presents to your office for full dentures. As is your practice, you take complete radiographs before commencing the dentures. You find this asymptomatic radiopacity indicated by the arrow. What is the *most* correct approach?

   a. Don't tell the patient that you found it.

   b. Inform the patient of its presence, make a diagnosis, and explain that it would cause more harm to remove it than to leave it.

   c. Refer the patient to a competent otolaryngologist for diagnosis and removal of the radiopaque mass.

   d. Remove it yourself surgically and submit the specimen for microscopic study.

   e. Order radiographs of the skull.

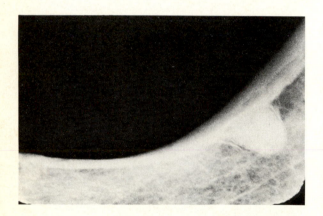

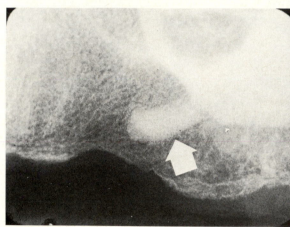

11. On routine radiographs of a 42-year-old woman, you notice this peculiar periapical appearance at the apices of the incisor teeth. The *most* important step in making the correct diagnosis in this case is to:
    a. obtain serum chemistry values.
    b. complete careful pulp tests on these teeth.
    c. test the teeth with percussion.
    d. look for similar lesions in the skull radiographs.
    e. do a test cavity without local anesthesia on the right lateral incisor in order to be certain of its vitality.

12. A. This 43-year-old patient presents in mild distress for treatment of a painful mass on the palate that is rubbery, fluctuant, nonemptiable, and painful to the touch. The mass *most* likely is:
    a. a chondrosarcoma.
    b. a palatal space abscess of odontogenic origin.
    c. a globulomaxillary cyst.
    d. a minor salivary gland tumor.
    e. fibrous dysplasia.
    B. The patient is quite poor and goes to the dentist only for relief of pain. The *most* considerate initial management of this case would be to:
    a. extract the tooth immediately.
    b. open into the pulp chamber of the premolar tooth in order to accomplish drainage.
    c. place the patient on high doses of oral penicillin V and when the abscess regresses, extract the tooth.
    d. place the patient on high doses of oral penicillin V and when the abscess regresses, commence root canal therapy.
    e. refer the patient to her physician for control of the infection.

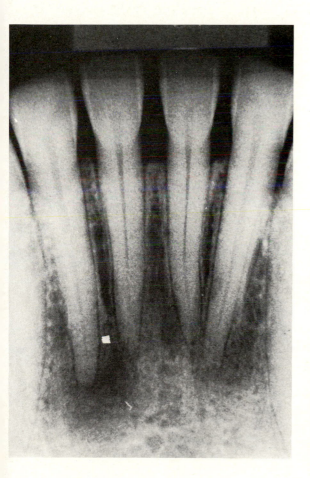

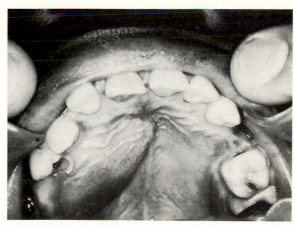

13. A mother brings her 13-year-old boy whom you consider to be in mild distress because he has difficulty in opening his mouth as widely as usual. This is what you see when you examine him. Suitable radiographs are also available. He has no swelling in the upper neck except for one or two tender nodes. Intraoral examination reveals that the oropharynx or soft palate is not involved in this process. What is the correct step to take in treating this emergency?

a. Extract the second molar tooth now.

b. Widely excise the swollen tissue on the posterior of the ridge.

c. Incise and drain the abscess, running the drain right through to the external skin surface.

d. Obtain a specimen for culture and sensitivity tests, and start the patient on high doses of penicillin V every 6 hours and copious rinse with hydrogen peroxide mouthwashes.

e. Hospitalize him immediately because of the imminent danger of airway obstruction.

14. A new patient presented for a routine check of her dentures, which she has had for 5 years. The examination reveals that the dentures seem to be fitting well, but radiographs reveal this solitary asymptomatic lesion. What would your approach be to this case?

a. Immediately order skull radiographs.

b. Advise the patient of the presence of the lesion, of your diagnosis, and of your plan to radiograph the region periodically.

c. Order serum acid phosphatase tests.

d. Surgically enucleate the lesion and send the specimen for microscopic study.

e. Recommend that the patient have a complete physical examination right away.

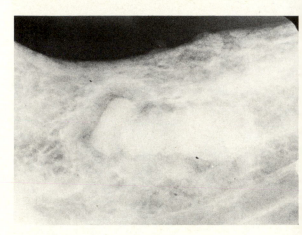

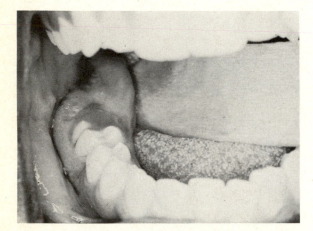

15. A 21-year-old black man presented for treatment of this solitary ulcerated lesion on the labial gingiva. His oral hygiene is unusually good and no gingival pockets are present. One of the *most* pertinent laboratory tests to order is:
a. a sickle cell preparation.
b. a culture and sensitivity test.
c. a platelet count.
d. a prothrombin time test.
e. exfoliative cytology.

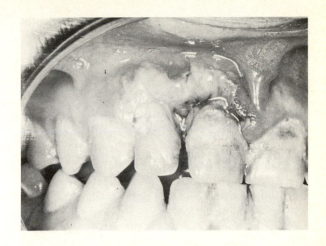

16. This nervous 31-year-old woman presents with a painful swelling in the anterior vestibule in the anterior maxillary region. The right central incisor is very painful to percussion and to hot stimuli. The most humane management of the acute phase would be to:
a. remove the root canal filling in order to establish drainage and follow closely.
b. place the patient on 500 mg of oral penicillin V q.i.d. after ascertaining that she is not allergic to it.
c. incise and drain the abscess immediately through the vestibular swelling.
d. extract the tooth under a local anesthetic.
e. not disturb the root canal filling because the swelling and radiolucency is most likely caused by an infected incisive canal cyst.

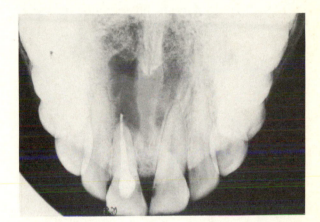

17. During examination of this 25-year-old patient, you discover these firm, yellowish-white areas on the left tonsil. You should:
a. perform culture and sensitivity tests and administer the indicated antibiotic in correct dosage.
b. prescribe nystatin.
c. advise the patient that this condition does not require treatment.
d. refer the patient to the local tumor board for evaluation and treatment.

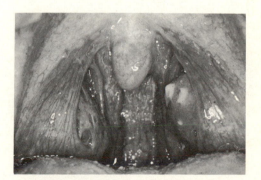

18. You should advise this healthy 25-year-old woman that:
   a. if the odontoma is removed, the central incisor will likely erupt into position without aid.
   b. the odontoma and tooth should both be removed because of the dentigerous cyst presently associated with the impacted incisor tooth.
   c. if the odontoma is removed, it may be possible to bring the impacted tooth into position with an orthodontic appliance.
   d. the odontoma and tooth should be left alone because they are fully developed, and so an additional associated pathologic condition will not occur.
   e. the impacted tooth should not be removed until it becomes infected.

19. A healthy 58-year-old man who has been having repeated problems with a painful ulcer on the crest of the ridge in the left mandibular molar region comes to you for help. You take this radiograph and find this radiopacity. What is the best definitive treatment?
   a. Relieve the occlusion on this side.
   b. Relieve the inside of the denture in this region.
   c. Tell the patient to leave the denture out for a week or so.
   d. Reline the denture with Coe Comfort.
   e. Remove the root tip and reline the denture if necessary.

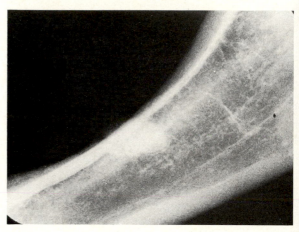

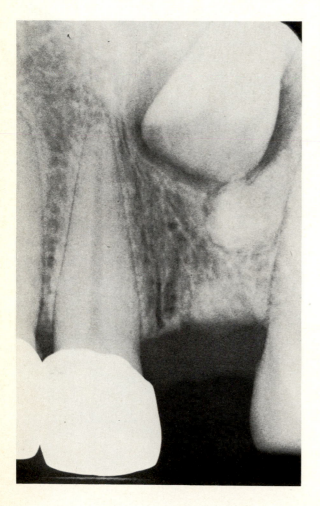

20. When this man presents with denture problems, you notice that he has petechiae on the oral mucosa and skin. Which one of the following laboratory tests would be *most* appropriate to order?
a. prothrombin time.
b. partial thromboplastin time.
c. clotting time.
d. platelet count.
e. Bence Jones test.

21. What is the correct approach to this asymptomatic red patch found on the posterior right border of the tongue in this 64-year-old man who has smoked heavily all his life?
a. Inform the patient that it is of no concern.
b. Prescribe topical cortisone preparations.
c. Refer him immediately for complete excision of the lesion and microscopic study.
d. Prescribe nystatin medication.

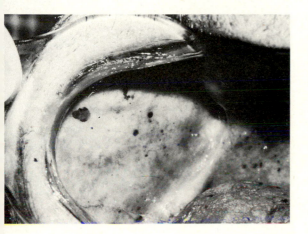

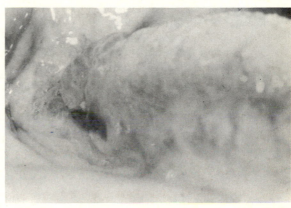

22. A. Which one of the following is *not* a correct approach to this painful fluctuant swelling of 4 days' duration?
   a. Examine the patient carefully intraorally.
   b. Radiograph the teeth on the affected side.
   c. Question the patient carefully concerning the onset and course of the condition.
   d. Prescribe high doses of tetracycline.
   e. Pulp test the teeth on the affected side.

   B. If you decide that the lesion is infectious and tooth related, what should be your next step?
   a. Have the patient return tomorrow to see if it has improved.
   b. Obtain a specimen for culture and sensitivity.
   c. Refer the patient to her physician for treatment of the swelling.
   d. Prescribe analgesics for pain.

   C. Which one of the following is indicated?
   a. Open only into the pulp chamber and canal of the offending tooth.
   b. Prescribe systemic penicillin (if the patient is not allergic); do an incision and drainage.
   c. Extract only the offending tooth.
   d. Only tell the patient to use hot compresses.

23. Which one of the following is indicated on finding this soft, fluctuant, painless swelling in the anterior maxilla?
   a. Order serum chemistries.
   b. Order a chest radiograph to check for bifid ribs or missing clavicles.
   c. Order an maxillary occlusal radiograph.
   d. Order a 2-hour postprandial serum glucose test.

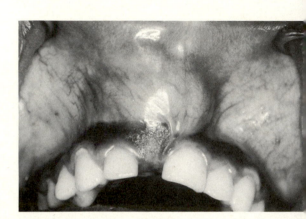

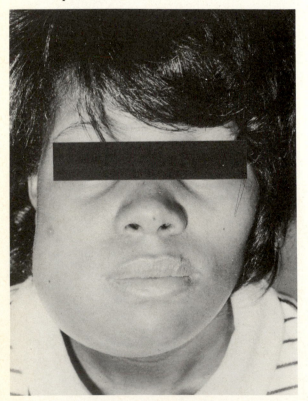

24. What advice would you give a 70-year-old woman who has this defect? Her speech and swallowing appear to be within normal limits.
    a. Do nothing.
    b. Have the cleft repaired so that the pharynx will not dry out.
    c. Have a prosthetic appliance fabricated to close the defect.
    d. Tell her that if she has children, there is an increased possibility that they will have clefts.

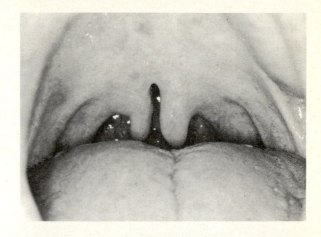

25. A. An incisional biopsy of this white lesion of the palate, which cannot readily be scraped off, in a 68-year-old man who wears his dentures constantly would *most* likely show:
    a. invasive squamous cell carcinoma.
    b. increased keratotic layer and *Candida albicans*.
    c. carcinoma in situ.
    d. changes compatible with nicotine stomatitis.
    B. The best initial treatment approach in this patient who has frequent attacks of ankle edema is to:
    a. perform a complete excision of the involved palatal mucosa.
    b. perform several representative incisional biopsies.
    c. prescribe nystatin ointment to wear in the maxillary denture and have the patient soak dentures at night in a nystatin solution.
    d. prescribe cortisone preparation to wear in the maxillary denture and tell the patient to soak denture in a penicillin suspension at night.

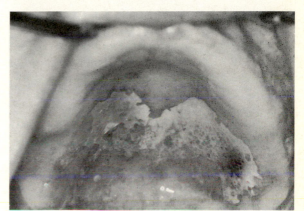

26. What is the indicated treatment for this painless ulcer that has been present in this 72-year-old farmer for at least 7 weeks?
    a. Prescribe sun screen.
    b. Perform an incisional biopsy.
    c. Have the patient return in 2 weeks for reexamination of the lesion.
    d. Refer the patient for definitive diagnosis and treatment of a probable malignancy.

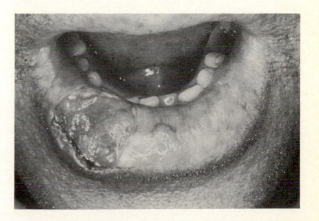

27. What is the correct management approach for the radiolucency indicated by the arrow?
   a. Perform root canal therapy on the retained root segment.
   b. Extract the root segment.
   c. Do nothing now but re-radiograph in 6 months.
   d. No treatment is necessary.

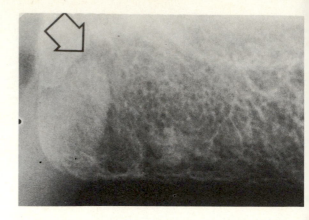

28. You find the asymptomatic radiolucency *(arrow)* just distal to the asymptomatic second molar. The third molar was removed 5 years ago. Clinical examination is negative. What should you do next?
   a. Order a Waters' radiograph.
   b. Open into the area surgically.
   c. Re-radiograph in 6 months.
   d. Compare with the appearance on the opposite side.
   e. c and d.

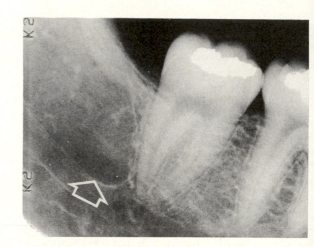

29. When shift shots were taken in this asymptomatic 42-year-old woman, the image of the supernumerary tooth *(arrow)* did not move significantly in relation to the image of the right central incisor. What is the best treatment?
   a. Remove the supernumerary tooth surgically.
   b. Do nothing but re-radiograph occasionally.
   c. Remove No. 8, and bring the supernumerary tooth into place orthodontically.
   d. Work up the patient for cleidocranial dysostosis.

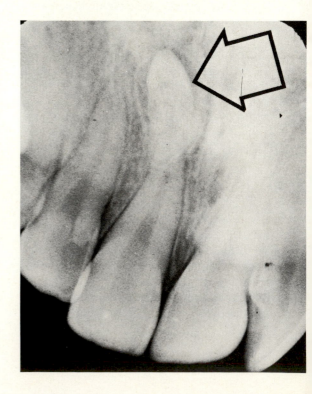

30. What would you do in this instance when the treatment plan calls for a mandibular partial denture in this 58-year-old patient who expresses much apprehension regarding oral surgery?
   a. Leave the roots in place and terminate the saddle mesial to the roots.
   b. Leave the roots in place and carry the saddle over the region in the normal manner.
   c. Leave the roots in place and carry the saddle over the region and relieve the saddle over the roots.
   d. Insist on removal of the roots.

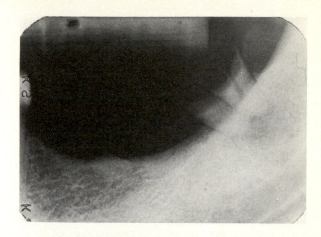

31. What is the best treatment for this asymptomatic finding in this 63-year-old man whose full dentures are functioning quite satisfactorily?
   a. Do nothing.
   b. Radiograph occasionally.
   c. Surgically remove the tooth with surrounding pathology and send for microscopic study.
   d. Remove the tooth and surrounding pathology by block resection and send for microscopic study.

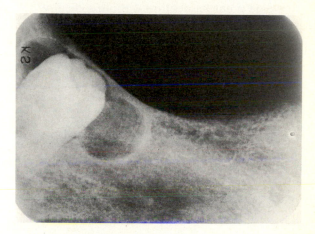

32. What is the best treatment for this firm, but not bony-hard, painless mass on the palate of this 38-year-old woman who noticed it first 2 weeks previously?
   a. Refer her immediately to a competent specialist for complete removal and microscopic study.
   b. Do nothing but reexamine periodically.
   c. Remove the mass if it becomes chronically traumatized.
   d. Incise, drain, and cover with penicillin.

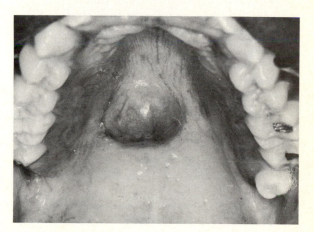

33. Prior to this surgical procedure, what is the most crucial information that the surgeon should give the patient?
   a. There will be considerable postoperative swelling.
   b. There may be a temporary or permanent numbness of the lip.
   c. There may be a fracture or fractures of the jawbone.
   d. There will be some postoperative bleeding.
   e. b and c.

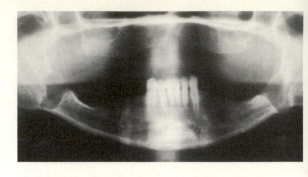

34. What is the correct management of this asymptomatic radiopacity in this patient who wears a partial denture without difficulty?
   a. Order serum chemistries.
   b. Do nothing but re-radiograph occasionally.
   c. Surgically remove the radiopacity and send for microscopic study.
   d. Take skull radiographs.

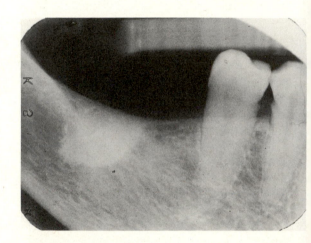

35. Which of the following are correct steps in the workup and management of this 54-year-old man, who has swelling of this region of the mandible and intermittent purulent drainage from the inferior aspect of the lower border of the mandible 6 weeks after a fracture of the jaw?
   a. Work up for diabetes.
   b. Perform a culture and sensitivity.
   c. Use hyperbaric oxygen.
   d. Administer the indicated antibiotics in adequate dosage.
   e. All the above.

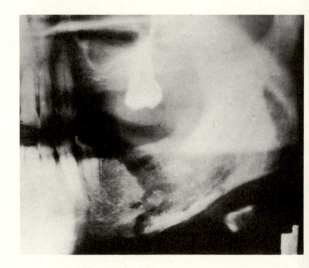

36. This patient has right side facial pain of long standing. The pain exacerbates during jaw movements, which are restricted. The proper approach is to:
a. refer the patient to have a workup for angina pectoris.
b. refer the patient to an endodontist.
c. refer the patient for management of severe osteoarthritis of the right temporomandibular joint.
d. fabricate an occlusal splint to alleviate muscle spasms.

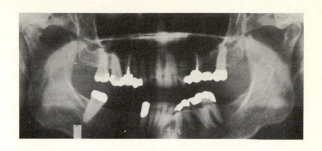

37. What is the indicated management in this 21-year-old woman who presents with this loss of tooth tissue on the lingual surfaces of the maxillary teeth?
a. full crown restorations only.
b. psychiatric counseling.
c. mouthwashes with special buffering capacity.
d. fabrication of an occlusal splint.
e. b and c.

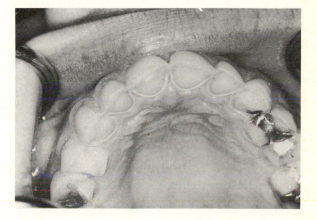

38. What is the correct management of this radiopacity *(arrow)*?
a. Remove it, because if it remains it will probably produce bone loss to distal of second molar.
b. Do nothing.
c. Do nothing but inform the patient of its presence.
d. Remove it because of the surrounding pathologic condition.

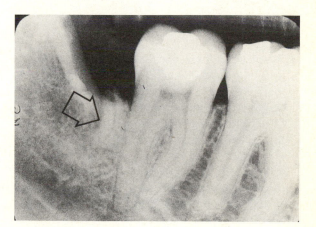

39. What is the best management of this problem involving the second and third molars in this 24-year-old patient whose other three arches have a full complement of teeth in good position?

a. Extract both the second and third molar.

b. Extract the second molar, and see if the third molar will erupt into position.

c. Extract the third molar only.

d. Extract the third molar, hemisect the second molar, do a root canal filling on the mesial root, and place a small crown.

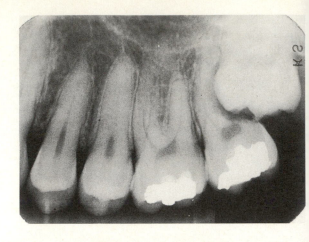

40. You find this asymptomatic radiopacity *(arrow)* during a complete examination of a 55-year-old man who is a new patient. Shift shots do not cause the image to move. Which one of the following is *most* correct?

a. Remove it surgically because of the surrounding pathology.

b. Do nothing.

c. Inform him of its presence and re-radiograph occasionally.

d. Work up the patient for general skeletal disease.

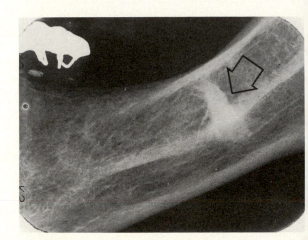

41. What is the best approach to this red lesion in a 26-year-old woman who is 2 months' post partum?

a. Exercise the lesion and send for microscopic study only.

b. Order a 2-hour postpradial blood glucose test.

c. Investigate the region for a local irritant, such as caries, overcontoured restoration, calculus, or foreign body; eliminate the irritant; follow with a.

d. perform a workup for AIDS.

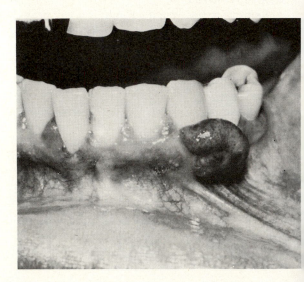

42. What is the correct treatment for this condition of the tongue?
a. nystatin.
b. penicillin.
c. hydrogen peroxide mouth rinses.
d. improved tongue hygiene.

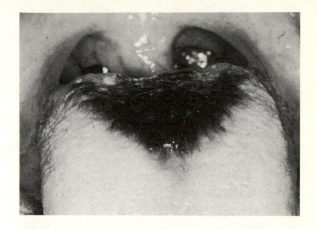

43. This painless, solitary, red-and-white mass in the floor of the mouth was found in a 64-year-old man who informs you that he noticed it first about 6 weeks ago. He has smoked heavily for many years. The best treatment is most likely to:
a. prescribe nystatin.
b. prescribe penicillin.
c. refer the patient for treatment of squamous cell carcinoma.
d. have the patient discontinue smoking, and reexamine in 2 weeks.

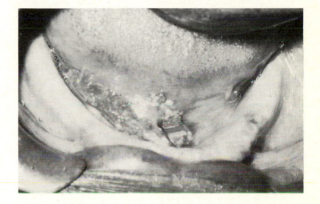

44. What is the best approach to this 21-year-old woman's gingival problem? She has experienced fever for several days along with very sore gums.
a. Prescribe penicillin.
b. Prescribe a cortisone mouth rinse.
c. Prescribe a tetracycline mouthwash.
d. Prescribe nystatin lozenges.

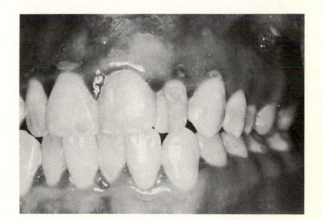

45. A. One of the *most* important steps in managing this case is to:
   a. perform a preliminary prophylaxis and superficial root planing.
   b. instruct the patient to use a differently designed toothbrush.
   c. place the patient on hydrogen peroxide mouth rinses.
   d. determine which teeth are mobile and extract them.
   e. work the patient up for the presence of systemic disease.

   B. The following laboratory values were obtained for this patient: total RBC, 4.9 million; hemoglobin, 14%; total WBC, 8500; differential: neutrophils, 55%; lymphocytes, 37%; monocytes, 7; eosinophils, 1; basophils, 0; 2-hour postprandial blood glucose, 220 g%; serum calcium, 9 mg%; serum phosphate, 3 mg%; serum alkaline phosphatase, 3 Bodansky units. From these results, one would suspect:
   a. diabetes mellitus.
   b. hyperparathyroidism.
   c. thalassemia.
   d. cyclic neutropenia.
   e. leukemia.

46. This 54-year-old patient presents for treatment of an advanced periodontal condition. When you question him about his limp, he says he has been bothered recently with large foot ulcers that are slow to heal. Before dental treatment is begun, it is essential that the patient be particularly worked up for:
   a. leukemia.
   b. foot-and-mouth disease.
   c. diabetes.
   d. congestive heart failure.
   e. subacute bacterial endocarditis.

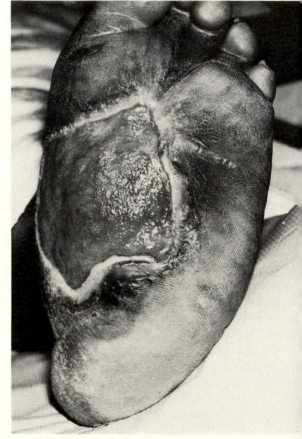

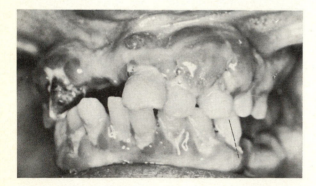

47. How would you approach this asymptomatic radiopacity *(arrow)* in a healthy 65-year-old man?

a. Remove the lesion and send for microscopic study.

b. Advise him of its presence and identity, and re-radiograph occasionally.

c. Advise him that it will have to be removed before the denture is relined.

d. Order a serum acid phosphatase test.

e. Order lateral skull radiographs.

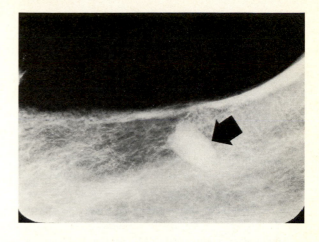

48. A concerned patient who has lived in the same locality all his life asks you what caused the staining of his teeth. The 6-year molars appear normal. Which of the following explanations is *most* likely correct in this case?

a. local trauma to the deciduous teeth.

b. excess fluoride in the drinking water.

c. tetracycline administration.

d. pulpal hemorrhage.

e. severe illness during the first year of life.

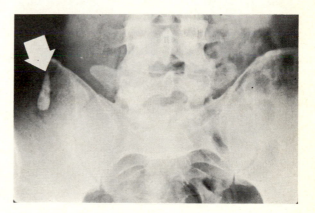

49. Which one of the following statements is correct in relation to the complication of dental work illustrated in this radiograph *(arrow)*?

a. This problem could have been prevented by employment of a rubber dam.

b. It is unnecessary to take further radiographs of the lost object once the dentist has ensured that the object in question has not been aspirated.

c. The statement in b is true because smooth objects such as the one illustrated here will pass through the gastrointestinal tract without mishap.

d. From both a legal and moral point of view, while providing dental services, it is always necessary to take follow-up radiographs of the chest and abdomen after an object is lost and disappears from view down the pharynx.

e. Use of a nasotracheal tube while giving a general anesthetic for oral surgical procedures would prevent this mishap.

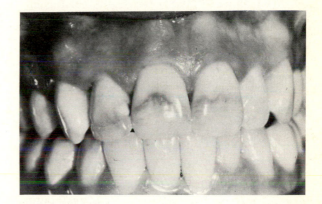

50. You extracted a painful, abscessed first premolar tooth for this patient 2 days ago. During the present postoperative visit, she says she is feeling much better but the canine tooth is somewhat sensitive to bite on. In response, you take this radiograph to reevaluate the situation. The correct treatment at present is to:

a. perform an immediate pulpectomy on the canine.

b. inform the patient that you would like to reexamine her after the extraction site has completely healed.

c. extract the tooth immediately.

d. double the antibiotic dosage.

e. prescribe diazepam (Valium).

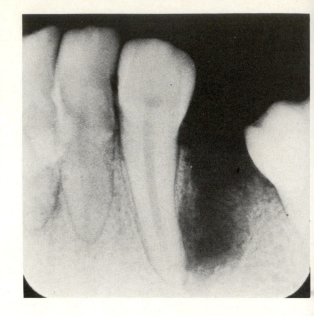

■ SECTION B

Periodontics

51. The full-mouth radiographs of this 45-year-old patient reveal varying degrees of periodontal bone loss. The lower incisors have minimal to moderate mobility. All these teeth test vital. What treatment is indicated for the obviously painful gingival lesion?

a. excisional biopsy of the lesion because it is probably squamous cell carcinoma.

b. therapeutic root planing and prophylaxis only.

c. antibiotics and curettage with possible flap surgery later.

d. oral hygiene instruction only.

e. antibiotics and gingivectomy.

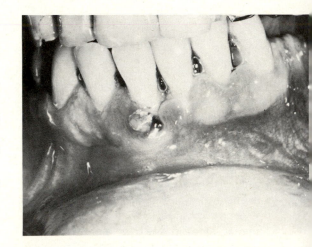

Dr. Joseph Keene authored questions 52 through 55.

52. The *most* suitable management of the condition shown here is to:
  a. teach the patient the importance of proper oral home care, and perform a prophylaxis and therapeutic root planing.
  b. prescribe antibiotics and hydrogen peroxide rinses.
  c. advise the patient to change toothpaste.
  d. complete a full-mouth gingivectomy.
  e. eliminate the systemic disease that is obviously contributing to the problem.

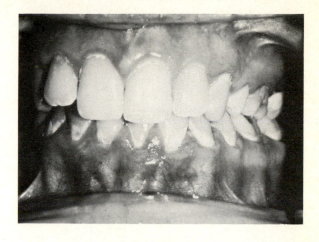

53. The procedure illustrated here is called:
  a. excisional biopsy.
  b. split-thickness flap surgery.
  c. full-thickness flap surgery.
  d. gingivectomy.
  e. incisional biopsy.

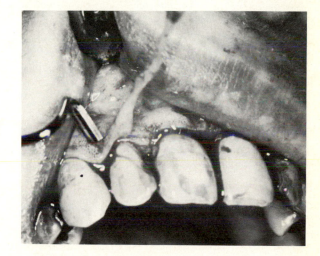

54. This procedure is called:
  a. therapeutic root planing.
  b. excisional biopsy.
  c. incisional biopsy.
  d. split-thickness flap surgery.
  e. full-thickness flap surgery.

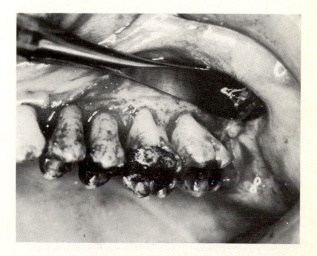

55. A. The gingival pattern indicated by the arrow is a good example of:
   a. McCall's festoon.
   b. fenestration.
   c. Stillman's cleft.
   d. a defect resulting from an attack of ANUG.

   B. This defect is best treated by:
   a. an apically repositioned flap.
   b. a laterally repositioned flap.
   c. gingivectomy.
   d. scaling followed by a free gingival graft.

56. Which is the correct treatment for the first premolar tooth?
   a. Correct treatment depends on the other oral findings.
   b. Extract the premolar tooth if the patient's health permits.
   c. Do therapeutic root planing only.
   d. Do flap surgery with bone grafting.
   e. Splint the premolar tooth to the canine tooth.

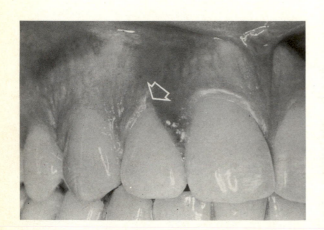

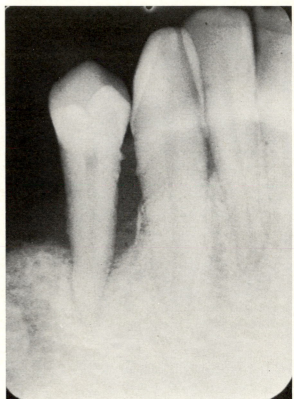

57. What is the *most* correct treatment for the radiolucent defect associated with the second premolar tooth? The patient has adequate funds and is genuinely interested in saving her teeth.
a. benign neglect.
b. flap surgery, curettage, and possible bone grafting, after occlusal adjustment.
c. extirpation of the pulp and root canal obliteration.
d. improved home care only.
e. extraction of the tooth because the situation is hopeless.

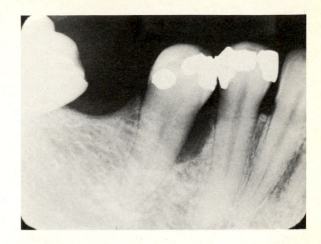

58. How would you treat the left central incisor for a patient who has the necessary funds and is genuinely interested in saving the tooth?
a. Perform a frenectomy only.
b. Perform a sliding flap procedure.
c. Complete a root canal filling.
d. Perform combined endodontic and periodontic techniques and splint the tooth to its neighbors.
e. Remove the tooth and place a fixed bridge.

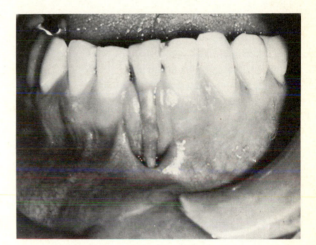

59. This 14-year-old boy presents with this gingival problem on the lower left quadrant (**A** and **B**). The crucial point in managing this problem is to:
a. order blood tests.
b. prescribe hydrogen peroxide mouthwashes and penicillin.
c. perform a gingivectomy on the lower left arch.
d. complete an extensive nutritional survey.
e. instruct the patient in proper toothbrushing techniques.

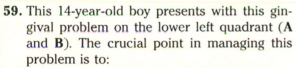

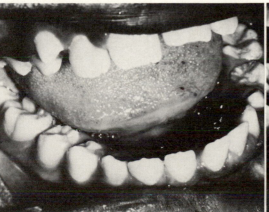

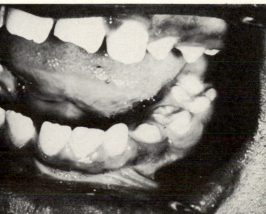

A

B

60. What is the correct management of the gingivitis in this patient?
   a. Consult with a otolaryngologist to see if the mouth-breathing habit is a result of a nasal obstruction.
   b. Reinforce home-care instruction.
   c. Perform a prophylaxis and superficial scaling.
   d. Replace the interproximal fillings.
   e. Instruct the patient to discontinue the use of birth control pills.

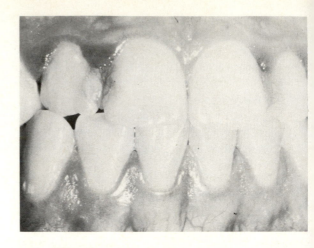

61. Which one is the *most* correct management of the gingival condition in this patient who is suffering from seizures?
   a. Reinforce home care.
   b. Gingivectomy.
   c. Request the physician to change the medication if possible.
   d. a, b, and c.
   e. Full-mouth extractions.

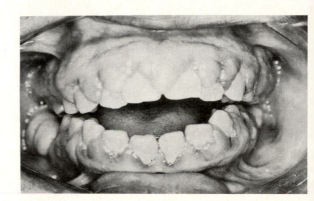

62. Which *one* of the following is not a suitable method of treatment for this painful gingival condition:
   a. administration of oral penicillin for at least 5 days.
   b. thorough and complete root planing at this stage.
   c. careful gross debridement.
   d. hydrogen peroxide mouthwashes.
   e. elimination of all predisposing gingival conditions after the acute phase has been eliminated.

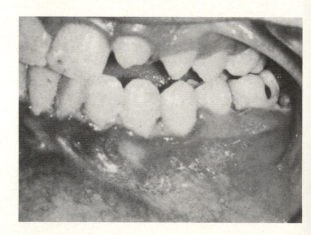

63. Which *one* of the following is indicated in this 35-year-old patient?
   a. tetracycline therapy.
   b. prophylaxis, scaling, and oral home-care instruction.
   c. gingivectomy.
   d. flap surgery.

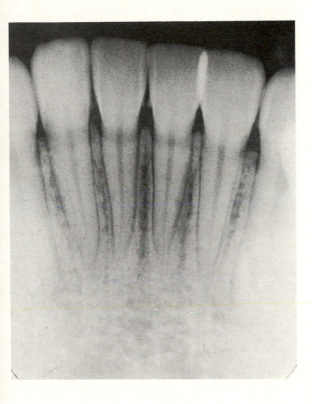

64. A 46-year-old woman who has adequate funds and does not want to lose any more teeth comes to you for treatment of the left central incisor. She is also insistent about having the diastema closed. With just the information you have from this picture, you should advise her that:
   a. the tooth will certainly require both extensive periodontal treatment and a root canal filling.
   b. an orthodontist could certainly close the space successfully if treatment begins immediately.
   c. as far as closing the diastema is concerned, it could be done quite successfully by placement of porcelain jacket crowns on the two maxillary central incisors.
   d. the diastema can best be eliminated by rubber bands worn around the two central incisors for approximately 2 weeks.
   e. the case must be worked up in its entirety, but it is unlikely that the left central incisor can be saved.

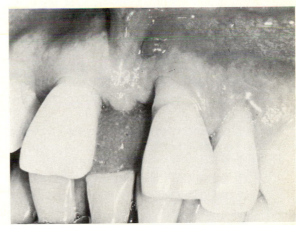

65. This woman has adequate funds and has expressed a fear of losing her teeth. The most correct approach for this painful and quite mobile second molar is to:

a. perform periodontal flap surgery and bone-grafting procedures.

b. extract the tooth.

c. hemisect the molar and endodontically treat the mesial root.

d. treat the tooth endodontically and with periodontal surgery, and splint to the first molar tooth.

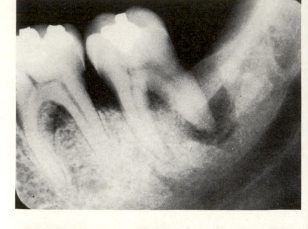

66. This 55-year-old woman presents with a periodontal abscess associated with this tooth. You have treated the abscess several times during the last 6 months on an emergency basis each time. She adamantly refuses to have any more teeth out. She has a full complement of teeth on the lower arch except for the left first and second molars. The premolars on this side are in good position. How should you manage this situation?

a. Give her a refillable prescription for penicillin and merperidine hydrochloride (Demerol) so that she will not bother you on evenings or weekends.

b. Go ahead and extract the tooth anyway.

c. Improve the mesial contour by building a bridge with a telescoping crown on the third molar.

d. Politely and courteously request that she find another dentist to take care of her problem.

e. Orthodontically upright the molar and build a 5-unit bridge.

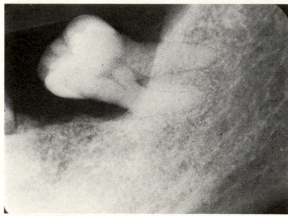

67. This 21-year-old woman presents with lassitude, malaise, and tender bleeding gums. There are some petechiae throughout the oral mucosa. She denies taking medication and claims she brushes and flosses three times a day. What is especially indicated for this patient?

a. hydrogen peroxide rinses and penicillin.

b. gross debridement and therapeutic root planing.

c. change of toothpaste.

d. gingivectomy.

e. an extensive workup to determine whether the patient has an underlying systemic disease.

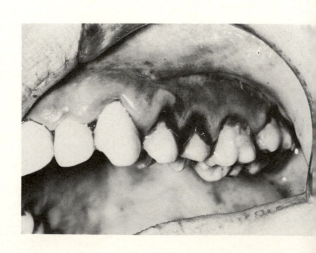

68. This 18-year-old youth presents with a mild complaint of tender and bleeding gums. The correct initial treatment is:
   a. extensive therapeutic root planing.
   b. gross debridement, hydrogen peroxide rinse, and penicillin V.
   c. a generalized gingivectomy.
   d. high doses of vitamin C.
   e. immediate bed rest.

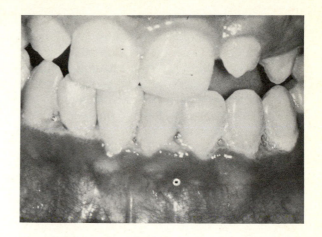

69. The periodontal probe in this photograph:
   a. shows a 7-mm pocket.
   b. shows a 5-mm pocket.
   c. is being used in a grossly improper manner.
   d. shows a 1-mm gingival crevice.
   e. shows a 2-mm gingival crevice.

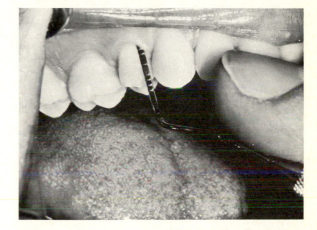

70. A 48-year-old man who has advanced periodontal disease and needs a large number of restorations is forced to come to you for treatment of this abscessed left central incisor tooth. He says he has $200 to spend on his teeth over the next 2 years. The best treatment of this tooth after the acute abscess has resolved is to:
   a. leave it alone.
   b. extract it without replacement.
   c. extract it and replace with a bridge.
   d. perform endodontic and periodontic therapy.
   e. extract it and replace with a temporary partial denture.

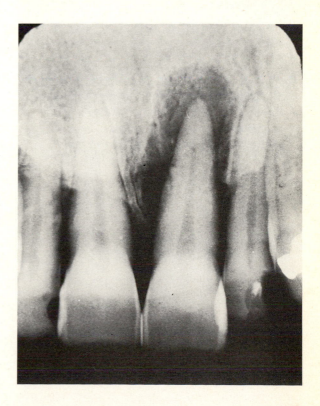

71. This 16-year-old boy presents with a complaint of burning and sore gingiva of 5 days' duration. He has a cervical lymphadenitis in the submandibular region bilaterally. All the gingiva is red with very small, roundish ulcers. Correct treatment to aid healing is to:
   a. prescribe tetracycline mouthwash.
   b. prescribe nystatin.
   c. prescribe cortisone in an emollient base.
   d. prescribe hydrogen peroxide mouth rinse.

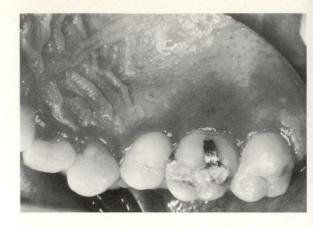

72. What treatment is indicated for this 30-year-old woman?
   a. gingivectomy.
   b. referral to an ENT specialist for establishment of the nasal airway.
   c. continued appraisal of oral home care.
   d. discuss the case with her obstetrician.

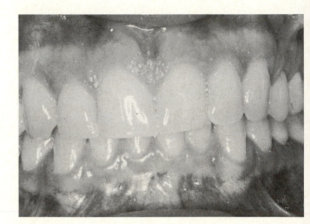

Dr. Alphonse Gargiulo authored questions 73 through 93.

73. Which of the following is the purpose of the noneugenol periodontal dressing as shown?
   1. allows for quicker gingival healing.
   2. promotes flap stabilization.
   3. gives protection against blood clots.
   4. acts as a disinfectant.
   5. stabilizes the teeth.
      a. 1.
      b. 2, 3.
      c. 1, 2, 3.
      d. 2, 3, 4.
      e. 1, 2, 3, 4, 5.

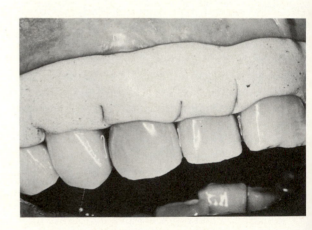

74. A. This mandibular left second molar demonstrated a Class V amalgam on the mesiobuccal root surface, which extended subgingivally. Upon gentle palpation of the buccal gingiva, purulent exudate was visible *(arrow).* The pulp tested within normal limits and a 7-mm pocket was demonstrated. What is your diagnosis?
   a. gingival abscess.
   b. periodontal abscess.
   c. herpetic stomatitis.
   d. strep infection of the gingiva.
   e. infected periodontal cyst.

B. What is your treatment of choice for the above described situation?
   a. Give palliative treatment only, because of viral etiology.
   b. Place the patient on an antibiotic for 5 days, then evaluate the situation.
   c. Flap the tissue, drain pus, thoroughly clean the root surface, and smooth alloy.
   d. Use Keyes' technique.
   e. Perform closed curettage.

75. A. This periapical radiograph of these mandibular anterior teeth represents:
   a. intracoronal splinting.
   b. wire splinting.
   c. extracoronal splinting.
   d. a and b.
   e. b and c.

B. What is the purpose of periodontal splints?
   a. distribution of occlusal forces.
   b. stabilization.
   c. patient comfort.
   d. all the above.
   e. none of the above.

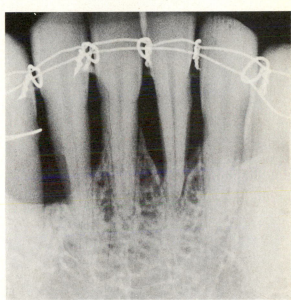

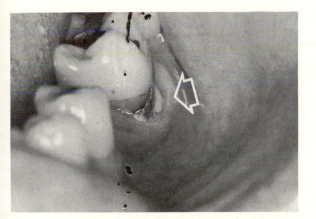

76. What is the most important feature in this incisal edge splint?
   a. the patient's easy access to interproximal areas for plaque control.
   b. conservative tooth preparation.
   c. it is only temporary.
   d. aesthetic quality.
   e. cuspid to cuspid splinting.

77. What would be the most ideal hygiene aid to clean this three-tooth intracoronal splint?
   a. waxed dental floss.
   b. a soft toothbrush.
   c. a rubber tip stimulator.
   d. Stim-u-Dent.
   e. Proxabrush.

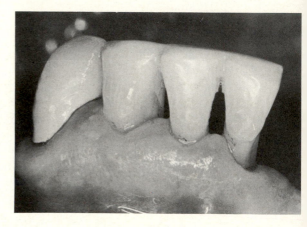

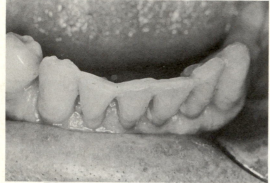

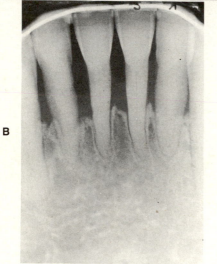

78. What is wrong with this extracoronal wire splint?
   a. It is positioned too far gingivally.
   b. It is causing localized papillary overgrowth.
   c. It appears too loose to maintain tooth stability.
   d. All the aboe.
   e. None of the above.

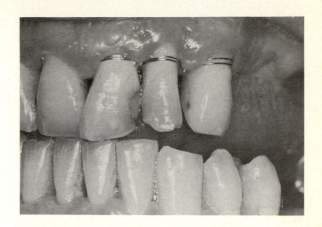

79. What is the name of the procedure used to remove this maxillary buccal exostosis (**A** and **B**)?
   a. osteoplasty.
   b. ostectomy.
   c. alveolectomy.
   d. gingivectomy.
   e. odontoplasty.

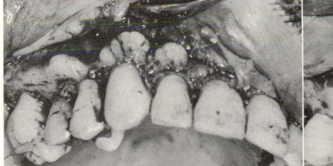 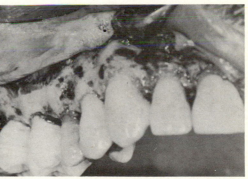

A   B

80. A mandibular right periapical view of a first molar and second premolar was taken during routine full-mouth radiography. What is the radiopaque mass seen at approximately the midroot of the second premolar?
   a. osteosarcoma.
   b. ossifying fibroma.
   c. synthetic bone material in a previously treated periodontal bone defect.
   d. crestal apposition of bone.
   e. none of the above.

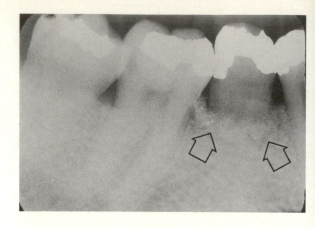

81. At this point in this bone-grafting procedure, what is of utmost importance?
   a. irrigation with copious amounts of sterile saline.
   b. primary closure of buccal and lingual flaps.
   c. placement of a noneugenol dressing.
   d. all the above.
   e. none of the above.

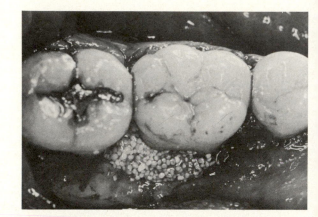

82. How would you describe this type of wound healing?
   a. slow and inadequate.
   b. secondary intention.
   c. primary intention.
   d. healing with an abundance of proud flesh.
   e. normal healing for 1 week after surgery.

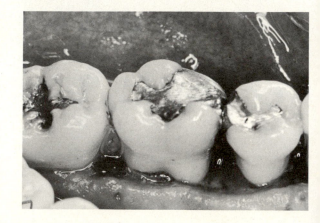

83. What is the best term for the bone graft, as seen in this picture, that will be utilized in its own host?
  a. osseous coagulum.
  b. autogenous bone.
  c. synthetic bone.
  d. alloplastic bone implant.
  e. allograft.

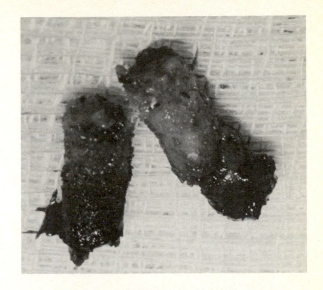

84. What type of periodontal therapy is being performed in this patient?
  a. soft tissue curettage.
  b. root curettage.
  c. root planing.
  d. gingivectomy.
  e. none of the above.

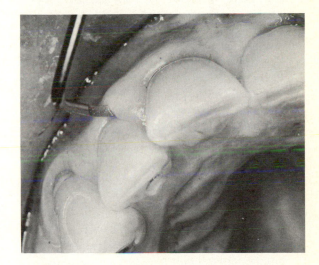

85. Describe the type of suturing used in this periodontal flap procedure. Note that the sutures can be seen around the lingual surfaces of the teeth.
  a. interrupted.
  b. saddle.
  c. continuous.
  d. noncontinuous.
  e. mattress.

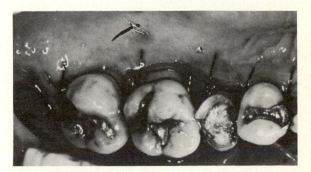

86. Citric acid may be used in root preparation during periodontal surgery. How long and at what approximate pH is it used?
   a. 2 to 3 min at an approximate pH of 8.
   b. 2 to 3 min at an approximate pH of 1.
   c. 5 min at an approximate pH of 1.
   d. 10 min at an approximate pH of 1.
   e. 1 min at a pH of 4.

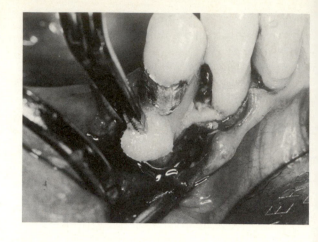

87. What is your choice of therapy if you wish to thoroughly prepare the root surface associated with this periodontal pocket?
   a. Keyes' technique with scaling and root planing.
   b. scaling and root planing only.
   c. antimicrobial therapy.
   d. gingivectomy.
   e. a full-flap procedure, allowing full visible access to the entire root surface.

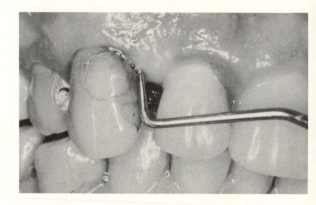

88. After completion of root preparation and suturing of this labial full-thickness flap at its approximate original position, what type of junctional epithelium is likely to develop?
   a. a long junctional epithelium.
   b. a short junctional epithelium.
   c. a similar junctional epithelium prior to pocket formation.
   d. none because the junctional epithelium does not redevelop after surgery.
   e. none of the above.

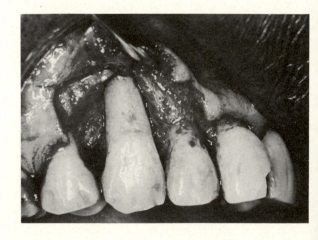

89. What surgical procedure is being performed in this patient?
   a. free gingival graft.
   b. occlusal repositioned graft.
   c. open-flap curettage.
   d. double papilla sliding flap.
   e. lateral sliding pedicle flap.

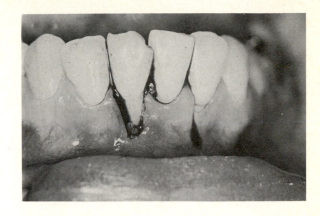

90. Which of the graft procedures shown has the *most* predictable outcome?
   a. Figure **A.**
   b. Figure **B.**

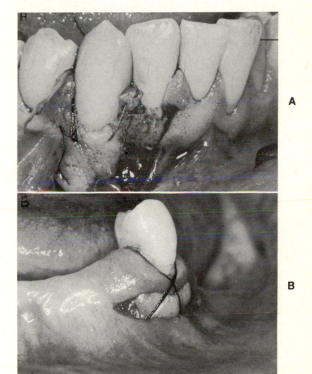

91. What type of periodontal surgical procedure is demonstrated in this patient?
   a. double papilla sliding flap.
   b. lateral pedicle sliding flap.
   c. free gingival graft.
   d. apically repositioned graft.
   e. none of the above.

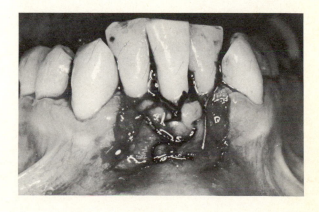

92. This 55-year-old man presented with a mucogingival defect on the labial surface of the mandibular right first premolar. A treatment plan suggested a full coverage restoration. What indicated surgical procedure will provide the *most* favorable clinical results for this area of the mouth?
a. apically repositioned flap.
b. free gingival graft.
c. lateral sliding pedicle flap.
d. alveolar ridge augmentation.
e. closed curettage.

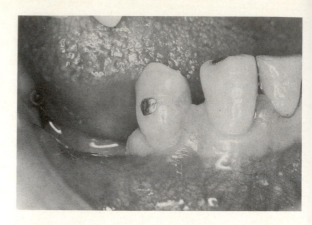

93. How would you treat this localized vertical bone defect?
a. root planing and closed curettage.
b. periodontal flap procedure, root planing, osteoplasty, and ostectomy procedure to remove supporting bone on the adjacent tooth in order to eliminate the intrabony defect.
c. tetracycline-impregnated hollow fiber, placed in the periodontal pocket for 24 hours.
d. periodontal flap procedure, root planing, and bone grafting to regenerate lost periodontal supporting tissues.
e. gingivectomy.

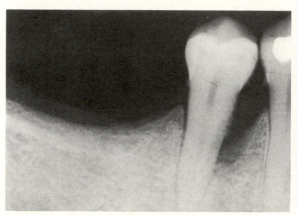

94. The *principal* cause of this developing periodontal problem should be addressed by:
a. gingivectomy.
b. alleviating the heavy occlusal stress on the anterior mandibular teeth.
c. therapeutic root planing only.
d. workup for scleroderma.

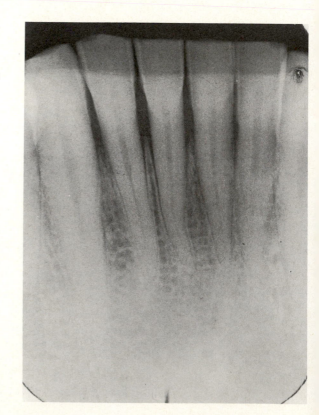

■ SECTION C

Endodontics

95. What is the treatment indicated for this 21-year-old woman?
   a. Use routine endodontics and fabricate a full crown.
   b. Use routine endodontics, section the roots, treat as two teeth, and fabricate two premolar crowns.
   c. Extract the permanent first molar tooth and replace with a three-unit fixed bridge.
   d. Extract the permanent first molar tooth and replace with a removable partial denture.
   e. Extract the tooth and transplant the developing third molar into its socket.

96. According to evidence revealed in this periapical radiograph of a healthy 28-year-old man, the correct management of this case should include:
   a. root canal therapy on the first molar with placement of a suitable restoration.
   b. placement of an occlusal restoration only.
   c. no treatment.
   d. a complete skeletal survey.
   e. ordering serum chemistry tests.

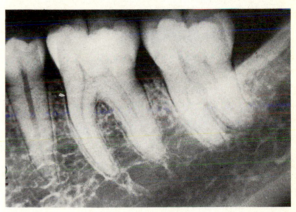

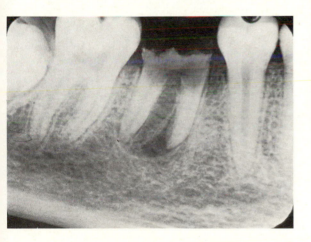

97. The correct treatment for the first premolar tooth as indicated by the radiograph is to:
a. place a DO restoration.
b. leave it alone.
c. complete root canal therapy and place a suitable restoration.
d. complete a pulpotomy and place a suitable restoration.
e. combine a root resection with root canal obliteration, send the specimen for microscopic study, and place a suitable restoration.

98. The best management for the vital asymptomatic incisor region is:
a. to evaluate the region periodically.
b. no treatment or surveillance.
c. to do conservative root canal fillings for all four incisors.
d. to do conservative root canal fillings for the central incisors only.
e. to do root resection and root canal filling for the two central incisors, and send the surgical specimen for microscopic study.

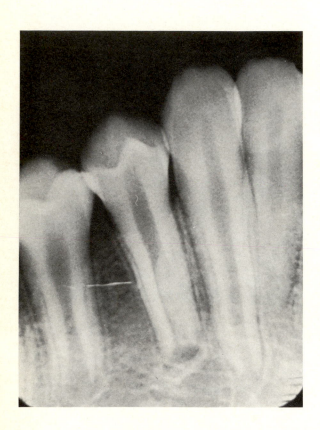

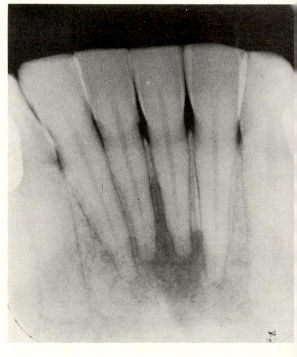

99. This patient has a good complement of the maxillary anterior ten teeth, which will require minimal treatment except for the lateral incisor. What is the treatment indicated for the lateral incisor if funds are sufficient and the patient agrees?

a. Extract the tooth and include it in a partial denture.

b. Extract the tooth and replace with a bridge.

c. Perform root canal therapy and place a crown and possible post and core.

d. Perform pulpotomy and place a mesial composite restoration.

e. Perform root canal therapy, do an apicoectomy, and place a crown.

100. What is the *most* correct treatment for the first molar tooth if the remainder of the examination fails to yield facts that would modify the findings illustrated here?

a. No further treatment.

b. Place a full crown only.

c. Extract the tooth without delay.

d. Perform root canal therapy if possible.

e. Perform root canal therapy if possible and place a full crown.

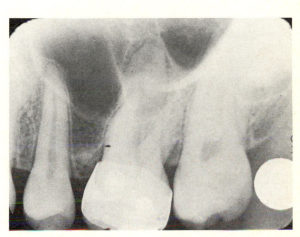

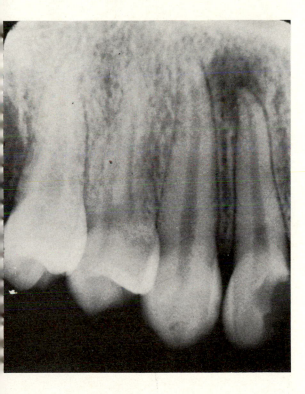

101. The indicated treatment for the second pre-molar tooth when the patient does not desire the first molar tooth replaced is to:
a. place a new MO restoration only.
b. equilibrate and place a new MOD overlay.
c. place a root canal filling and a MOD overlay.
d. advise that no treatment is needed.
e. perform a pulpotomy procedure and re-radiograph in 6 months.

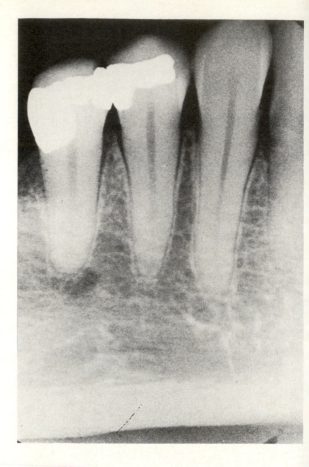

102. If the remainder of the examination does not reveal findings that would contraindicate it, the best approach for this man (**A** and **B**) is to:
a. extract the two roots and place a partial denture.
b. perform root canal therapy on both roots and build crowns on these teeth, using posts.
c. extract both roots, enucleate the periapical lesions, send the material for biopsy, and place a partial denture.
d. extract both roots, enucleate the soft tissue lesion in the vestibule, and place a partial denture.
e. institute no treatment at present but follow a program of benign neglect, planning to extract all the remaining teeth and place an upper denture when suitable deterioration has been achieved.

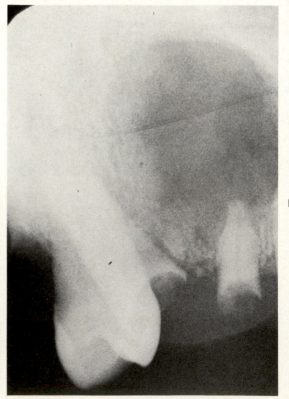

B

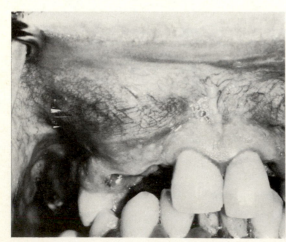

A

103. A mother on welfare with no dental benefits brings her 12-year-old son to you. The mandibular left first molar is best treated by:
a. extraction.
b. gingivectomy and placement of a stainless steel preformed crown.
c. pulpotomy and placement of a stainless steel preformed crown.
d. root canal therapy and placement of a stainless steel preformed crown.
e. root canal therapy, gingivectomy, and placement of a stainless steel preformed crown.

104. If the remainder of the oral findings are non-contributory in this 17-year-old son, and the premolar tooth is asymptomatic, it is obvious that the preferred approach is:
a. no treatment.
b. conservative root canal therapy on the premolar tooth and placement of a suitable restoration.
c. calcium hydroxide therapy followed by conservative root canal therapy.
d. a pulpotomy on the premolar and placement of a suitable restoration.
e. antibiotics and drainage by opening into the pulp chamber of the premolar.

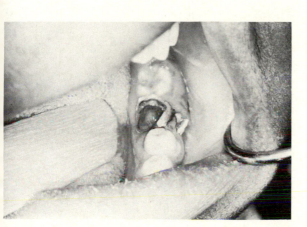

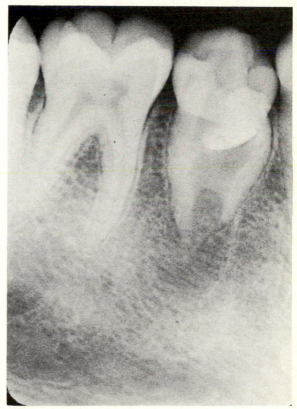

105. The findings of the other three quadrants are such that they will not modify the treatment approach to the tender mandibular right first molar tooth. Gingival probing fails to reveal the presence of pockets. The best approach for this healthy patient who has adequate funds is to:

a. place a DO amalgam restoration only.

b. place a three-quarter crown restoration only.

c. perform conservative root canal therapy and place a restoration that will adequately protect the cusps.

d. remove the temporary filling and replace it after first placing a eugenol dressing on the pulpal wall.

e. place a DO overlay only, making sure that the occlusion is correct.

106. The best approach to the problem associated with the right central incisor of this 68-year-old man who has had a recent hip prosthesis placed and who is dependent entirely on social security is to:

a. extract the tooth.

b. perform a pulpotomy procedure.

c. do a root canal filling.

d. do a root canal filling and place a Vitallium implant that extends through the apex into the bone.

e. do a root canal filling and splint the tooth to its neighbors.

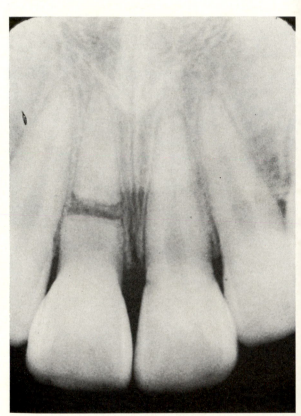

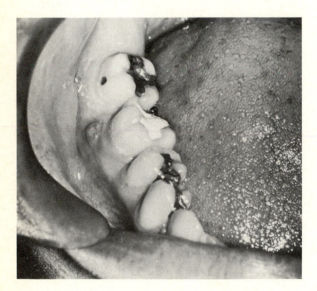

107. The correct treatment for the asymptomatic second premolar tooth of a person whose desires and adequacy of funds are satisfactory is to:
a. place a crown only.
b. perform a pulpotomy procedure and place a crown.
c. do a root canal filling and place a crown.
d. extract the tooth and perform a Caldwell-Luc procedure for the sinus problem.
e. treat the tooth and work up the patient for osteogenic sarcoma or scleroderma.

108. This 55-year-old man presents to you for consultation concerning the painful lateral incisor tooth. He tells you he had the tooth treated endodontically 5 years previously. The tooth carries a poor prognosis because of the:
a. internal resorption.
b. root fracture.
c. external resorption.
d. root perforation.
e. dilaceration.

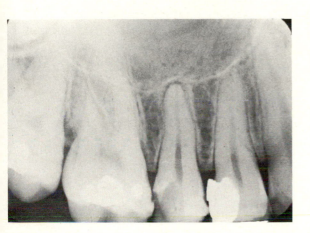

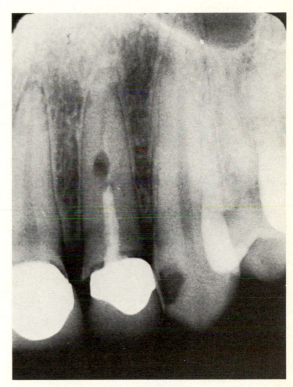

109. This 30-year-old man with adequate funds presents for a routine dental examination. If the complete workup corroborates the suggested radiographic diagnoses, what treatment would you recommend for him? He has a full complement of teeth in good health except for the problems illustrated here? These teeth are asymptomatic.

a. Perform conservative endodontics on the central incisor.

b. Perform conservative endodontics on the lateral incisor.

c. Do root canal fillings on both teeth and apicoectomies on both teeth.

d. Perform conventional endodontics on the central incisor and a retrofill on the lateral incisor, considering the likelihood that conventional endodontics cannot be completed on the lateral tooth.

e. Advise the patient not to have any treatment until the teeth become symptomatic.

110. You detect the radiolucency at the apex of the asymptomatic incisor tooth in a new patient. You request and receive the periapical radiograph of the tooth taken just before placement of the endodontic filling 5 years ago. The radiolucent lesion was about 2.5 cm in diameter at that time. The patient states that the tooth has not bothered him since it was endodontically treated. The *most* correct management at the present time is to:

a. remove the old root canal filling and refill.

b. search for a second canal.

c. place a crown on the tooth.

d. perform an apicoectomy and submit the specimen for microscopic study.

e. do nothing because the radiolucency is the image of the incisive canal.

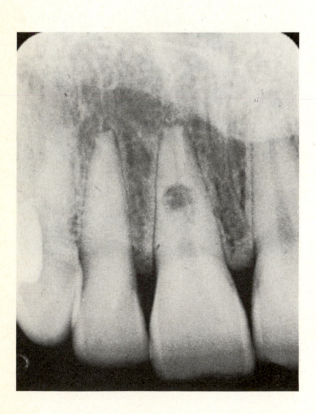

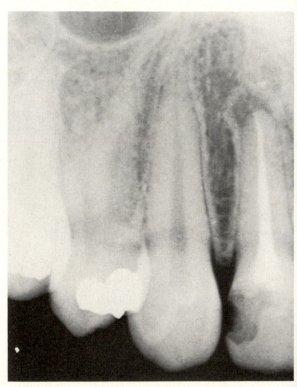

111. This radiograph is of a 62-year-old man who has spent considerable time and money over the previous 20 years in maintaining the central and lateral incisor teeth. He has now grown discouraged and weakly suggests that perhaps he wouldn't mind losing them. Except for these two teeth, the rest are in good health and relationship. The patient has suffered from diabetes for several years and has experienced some difficulty in keeping it under control in the last 6 months or so. The correct treatment in this case is to:

a. perform flap surgery on the mesial pocket of the central incisor.

b. extract the central incisor under antibiotic coverage and reevaluate No. 7 after the socket heals.

c. redo the endodontic fills in both teeth.

d. perform a root resection on both teeth only.

e. perform a root resection on both teeth and do flap surgery on the mesial pocket of the central incisor.

112. The canine is asymptomatic in this case and so is the patient. The correct treatment is to:

a. keep the periapical area under surveillance every year or so by re-radiographing.

b. keep the periapical area under surveillance but re-radiograph only if the tooth becomes painful.

c. treat with conservative endodontics.

d. do a root canal filling in conjunction with a root resection and send the specimen for microscopic study.

e. do nothing because there is no problem.

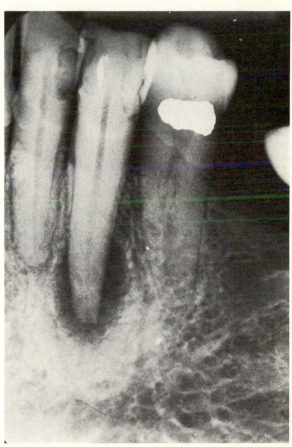

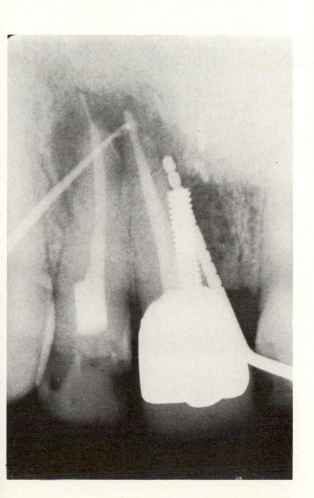

113. The correct treatment for the painful left central incisor of this patient who has limited funds is:

a. endodontic root fill with apicoectomy.
b. no treatment.
c. extraction of the tooth.
d. endodontic treatment in combination with a Vitallium implant passed through the apex into the periapical bone.
e. just splinting the tooth to its neighbors, using a fine-wire technique.

114. During radiographic examination of a new patient who is 68 years old, you find this seemingly inadequate root canal filling. The patient tells you he had the tooth treated about 20 years ago and that it has never bothered him since. The correct approach is to:

a. leave it alone.
b. remove the bridge and redo the filling.
c. leave the bridge in place and redo the filling.
d. do a root resection and try to seal the apices under direct vision.
e. extract the tooth.

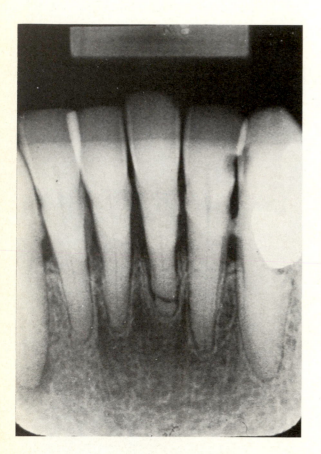

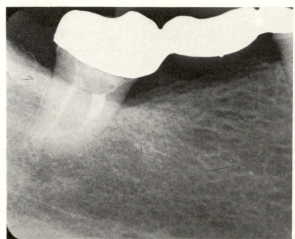

115. A. This vertical fracture in the second molar tooth *most* likely occurred because of:
   a. failure to remove all the decay from the crown.
   b. improper root canal filling techniques.
   c. a peridontal bifurcation involvement.
   d. failure to protect the cusps with a suitable restoration.
   e. a developmental defect in the crown.

 B. This patient is very interested in saving all her 28 teeth and practices good oral hygiene. What is the best way to manage the situation?
   a. The situation is hopeless; extract the tooth and place a partial denture.
   b. Extract the tooth and place a cantilever bridge with multiple abutments.
   c. Extract the tooth but do not replace it.
   d. Bring the two segments together with a circumferential wire.

116. Although all the details of the examination are not available to you, what is the *most* likely correct approach to the asymptomatic radiolucency in this 15-year-old girl?
   a. Do a root canal filling on the lateral incisor.
   b. Do a root canal filling on the lateral incisor and the canine.
   c. Perform surgical exploration of the radiolucency and submit the specimen for microscopic study.
   d. No treatment.

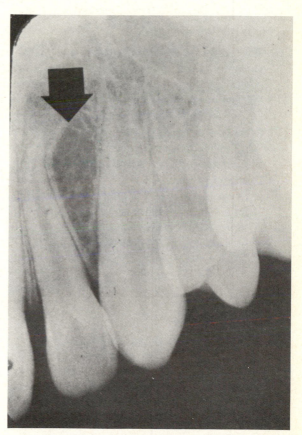

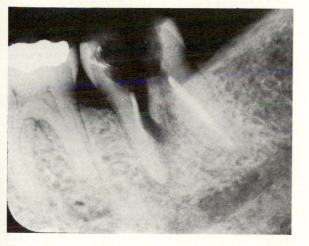

117. What is *most* likely to be the correct treatment for this radiopacity *(arrow)* in the antrum?
   a. Remove the palatal torus.
   b. Investigate surgically using a Caldwell-Luc approach.
   c. Do nothing but re-radiograph in 6 months.
   d. Extract the premolar tooth.
   e. Perform endodontics on the premolar tooth.

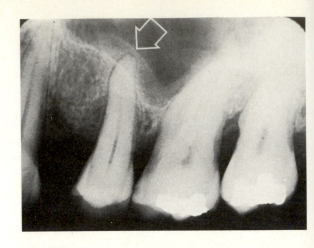

118. The premolar tooth was root canal filled 1 week ago after a history of chronic pain and sensitivity to percussion. What is the correct management of the antral shadow indicated by the arrow?
   a. Radiograph occasionally; it is most likely pulpal in origin.
   b. Radiograph occasionally; it is most likely a benign mucosal cyst.
   c. Do nothing; it is most likely a shadow cast by a buccal exostosis.
   d. Refer for an extensive workup; it is probably cancer of the maxillary sinus floor.

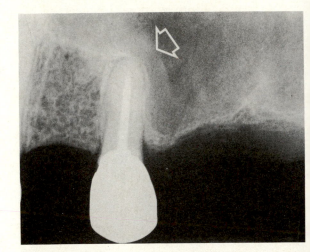

119. The 62-year-old patient wants to save this molar tooth, which has some sensitivity, and it would be very beneficial to the overall treatment plan if the tooth could be saved. What is the indicated approach?
   a. Extract the tooth and take a biopsy of surrounding bone because of probable malignancy.
   b. Do a root canal filling on the tooth.
   c. Order a serum alkaline phosphatase test because the patient probably has Paget's disease.
   d. Perform periodontal flap surgery.

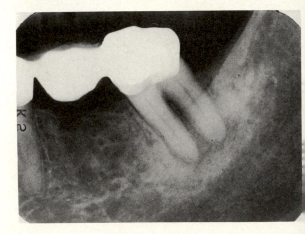

120. After the radiolucency *(arrow)* in this 14-year-old boy's radiographs is noticed, the most helpful step in the examination is to:
   a. pulp test the canine tooth.
   b. pulp test the lateral tooth.
   c. clinically examine the labial alveolus to determine whether an anatomic depression is present in the area (the incisive fossa).
   d. attempt to aspirate the radiolucency because it is most likely a globulomaxillary cyst.

121. You notice this radiolucency in the radiographs of a 23-year-old patient. After a complete workup, which one of the following approaches is *most* likely indicated?
   a. root canal therapy on tooth No. 7.
   b. root canal therapy on tooth No. 6.
   c. surgical removal of a globulomaxillary cyst.
   d. block resection for malignancy.

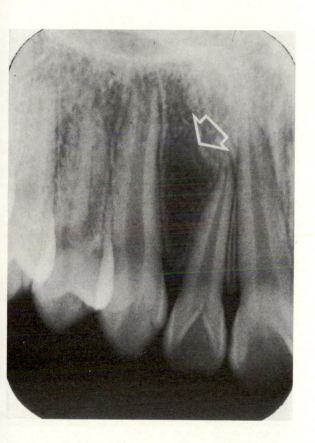

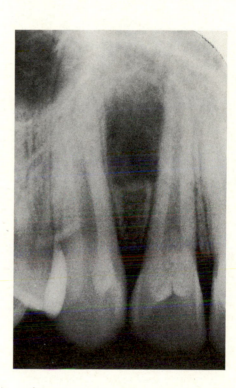

122. In addition to the periodontal problem involving the second premolar and first molar teeth, a radiopacity *(arrow)* is seen in the periapex of the second premolar. What is the *most* likely treatment necessary in relation to the premolar and the radiopacity?
a. No treatment, because the radiopacity is a cementoma.
b. Endodontics on the second premolar.
c. No treatment, because the radiopacity is a torus.
d. A block resection because the lesion is probably an osteogenic sarcoma.

123. What is the indicated treatment for the left central incisor *(arrow)*, which is tender to percussion?
a. Extract No. 9 because of the lack of root strength.
b. Extract No. 9 because the canal will probably be nonnegotiable.
c. Extract No. 9 because of the degree of periodontal bone loss.
d. Perform an apicoectomy in combination with retreatment of the tooth.

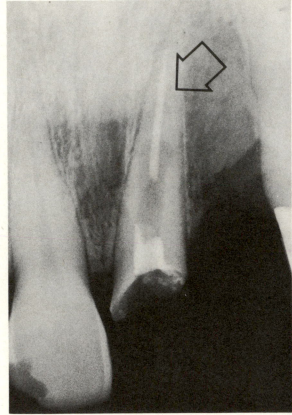

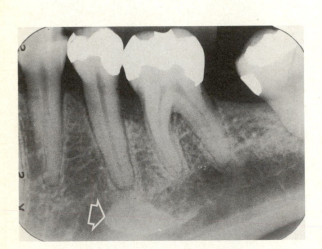

124. What is the indicated treatment for the left central incisor tooth?
   a. Perform conservative root canal therapy.
   b. None.
   c. Inform the patient of the entity at the apex, and re-radiograph occasionally.
   d. Perform root resection in combination with root canal filling and microscopic study of the specimen.

125. What treatment is most likely indicated for the first molar tooth?
   a. occlusal adjustment.
   b. only a MOD restoration.
   c. a pulpotomy and a suitable restoration.
   d. conservative root canal therapy and a suitable restoration.

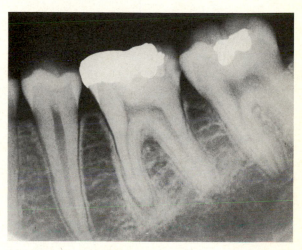

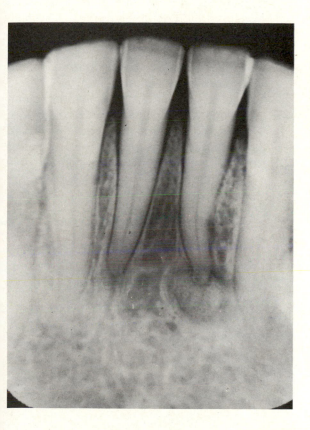

Dr. Gary Taylor authored questions 126 through 137.

126. This radiograph was made of the mandibular first molar just before cementation of a porcelain-fused-to-metal crown as a check of marginal adaptation. The patient has no history or pain from this tooth, and all vitality tests are within normal limits. Which of the following is the *most* correct treatment for this patient?

a. final cementation of the crown.

b. temporary cementation of the crown and observation.

c. temporary cementation of the crown, warning the patient that internal resorption may be present.

d. intentional endodontic therapy and final cementation of the crown.

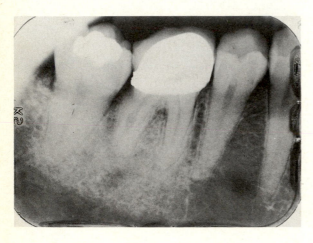

127. This 53-year-old woman complains of a "pus bag" draining from the gingival sulcus near the bifurcation of the mandibular first molar. Endodontic therapy was completed through the existing crown approximately 6 months ago. The opposite dental arches are intact and the opposing maxillary quadrant is missing only the second molar. No other endodontic or periodontic condition is present. The *most* reasonable course of treatment, considering the amount of alveolar bone loss, the condition of the root canal system, limited finances, and the intactness of the dental arches is:

a. hemisection and bicuspidization, retaining both roots with new crowns.

b. hemisection and root amputation, retaining one root included into a fixed bridge extending onto first and second premolar.

c. removal of the tooth and a fixed cantilever bridge extending onto both first and second premolars.

d. tooth extraction and replacement with a removable partial denture.

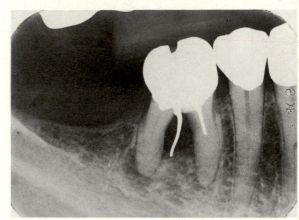

128. This 39-year-old man reports acute distress for the past 24 hours when any occlusal contact occurs involving the mandibular first molar. The crown has been in place for 2 years, appears intact, is free of caries, and is not mobile. The patient is *best* treated by:
a. referral to an endodontist.
b. written prescription for an oral antibiotic and analgesic with observation.
c. written prescription for an oral antibiotic and analgesic with observation, and appointment for endodontic therapy by a general dentist.
d. occlusal equilibration.
e. pulpotomy.

129. This 22-year-old woman is seen as a new patient, and routine full-mouth radiographs reveal the following radiolucency. She is asymptomatic and all teeth respond within normal limits to vitality tests. She reports removal of her "wisdom" teeth 6 months ago by an oral surgeon, who also performed additional surgery a month later. Developing a treatment plan should include all the following *except:*
a. obtaining a more detailed history of the recent surgery.
b. contacting the oral surgeon about the nature of the surgery.
c. beginning immediate intentional endodontic therapy.
d. requesting the oldest existing radiographs available.

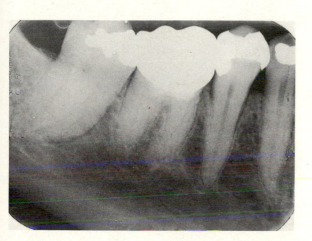

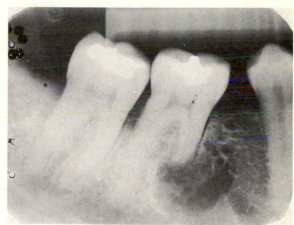

130. A 28-year-old man presents with facial swelling that began the previous evening in the area of the canine fossa and has extended to the periorbital soft tissues, closing his eye. The maxillary central, lateral, and canine are all mobile and respond positively to percussion. There is no discoloration of any tooth. Electrical pulp tests are inconclusive. Cold tests are positive on the canine and lateral incisor but negative on the central incisor. **A** is the radiograph taken at the present visit. **B** shows the region 12 months after definitive treatment. Without the benefit of the view in **B,** appropriate endodontic therapy would have been to:

a. open both lateral and central incisors for drainage.

b. give second-division block anesthesia and access cavity preparation on the lateral incisor.

c. access cavity preparation on the lateral incisor without anesthesia.

d. test cavity (access to dentin only) first on the central incisor without anesthesia.

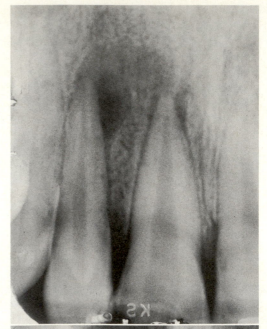

A

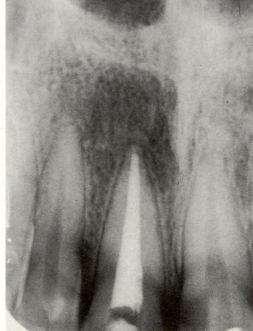

B

131. A 63-year-old man had endodontic therapy completed through an existing crown on tooth No. 7 within the previous year. The restoring dentist cemented a post in the canal to increase retention of the crown, which dislodged during treatment. The tooth is now chronically tender in an apical direction. Which of the following should be the *first* treatment option?

a. surgical intervention with apicoectomy and reverse (retro) filling of the root canal.
b. extraction and replacement with a three-unit fixed prosthesis.
c. removal of the crown and post with conventional treatment of the root canal space.
d. oral antibiotic therapy for 5 days.

132. A 44-year-old woman complains of a draining sinus tract just distal to the apex of the maxillary second premolar. Her previous dentist had been endodontically treating the tooth for 3 months. Which of the following is the *most* appropriate treatment?

a. conventional retreatment of the root canal space.
b. calcium hydroxide therapy after removal of the existing endodontic filling.
c. surgical intervention including apical reverse filling.
d. tracing the path of the sinus tract and performing vitality tests on adjacent teeth.

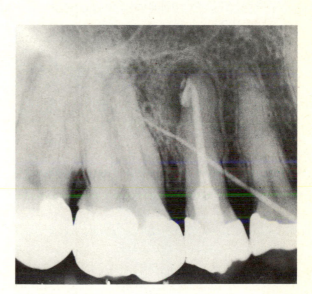

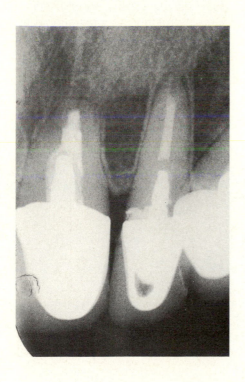

133. A 27-year-old man has an indurated expansion of the alveolar cortical plate near the apex of the maxillary right central incisor. The tooth had conventional endodontic therapy following carious exposure 5 years ago, and a surgical procedure was performed to correct a nonhealing endodontic periapical lesion 3 years later. The patient has been asymptomatic until the present problem occurred 2 weeks ago. Which of the following diagnosis and treatment options is *most* likely correct?

a. The root is fractured and the tooth should be extracted.

b. The original bony lesion was a cyst not completely enucleated and surgery should be redone.

c. Excess particles of amalgam distant from the root end filling have caused a foreign body reaction and require surgical removal.

d. The conventional and surgical endodontic procedures were improperly done and surgery should be redone.

134. A 43-year-old woman has tenderness and slight gingival swelling associated with the embrasure space between the mandibular canine and first premolar. Her chief complaint is chronic soreness when brushing and flossing in this area. Despite the appearance of the radiograph, the interproximal area does not probe more than 3.0 mm at any position. Which of the following is *most* correct?

a. This is a lesion of periodontal origin and will require flap surgery.

b. This is an alveolar defect caused from the occlusal stress of the cantilever bridge and will require only equilibration and observation.

c. This is possibly a lesion of endodontic origin only and a test cavity should be done to determine vitality. If pulpal necrosis exists, endodontic therapy should be completed and the area observed radiographically.

d. This is a combined endodontic-periodontic lesion requiring both endodontic therapy and surgical periodontics.

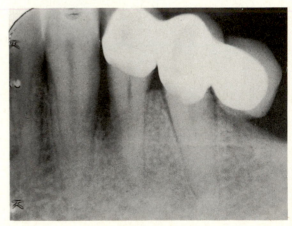

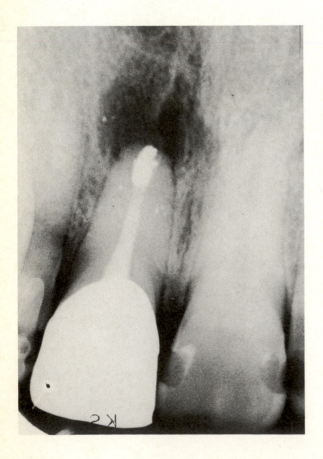

135. A 23-year-old woman was instructed to have endodontic therapy 4 years ago following an acute alveolar abscess and neglected to do so. The tooth is still asymptomatic but requires treatment. The treatment of choice should be:

a. extraction, considering the duration and size of the periapical lesion.

b. conventional endodontic therapy.

c. conventional endodontic therapy combined with placement of intracranial calcium hydroxide for several months prior to final condensation of gutta-percha.

d. conventional endodontic therapy with immediate surgical curettage of the periapical area.

136. An 11-year-old girl has a history of trauma to the face 2 years ago. The central incisor is discolored and does not respond to vitality tests. The *most* favorable treatment is:

a. observation for continued apical closure.

b. routine endodontic therapy.

c. apexification.

d. apexogenesis.

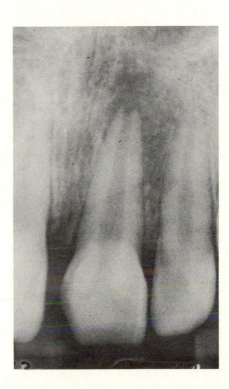

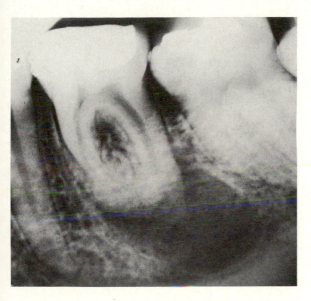

137. This 27-year-old woman had intentional endodontic therapy completed 5 years ago following coronal fracture as a result of anterior facial trauma. The procedure was uneventful, but the existing crown, including the core and dowel, has loosened at least 10 times on the right central incisor, requiring recementation. It is now loose again, but a large parulis is present over the root on the labial surface. The anterior segment has a normal overjet and overbite but very heavy contact of the incisal edges during protrusive movements. Contact is particularly extreme on the right central incisor. What are the most probable diagnosis and treatment?

a. The restoration has simply loosened and should be recemented.

b. The restoration has simply loosened and should be recemented, but the incisal contact should be reduced.

c. The excessive physical contact has caused breakdown of the surrounding periodontal structures, causing the parulis, which will spontaneously heal after incisal adjustment.

d. The excessive contact has resulted in vertical radicular fracture along the length of the dowel, and the tooth must be extracted.

138. Which item gives the greatest concern in this radiograph?

a. the three roots on the second molar.

b. there is no rubber dam in place.

c. the "downhill" lie to the radiograph.

d. instrumentation has progressed into the periapical tissue.

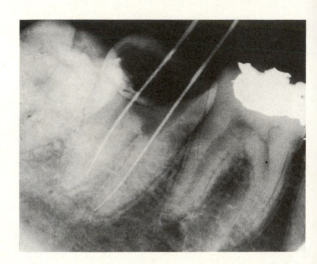

■ SECTION D

Operative dentistry

Dr. Vickyann Chrobak authored questions 139 through 152.

139. What is the best approach for restoring the asymptomatic mandibular first molar tooth in this healthy patient who has adequate funds? Findings in the other three quadrants are noncontributory.
a. Place an occlusal amalgam.
b. Place an MO overlay in proper occlusion.
c. Place a suitable core and dowel and a restoration that will adequately protect the cusps.
d. Place a suitable core and dowel and a three-quarter crown.
e. This tooth is not restorable.

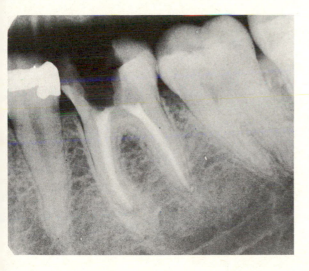

140. A. This bite-wing radiograph is of a 36-year-old woman who maintains reasonably good home care and presents every 6 months for a periodic dental examination. Which of the following treatments would you recommend at this time for the mandibular first molar and second molar, respectively?
a. an MOD restoration on the first and second molar.
b. an MOD restoration on the first molar and an MO restoration on the second molar.
c. a DO restoration on the first molar and an MO restoration on the second molar.
d. an MOD restoration on the first molar only.
e. an MO restoration on the first and on the second molar.

B. Regarding the same bite-wing radiograph, the correct treatment for the second maxillary premolar tooth as indicated by the radiographic features is to:
a. place a DO restoration.
b. perform a pulpotomy and place a suitable restoration.
c. complete root canal therapy and place a suitable restoration.
d. leave it alone.
e. place an MOD restoration.

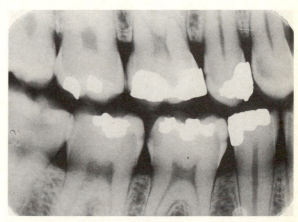

141. What is the *most* correct plan of treatment for the mandibular first molar, which has been painful to bite on recently in this 47-year-old patient?
  a. Extract the tooth and place a three-unit bridge.
  b. Place a stainless steel crown.
  c. Place an MOD amalgam restoration and perform a pulp-capping procedure if necessary.
  d. Perform root canal therapy and crown the tooth.
  e. Prescribe pain medication and see if the pain subsides.

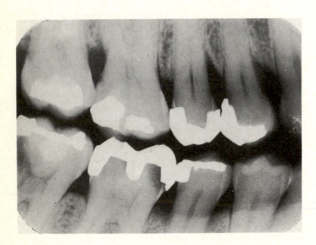

142. A. Which one of the following statements is *most* correct concerning this 35-year-old women who had all these restorations placed 12 years ago?
  a. Excellent cavity form has been followed for all restorations.
  b. Some of the cavity preparations were too shallow.
  c. Failure to follow the usual concepts of cavity design has been disastrous for this patient.
  d. The DO amalgam restoration has a marginal overhang.
  e. All the restorations should be replaced.
  B. According to this bite-wing radiograph, the *most* correct treatment for the maxillary teeth would be:
  a. placement of a DO restoration only.
  b. a complete workup of serum chemistry before initiating restorative work.
  c. placement of an MOD restoration only.
  d. placement of two amalgam restorations.
  e. no treatment.
  C. One would expect that the surfaces of human permanent teeth *most* frequently found to become carious first are:
  a. proximal surfaces of maxillary first molars.
  b. occlusal surfaces of maxillary first molars.
  c. proximal surfaces of mandibular first molars.
  d. occlusal surfaces of mandibular first molars.
  e. occlusal surfaces of maxillary second molars.

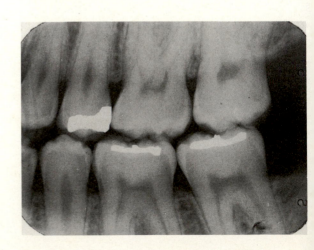

143. A. When there is a major loss of dentin in a cavity preparation not involving pulp conditions, a base is required for:

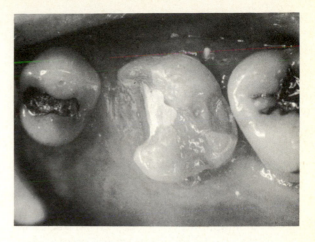

   a. temporization, protection, and economics.
   b. therapy, efficiency, and insulation.
   c. protection of the pulp only.
   d. insulation, strength, and retention.

B. The internal mortise form for the cavity preparation on the maxillary first molar is developed by use of:
   1. the dentin of the tooth.
   2. zinc phosphate cement.
   3. Copalite.
   4. calcium hydroxide.
      a. 2, 3, 4.
      b. 1 and 2.
      c. 2 and 4.
      d. 1, 3, 4.
      e. none of the above.

C. Your patient is a 45-year-old male TV salesman. If the zinc phosphate base you just placed in a large MOD preparation on this maxillary first molar falls out before you have inserted the amalgam, which of the following problems should you consider?
   1. There was inadequate retention for the base.
   2. There was caries remaining in the tooth.
   3. You forgot to use Copalite first.
   4. The zinc phosphate base was old.
      a. 1 only.
      b. 1 and 3.
      c. 1 and 2.
      d. 2 and 4.
      e 1, 3, and 4.

D. When planning treatment for the use of a base in a large cavity preparation, one must consider that a cement base can be placed on:
   a. buccal wall irregularities.
   b. gingival floor concavities.
   c. a pulp exposure.
   d. pulpal and axial walls only.
   e. all the above.

E. On a periapical radiograph, the cement base placed in the mesial of the maxillary first molar will:
   a. appear less opaque than amalgam.
   b. appear similar in opacity to caries.
   c. appear similar in opacity to amalgam.
   d. appear more opaque than amalgam.
   e. not be able to be seen.

144. A. A portion of the progressive destruction of the periodontal tissues following restorative procedures as indicated by this bite-wing radiograph can be attributed to:
   a. the type of material used.
   b. rough surfaces and ill-fitting margins.
   c. retraction strings and impression techniques for cast restorations.
   d. the degree of trauma caused by tooth preparation.

   B. This 58-year-old woman presented with a chief complaint of soreness in the gum tissue. As indicated by this bite-wing radiograph, a poorly adapted matrix band for a dental amalgam restoration of a Class II cavity may result in:
   1. an overhang.
   2. short margins.
   3. improper condensation of the restoration.
   4. improper contact with the adjacent tooth.
   5. inadequate proximal contour in the amalgam restoration.
      a. 1, 2, and 3.
      b. 1, 3, and 5.
      c. 2, 4, and 5.
      d. 3, 4, and 5.
      e. all the above.

145. After placing an MO and OL amalgam restoration in the maxillary first molar and an MO restoration in the maxillary second molar, the patient returns several days later with pain between teeth Nos. 13 and 14. The *most* likely cause of this pain would be:
   a. hyperocclusion.
   b. inadequate pulpal protection with base or liner.
   c. reaction to local anesthesia.
   d. inadequate interproximal contact.
   e. fractured restoration.

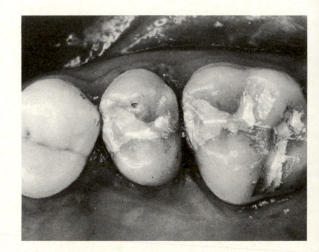

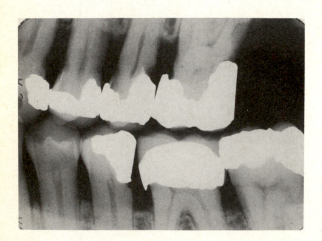

146. A 49-year-old man presents to your office with constant pain in the mandibular premolar region. He states that another dentist placed an amalgam restoration in that tooth several weeks ago. In reviewing this periapical radiograph, the proper choice of treatment at this time would be to:

a. leave it alone.

b. replace the amalgam because it has an open margin.

c. remove the existing amalgam and pin, if possible, and initiate root canal therapy.

d. provide a full crown, although the existing amalgam and pin are fine.

e. remove the existing amalgam and pin, if possible, and place a full crown with appropriate cement base.

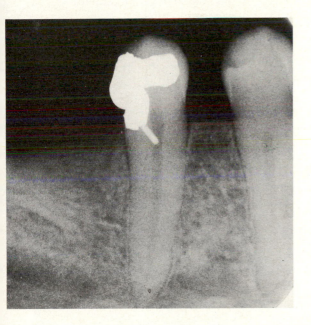

147. A. Concerning polishing amalgams, all the following are true *except:*

1. Preliminary smoothing and finishing is achieved with tin oxide.

2. The key to finishing and polishing an amalgam restoration is a well-carved amalgam.

3. Improper use of green stones can result in loss of tooth structure.

4. Reshaping the amalgam restoration is done with round and flame-shaped burs at high speed.

5. When using the Shofu system of polishing, finishing burs are not necessary because the brown point takes their place.

6. During the margination step of polishing, we strive to achieve continuity between tooth structure and restorative material.

7. The functional life of the restoration can be extended with proper polishing.

   a. 1, 3, 4.

   b. 1, 4, 5.

   c. 1, 5, 6.

   d. 2, 3, 6, 7.

   e. 4, 5, 6.

B. A 35-year-old patient presents to your office with these two restorations already in place. The remaining 30 teeth have no restorations. The only defects are deep, stained grooves in the posterior teeth. The explorer catches in the grooves, but there is no evidence of softness. The treatment of choice at this time is:

a. application of a topical fluoride compound.

b. cyanoacrylate pit and fissure sealant.

c. prophylactic odontotomy.

d. amalgam restorations in the occlusal portion of all teeth with deep grooves.

e. no treatment, but periodic examination is necessary.

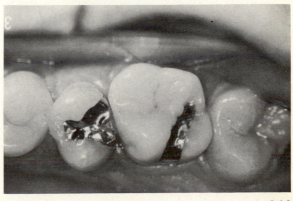

148. A. In this radiograph of a 23-year-old patient, the radiolucency seen on the mesial of tooth No. 23 and the radiolucency seen on the mesial of tooth No. 25 can be compared as follows:

    a. Both are carious lesions.

    b. Radiolucency on tooth No. 23 is a carious lesion only, whereas the radiolucency on the mesial of tooth No. 25 includes an existing tooth-colored restoration.

    c. Radiolucency on the mesial of tooth No. 25 is a carious lesion only, whereas the radiolucency on the mesial of tooth No. 23 includes an existing tooth-colored restoration.

    d. Both areas include tooth-colored restorations.

    e. A tooth-colored restoration cannot be distinguished from caries on a radiograph.

  B. In your treatment plan for this 27-year-old woman, the best choice for restoring the carious area on the distal of tooth No. 26 would be:

    a. a composite restoration.

    b. an amalgam restoration.

    c. a gold foil restoration.

    d. a cast gold restoration.

149. A. This 26-year-old woman presents with a recurrent carious lesion on the mesial on tooth No. 7. You should anticipate doing which one of the following on the mesial of this tooth?

    a. a Class III amalgam restoration.

    b. a Class IV direct gold restoration.

    c. a Class III tooth-colored composite restoration.

    d. a Class IV tooth-colored composite restoration.

    e. a Class IV silicate restoration.

  B. In this periapical radiograph, the most likely explanation for the very radiopaque areas on tooth No. 7 and tooth No. 8 is:

    1. calcium hydroxide liner material.

    2. copal resin varnish.

    3. zinc phosphate cement base.

    4. zinc oxide eugenol cement.

    5. recurrent caries.

      a. could be any of the above.

      b. 1 and 2.

      c. 1 and 3.

      d. 1, 3, 4, 5.

      e. 1, 2, 3.

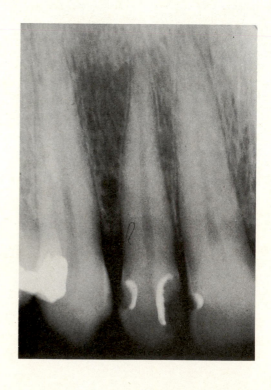

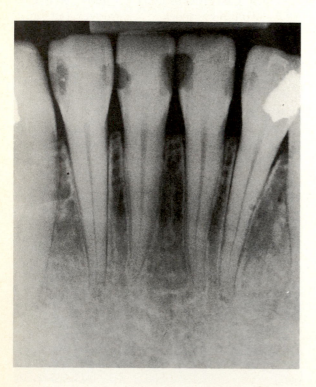

150. A. This bite-wing radiograph is of a middle-aged man who has come to your office with a toothache on the lower arch. He states that finances are no problem, and he is very interested in saving all his teeth. The best approach for treatment of tooth No. 31 is therefore to:

a. leave it alone.

b. extract it without replacement.

c. place an MOD amalgam and cap the pulp, if necessary.

d. do a conservative root canal filling and place a stainless steel crown.

e. do a root canal filling and restore with suitable core and dowel and full coverage restoration.

B. Suppose that this is a radiograph of a 47-year-old man with limited finances. Tooth No. 31 has already been extracted. The patient is still having toothache, and radiographs show a deep carious lesion on tooth No. 4. There is no detectable pulpal exposure upon excavation of all decay. The tooth tests vital. The *best* treatment at this time is:

a. direct pulp cap.

b. root canal therapy.

c. a permanent restoration after placing a suitable base.

d. placement of a zinc phosphate cement temporary restoration.

e. placement of two coats of cavity varnish and an amalgam restoration.

151. One week after cementation of a cast gold restoration on the maxillary first premolar adjacent to an existing DL amalgam, the patient reports to your office with sensitivity to cold and pressure from the tooth. The *most* likely cause is:

a. hyperocclusion.

b. chronic pulpitis.

c. galvanic response.

d. maxillary sinusitis.

e. minute pulpal exposure.

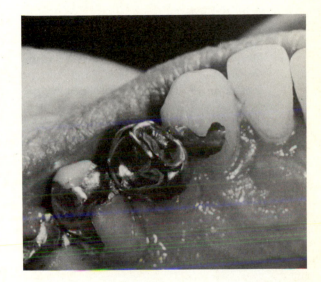

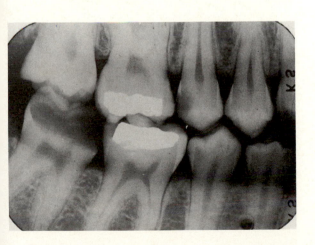

152. A. This 21-year-old woman presented to your office with minimal interproximal caries on the distal of the second premolar. She said she wanted a "tooth-colored" restoration placed because of aesthetics and because she felt amalgam was "unsafe." After placing the DO posterior composite, which areas will you be especially concerned about checking on 6-month recall examination?

a. interproximal contact area.
b. occlusal wear.
c. marginal ridge wear.
d. all the above.
e. b and c only.

B. In restoring the distal surface of the mandibular second premolar *(arrow)*, how should the distal marginal ridge be restored in relation to the mesial marginal ridge of the mandibular first molar, provided that the teeth are ideally shaped and aligned?

a. lower.
b. higher.
c. same height.
d. marginal ridges are unrelated.

153. This bite-wing radiograph is of a 40-year-old man who maintains excellent home care and presents every 6 months for a periodic dental examination. Which one of the following treatments would you prescribe at this time for the mandibular teeth?

a. an MO restoration on second molar, an MOD restoration on first molar, and a DO restoration on the second premolar.
b. an MOD restoration on the first molar only.
c. an MOD restoration on the first molar and a DO on the second premolar.
d. an occlusal restoration on the second molar and a DO restoration on the first molar.
e. a DO restoration on the first molar only.

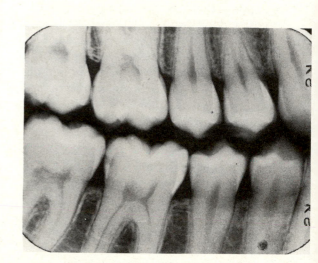

154. This periapical radiograph is representative of the other 13 films of a man from a middle-class home who is working his way through college. What is the best approach to this case?
    a. full-mouth extractions and complete dentures.
    b. fluoride treatments.
    c. advise the student to obtain a bank loan so that you can do extensive crown and root canal work.
    d. treatment as a caries-control case; instruct in home care and nutrition and restore teeth temporarily with amalgams and composites.
    e. extraction of most of the teeth but retention of a few of the best ones to support partial dentures.

155. Which is the correct treatment for the second premolar tooth if we agree that the first and second molars can be successfully crowned?
    a. No treatment is necessary.
    b. Place an MO restoration only.
    c. Place a DO restoration only.
    d. Place an MOD restoration only.
    e. Place an MOD overlay restoration.

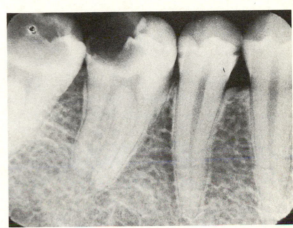

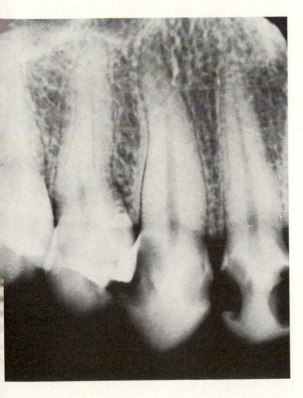

Dr. Peter Hasiakos authored questions 156 through 168.

156. You have just performed endodontic therapy on the mandibular central incisor. The only tooth structure missing is the conservative access cavity in the lingual surface. The patient is 70 years old and enjoys good health. Restorative treatment of this tooth may be to place:
   a. a lingual composite or amalgam restoration.
   b. a postamalgam buildup.
   c. cast core and dowel and crown.
   d. a Class I occlusal inlay.

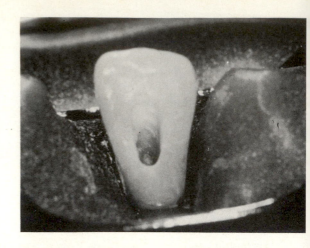

157. This 15-year-old patient has severe discolorations of the labial surfaces of maxillary anterior teeth. The parents and patient desire a predictable cosmetic result. He has a Class I occlusion, and the teeth suffer from no other maladies. Treatment will *most* likely involve:
   a. vital tooth bleaching.
   b. porcelain or composite bonded veneers.
   c. porcelain-fused-to-metal crowns.
   d. porcelain jacket crowns.
   e. reassuring those involved that at this time no such treatment need be initiated.

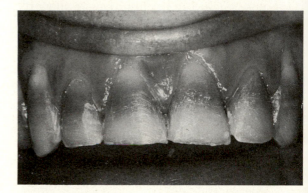

158. The mode of treatment exemplified in treating the patient depicted in **A** and **B** is:
   a. porcelain jacket crowns.
   b. porcelain-fused-to-metal crowns.
   c. porcelain-bonded veneers.
   d. vital tooth bleaching.
   e. castable ceramic crowns.

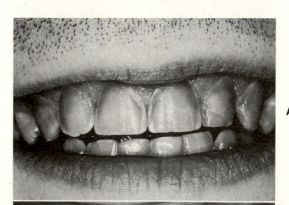

A

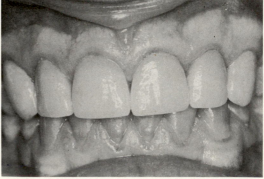

B

159. This 14-year-old patient who suffers from amelogenesis imperfecta (**A** and **B**) had been treated to enhance her dental condition as depicted by use of composite restorative material. This is an acceptable means of restoration because of the following:

a. the patient's age.
b. consideration of placement of permanent crown margins.
c. the size of the pulpal tissue involved.
d. inexpensiveness.
e. all the above.

160. The gingival margin of this complete veneer gold crown, which was placed 1 year ago, is slightly sensitive to cold air and to mechanical stimulation. No dental caries is evident clinically. Initial treatment *may* be to:

a. place a gold foil restoration at the crown margin.
b. place an amalgam restoration at the crown margin.
c. treat the area with a series of office topical fluoride applications along with home fluoride applications for 2 months, and follow the progress of symptoms.
d. reassure the patient that the situation is normal and that the sensitivity will go away.

A
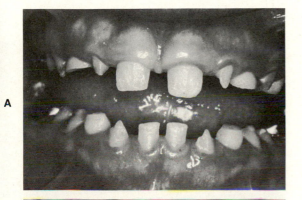

B
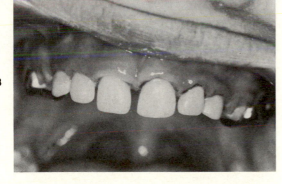

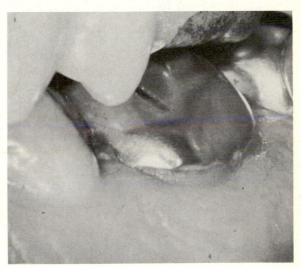

161. This 19-year-old man comes to your office and requests restoration of the spacing that exists between the maxillary incisors. Conservative treatment of choice for this Class I dentition can be:
a. placement of bonded porcelain or composite veneers.
b. placement of porcelain-fused-to-metal crowns.
c. placement of porcelain jacket crowns.
d. informing the patient that the spaces are too large for aesthetic treatment with any of the above restorations.
e. referring the patient to an orthodontist.

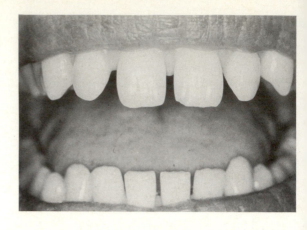

162. The completed orthodontic case depicted in this photograph resulted in some spacing of the mandibular incisors that could not be avoided. Treatment to preserve the existing arch length and tooth positions consists of:
a. placement of a Class IV bonded composite restoration on the incisors.
b. placement of an orthodontic composite retained lingual retainer.
c. placement of porcelain jacket crowns on the mandibular incisors.
d. a and b.
e. none of the above.

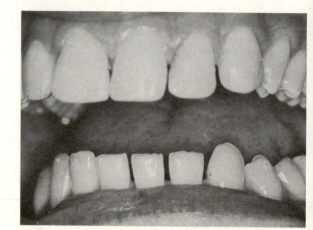

163. The maxillary left central incisor of this 16-year-old patient was traumatically avulsed and could not be successfully replanted. It was replaced using the prosthesis shown in **B.** The advantages of this method for replacing the lost tooth are:
1. minimal tooth reduction.
2. supragingival margins.
3. lack of pulpal involvement.
4. minimal to no anesthesia.
5. reduced cost.
   a. 1 and 2 only.
   b. 2, 4, and 5.
   c. 3, 4, and 5.
   d. 2, 3, 4, and 5.
   e. all of the above.

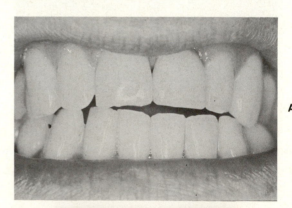

A

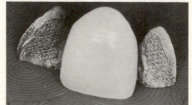

B

164. A 13-year-old patient comes to your office for a dental examination. Teeth Nos. 18 and 31 have just erupted into the oral cavity. They both have occlusal sticks with the tine of the explorer. No other dental carious lesions are noted and there are no other restorations in the patient's mouth. Your treatment plan should be to:
   a. place occlusal sealants.
   b. place occlusal amalgam restorations.
   c. place occlusal composite restorations.
   d. treat only with topical fluorides.

165. You have cemented a complete gold crown on tooth No. 19. The next day your patient complains of sensitivity upon chewing. You should first:
   a. refer the patient to an endodontist.
   b. tell the patient to wait another week.
   c. check and adjust the occlusion.
   d. suspect pulpal involvement.
   e. grind the opposing tooth.

166. Treatment sequencing ensures that:
   a. the most serious dental problems are treated first.
   b. incipient anterior restorations are completed first for better aesthetics.
   c. conditions that affect the outcome of future treatment are completed prior to most other procedures.
   d. a and c.
   e. all of the above.

167. You have just placed a dark shade photo-cured composite restoration. After examining the surface texture you determine that the material is soft. The *most* likely cause of this is:
   a. not exposing the composite to light for a long enough time.
   b. using material that has had its shelf-life expire.
   c. the material having been contaminated with saliva as a result of improper rubber dam application.
   d. none of the above.

168. Indicate the *most* correct sequence used in *most* direct restorative bonding procedures.
   1. acid-etching the enamel.
   2. placing the unfilled bonding resin.
   3. placing the filled bonding resin.
   4. pumicing the tooth.
   5. rinsing the tooth with water.
   6. finishing and polishing the restoration.
   7. selecting the proper shade.
   8. placing the rubber dam.
      a. 7, 8, 5, 4, 3, 5, 2, and 6.
      b. 4, 5, 7, 8, 1, 5, 2, 3, and 6.
      c. 1, 5, 3, 5, 2, 8, and 6.
      d. 5, 4, 1, 8, 5, 2, 5, 3, and 6.
      e. 7, 4, 1, 2, 3, and 6.

■ SECTION E

Fixed prosthodontics and occlusion

169. What is the *most* correct treatment for this 22-year-old woman (**A** and **B**) who has adequate funds? She has a full complement of teeth and is in good health in the other quadrants.

a. Perform a surgical exploration and biopsy of the soap-bubble lesion.

b. Order arteriograms of the mandible on this side.

c. Place a three-unit bridge replacing the first molar.

d. Orthodontically move the second molar forward into the first molar position.

e. Place a partial denture with a framework, designing it so that bilateral retention is employed.

170. This patient complains of pain in tooth No. 12 when he occludes. Before you remove the crown on No. 12, what *must* you tell the patient?

a. Careful oral home care is very necessary.

b. The tooth may fracture and have to be extracted.

c. Root canal therapy has a very high success rate.

d. The pain is probably caused by a maxillary sinus infection.

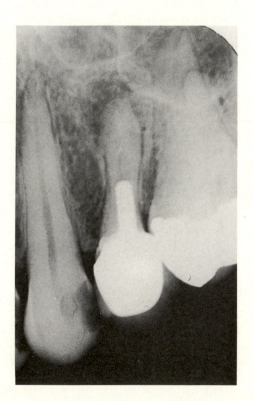

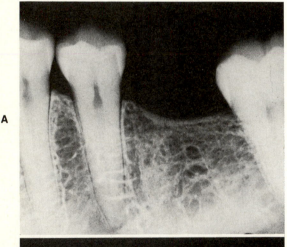

A

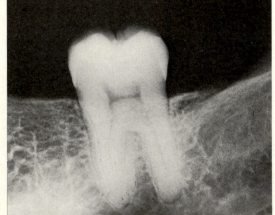

B

171. The *most* serious problem in this case is:
a. that the bridge span is too long.
b. the periapical lesion associated with the second molar tooth.
c. the overcontouring of retainer on the molar.
d. the contact between the premolar and the canine.

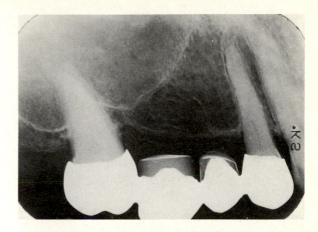

172. What is the *optimal* treatment in this case in which finances are not a problem? In the opposing quadrant the patient has a full complement of teeth in good health and in good position.
a. No treatment.
b. Place a routine three-unit bridge.
c. Place a three-unit bridge with a telescoping crown on the molar tooth.
d. Orthodontically upright the molar and place a three-unit bridge.
e. Move the molar foward orthodontically into the first molar position.

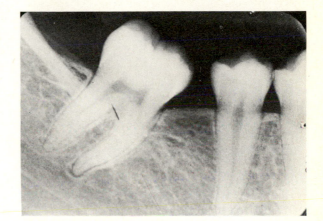

173. This 48-year-old man (**A** and **B**) presents with the myofascial pain syndrome. Which of the following is the *most* logical first step in treating this patient?
a. Extract the third molar tooth.
b. Place a bite plane.
c. Open the bite with full crowns.
d. Prescribe Valium.
e. Construct a three-unit bridge to replace the upper second premolar tooth.

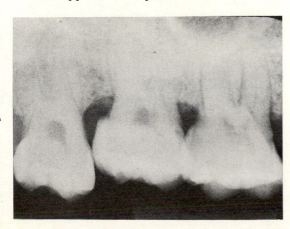

A

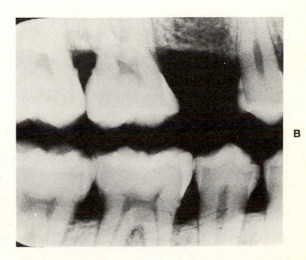

B

273

174. This man presents to you shortly after you graduate from dental school with the request that you cap his front teeth. The following approach would show the greatest discernment:
a. Fabricate porcelain jackets for him.
b. Use gold-acrylic crowns.
c. Use gold-fused-to-porcelain crowns.
d. Refer him to a practitioner who specializes in these types of problems.
e. Suggest that you try composite restorations.

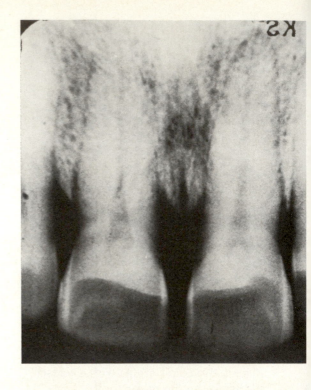

175. This occlusal problem in a healthy 18-year-old woman who has adequate funds is usually *best* managed:
a. by oral surgical procedures alone.
b. by orthodontic procedures alone.
c. by a combined surgical and orthodontic approach.
d. by advising the patient to learn to live with the problem.
e. by extracting the lower incisors and replacing them with a six-unit bridge.

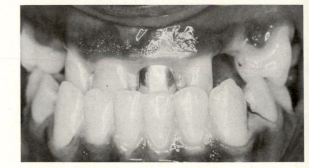

176. This patient presents with the myofascial pain syndrome. Correct dental treatment is to immediately:
a. perform a full-mouth rehabilitation, increasing the vertical dimension.
b. perform a full-mouth rehabilitation, decreasing the vertical dimension.
c. construct a night-guard appliance and re-evaluate the case.
d. recontour the cusps so that they will be more efficient.
e. replace the upper first premolar with a three-unit bridge.

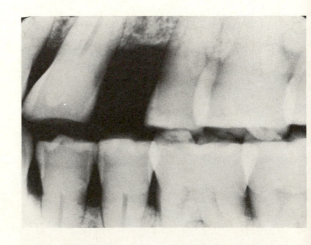

177. This 32-year-old healthy man presents for a periodic dental checkup. You find that some restorative work and minimal periodontal work will be required. What is the *best* method of reducing the patient's open bite, given that the photograph shows his teeth in centric occlusion?
  a. orthodontics.
  b. surgical resection.
  c. surgical resection in combination with orthodontics.
  d. extraction of the posterior teeth.
  e. reduction of the height of the posterior teeth using overlays and crowns.

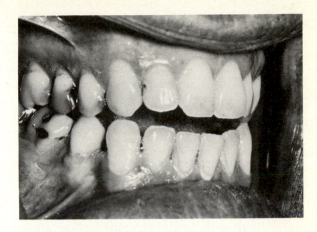

Dr. Martin Land authored questions 178 through 189.

178. What is the *most* likely cause of this miscast?
  a. incomplete burnout of wax.
  b. improperly vented wax pattern.
  c. inadequate heating of alloy and premature freezing.
  d. inadequate casting pressure.

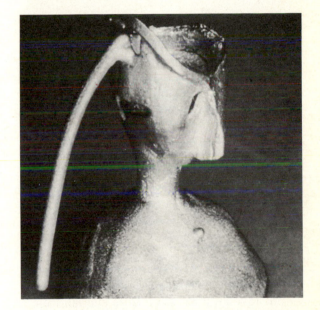

179. Assuming that the margins are satisfactory, why would you not use this polysulfide rubber base impression?
  a. Mixing appears to have been improperly done.
  b. Polysulfide rubber base is not suitable for this type of procedure.
  c. The impression should have been made in a custom tray.
  d. The edentulous areas have been inaccurately reproduced.

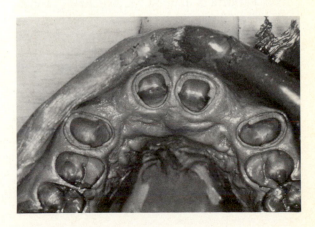

180. What is the *best* treatment approach to the loss of porcelain in this newly cemented bridge?
   a. Have the laboratory remake the bridge using proper standard procedures.
   b. Adjust for interferences and have the laboratory remake the bridge adding a thicker layer of porcelain on the canine crown.
   c. Adjust occlusion and working excursion; repair the bridge as a short-term solution; remake the bridge as a long-term solution.
   d. Adjust occlusion and working excursion; repair the bridge as a short-term solution; remake the bridge as a long-term solution, but include No. 10 as secondary abutment.

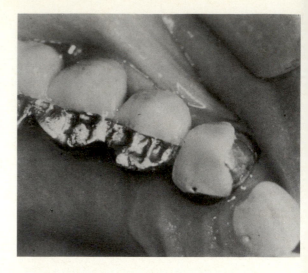

181. When replacing this fixed prosthesis, what special step should you take to ensure that this problem does not recur?
   a. Check working excursion carefully.
   b. Reduce the occlusal surface of the natural tooth more so that more bulk can be added to the crown.
   c. Use a cast metal prosthesis only.
   d. Instruct the patient not to chew on hard foods such as spare ribs.

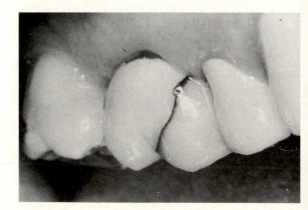

182. What is the *best* solution for the existing problem concerning No. 10?
   a. Take an impression as is and fabricate a permanent restoration.
   b. Perform a limited gingivectomy around No. 10.
   c. Fabricate satisfactory interim coverage and reassess after tissue recovery.
   d. Extract No. 10 and place a three-unit bridge.

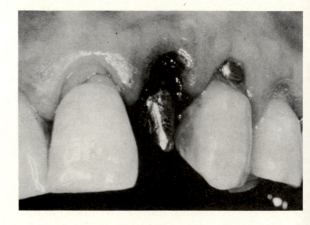

183. What is the correct management of this soft tissue problem that was discovered when the fixed prosthesis was removed?
a. Do CBC, WBC, and differential counts.
b. Do a sickle cell prep.
c. Fabricate a provisional three-unit fixed prosthesis with guidance in harmony with adjacent anterior teeth.
d. Radiograph the region of No. 8 to see if retained root is present.

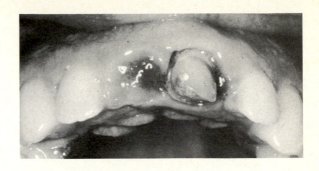

184. What concerns you *most* from a fixed prosthodontic standpoint in this patient?
a. lack of support provided for the porcelain through substructure design.
b. location of centric stops on the canine too close to the ceramometal interface.
c. the design does not permit maintenance and promotion of health of the supporting structures.
d. the connectors do not extend far enough incisally.

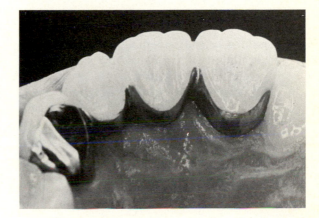

185. Which *one* of the following procedures *must* be done before making a three-unit bridge for this patient?
a. orthodontic repositioning of the canine tooth.
b. periodontal recontouring of soft tissue in the pontic area.
c. frenectomy.
d. crown lengthening of both the canine and central incisor.

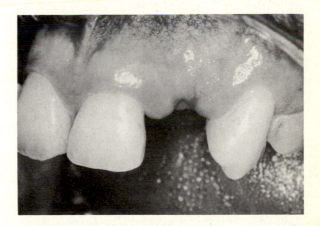

186. What is the *most* likely cause of porcelain fracture on this six-unit bridge?
a. traumatic occlusion.
b. inadequate tooth preparation.
c. use of no precious metals.
d. improper framework design.

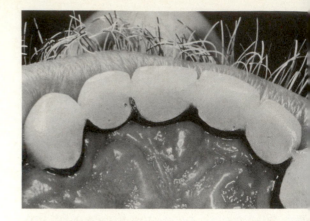

187. Which *one* of the following does *not* need to be done before cementation?
a. recontour the cervical region of the left central incisor crown.
b. relieve the internal aspect of the retainers to improve the seating of this fixed partial denture.
c. trim the pontics at the cervical regions to provide better aesthetics.
d. reglaze the appliance after adjustments.

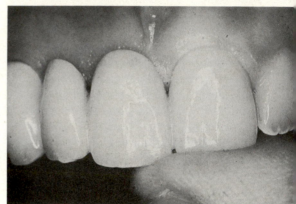

188. What is of concern about the crowned teeth in this radiograph?
a. the periapical region of the first premolar.
b. pin placement of buildup on the first premolar.
c. inadequate mesial marginal adaptation of the crown on the first premolar.
d. inadequate distal marginal adaptation of the crown on the second premolar.

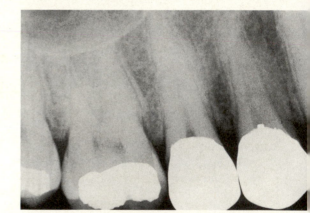

189. What is the *most* likely cause for this tissue irritation adjacent to tooth No. 8 *(arrow)*?
a. excessive flossing, brushing, and irrigation by patient.
b. response to rough Class V glass ionomer restoration.
c. poor contour of metal-ceramic restoration.
d. allergy to restorative material.

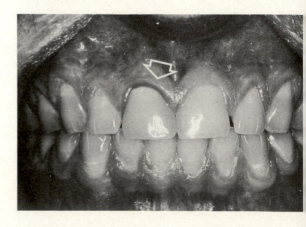

■ SECTION F

Removable prosthodontics

190. This 52-year-old man (**A, B,** and **C**) presents for an upper denture. He has a full complement of teeth on the lower arch, and although he needs some periodontal treatment, there are really no questionable teeth. The physical characteristics of the upper arch and palate are unremarkable. The teeth shown in these periapical radiographs are the only ones left in the maxilla. The canine tooth is nonvital, as is the lateral incisor. What would you advise as the *most* appropriate treatment for the maxillary arch?

a. a maxillary overdenture using the left canine and left central teeth.

b. a partial denture retaining and treating all the remaining teeth.

c. a full maxillary denture.

d. an acrylic partial denture treating and retaining the left canine and central incisor.

e. an acrylic partial denture treating and retaining the left canine and lateral and central incisors.

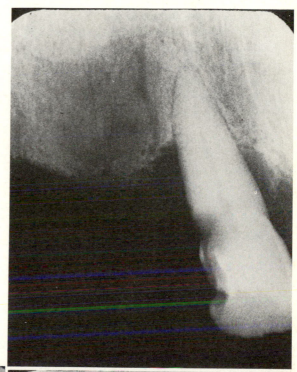

A

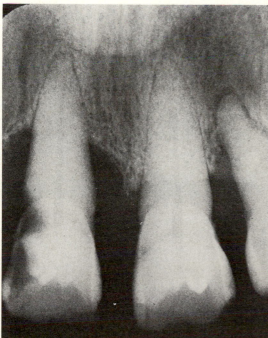

B

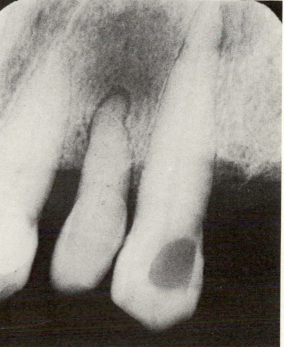

C

191. The correct management of this case is:
  a. to surgically excise and perform a biopsy of redundant tissue on the maxillary anterior ridge and fabricate a new upper denture.
  b. the same as a. but in addition to fabricate a mandibular lower partial denture and ensure that the patient wears it successfully.
  c. to rebase the upper denture only.
  d. to use a soothing liner in the present upper denture and later rebase the upper denture.
  e. to excise the redundant tissue and place a skin graft in the vestibule in conjunction with a ridge-extension procedure.

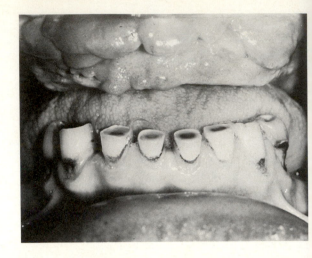

192. Which one of the following is *most* likely indicated in preparing this patient for maxillary and mandibular partial dentures?
  a. Open the bite.
  b. Extract all the remaining premolar teeth.
  c. Perform a bilateral reduction of bony tuberosities.
  d. Perform a bilateral reduction of fibrous tuberosities.

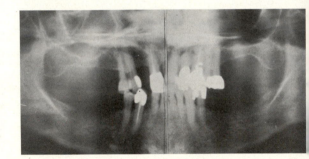

193. In preparing this arch for a partial denture, which of the following options is *most* likely necessary?
  a. removal of a retained root.
  b. reduction of fibrous tuberosity.
  c. reduction of bony tuberosity.
  d. closure of an oroantral fistula.

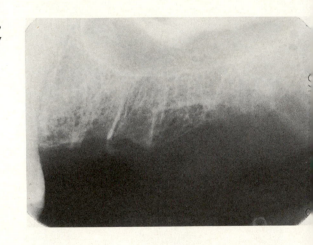

Dr. William Groetsema authored questions 194 through 240.

194. A. The exophytic mass indicated by the arrow in this edentulous maxilla is *most* likely the result of:
 a. a poorly fitting maxillary denture.
 b. advanced periodontal disease involving the maxillary anterior teeth prior to their removal.
 c. normal atrophic changes associated with loss of the natural teeth.
 d. never wearing a maxillary prosthesis after the natural teeth were lost.

 B. Before fabricating a new maxillary complete denture for this individual:
 a. no treatment is required to eliminate this redundant tissue.
 b. the flabby tissue should be surgically eliminated, and the existing prosthesis should be relined or a new denture remade to prevent recurrence.
 c. tissue-conditioning treatment should be given to improve the denture-bearing tissues.
 d. a multivitamin should be prescribed to improve the tissue consistency.

195. A. A thermoplastic material has been added to the borders of a custom impression tray. The material will allow the dentist to:
 a. correct areas of the tray that are grossly short of the desired denture borders.
 b. better retain the impression material in the custom tray.
 c. physiologically register the desired length and width of the denture flanges that will best complement each patient.
 d. overextend the tray flanges to ensure that all potential denture-bearing areas will be registered in the final impression.

 B. Border molding or muscle trimming:
 a. captures the denture border areas in an active functional state.
 b. involves the dentist's and/or patient's manipulating facial and oral structures to mold the thermoplastic materials to the desired shape.
 c. is done primarily to determine the correct posterior termination of maxillary dentures.
 d. if done well, will serve as a guide for posterior tooth position in the forthcoming prosthesis.
 e. a and b.
 f. b and c.

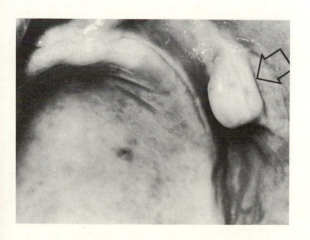

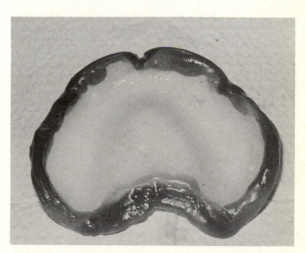

196. A. The line drawn along the posterior of this maxillary final impression is:
   a. the junction of the movable and immovable portions of the palate.
   b. the junction of the hard and soft palate.
   c. an aid to determine the occlusal plane.
   d. the posterior palatal seal and is essential in complete denture fabrication.
   e. all the above except c.

   B. Laterally, posterior to the maxillary tuberosities, this line will:
   a. be anterior to the hamular (pterygomaxillary) notches.
   b. be posterior to the hamular notches.
   c. continue through the hamular notches.
   d. continue through the fovea palatinae.

197. A. The line drawn on the final mandibular impression relates to which oral area?
   a. the oral vestibule.
   b. the oral pharynx.
   c. the alveolingual sulcus.
   d. the buccal shelf.

   B. The lingual border of this impression can be arbitrarily divided into anterior, middle, and posterior sections. During border molding, which muscle contributed most to forming the contour of the middle section?
   a. the genioglossus muscle.
   b. the mylohyoid muscle.
   c. the geniohyoid muscle.
   d. the palatoglossus muscle.

   C. The anterior lingual area of the impression and most mandibular complete dentures will include an obvious notch. What muscles associated with the mandible requires this notch?
   a. the genioglossus muscle.
   b. the mylohyoid muscle.
   c. the geniohyoid muscle.
   d. the palatoglossus muscle.

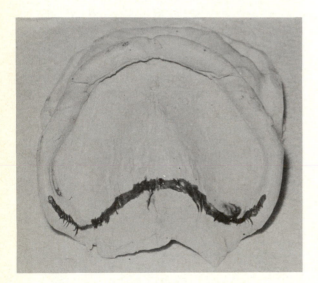

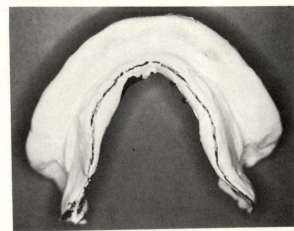

198. A. The firm-rolled tissues *(arrow 1)* registered on the anterior palatal area of this master cast are *most* likely:
   a. rugae.
   b. benign papillary hyperplasia.
   c. the result of a monilial infection.
   d. redundant tissues resulting from long-term use of an ill-fitting denture.

   B. These tissues require which mode of treatment before denture fabrication?
   a. oral nystatin rinses.
   b. surgical elimination.
   c. tissue conditioning.
   d. no treatment.

   C. The prominent bulbous areas *(arrow 2)* present bilaterally and distally on the edentulous alveolar ridge are called:
   a. retromolar pads.
   b. maxillary tuberosities.
   c. pterygomaxillary prominences.
   d. fovea palatinae.
   e. a and b.
   f. a, b, and c.

199. A. The line superimposed on the patient's face represents:
   a. the tragus-canthus line.
   b. the ala-canthus line.
   c. the Frankfort horizontal plane.
   d. the ala-tragus line.
   e. c and d.

   B. In complete denture prosthodontics this line serves to:
   a. help determine the condylar guidance.
   b. help establish the occlusal plane.
   c. help determine which type of posterior teeth are needed.
   d. develop acceptable anterior aesthetics.
   e. a and c.
   f. b and d.

   C. The patient's posture in this photograph is:
   a. sufficient to allow any procedure associated with complete denture prosthodontics to be performed.
   b. not ideal for maxillary impression procedures.
   c. too strained and upright for patient comfort.
   d. not correct for proper head support during denture-related procedures.

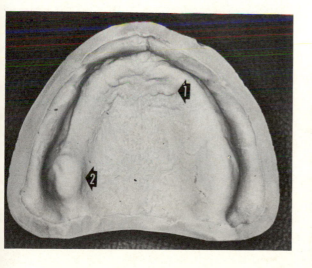

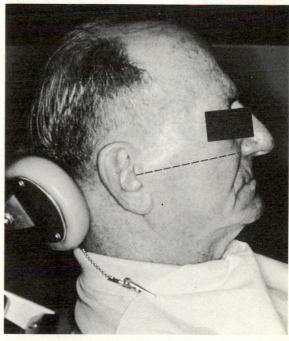

200. A. The circled anatomic landmark on this maxillary cast is:
   a. the fovea palatinae.
   b. the incisal papilla.
   c. the maxillary tuberosity.
   d. the result of trauma when the incisors were extracted.

   B. If a prosthesis presses too firmly on this area, a patient may experience:
   a. tingling or itching of the upper lip.
   b. difficulty when speaking.
   c. difficulty when swallowing.
   d. burning or tingling of the palate.
   e. a and d.

   C. This circled landmark serves as an aid for:
   a. placement of the maxillary anterior teeth.
   b. determining the best position for the incisal edges of the maxillary incisors.
   c. making a protrusive bite record.
   d. selecting the appropriate anterior teeth.
   e. a and d.

201. A. The articulator shown is typical of those used for many prosthodontic procedures. It is best described as:
   a. fully adjustable.
   b. average value.
   c. simple hinge.
   d. semiadjustable.

   B. To set the condylar guidance specifically for each patient would require:
   a. a face-bow transfer.
   b. an interocclusal jaw relation record.
   c. a protrusive bite registration.
   d. lateral bite registrations.
   e. c and d.

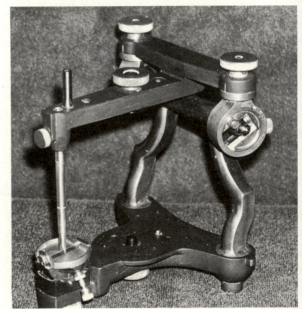

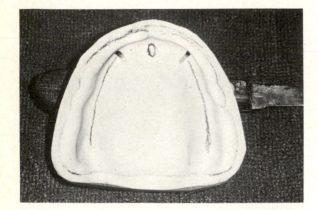

202. A. This knob *(arrow)* is used so that the articulator can be set to simulate which aspect of mandibular movement?
   a. simple hinge opening.
   b. protrusive excursions.
   c. lateral excursions.
   d. Bennett shift.
B. Failure to consider this mandibular movement will result in improper oral occlusal contacts when complete dentures are occluded:
   a. at the centric relation position.
   b. during working contact.
   c. during balancing contact.
   d. during protrusive contact.
   e. b and d.
   f. b and c.

203. A. This portion of the articulator functions to simulate:
   a. condylar guidance.
   b. Bennett movement.
   c. incisal guidance.
   d. protrusive guidance.
B. Adjusting this element of the articulator is done:
   a. before setting any prosthetic teeth.
   b. after setting the posterior teeth.
   c. after the denture is processed.
   d. during the setting of the posterior teeth to complement the many factors contributing to complete denture occlusion.

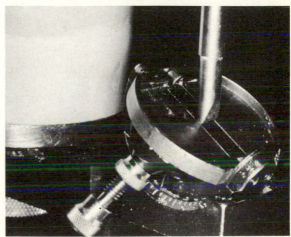

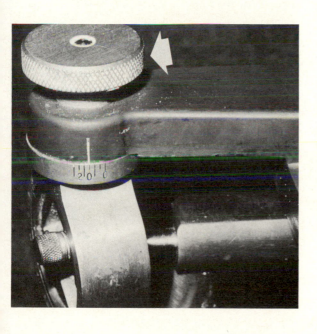

204. A. The major purpose for the instrument shown attached to the articulator is to:
   a. determine the intercondylar width.
   b. relate the maxilla to the opening/closing axis of the mandible.
   c. determine the occlusal vertical dimension.
   d. determine the axis of mandibular rotation.

B. This instrument can be best described as:
   a. an arbitrary face-bow.
   b. a kinesiologic face-bow.
   c. a physiologic face-bow.
   d. a pantograph.

205. A. By employing an infraorbital pointer:
   a. the patient's casts can be related horizontally on an articulator in the same manner as on the patient.
   b. the proper plane of occlusion is determined.
   c. facial height and vertical dimension of occlusion are readily determined.
   d. the casts will relate more symmetrically to the articulator.

B. Caution is required with the infraorbital pointer so that:
   a. the trial bases are not dislodged.
   b. the pointer does not injure the eye.
   c. freeway or interocclusal space is not eliminated.
   d. the condyles are confirmed to be at the centric relation position.

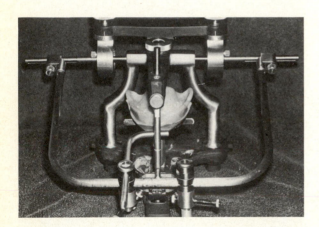

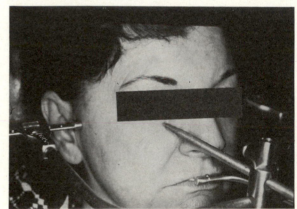

206. A. Which muscle of mastication inserts on this area of the mandible *(arrow 1)?*
   a. the lateral pterygoid muscle.
   b. the medial pterygoid muscle.
   c. the temporal muscle.
   d. the masseter muscle.

B. Which process of the mandible might interfere with the distobuccal flanges of maxillary complete dentures?
   a. the ramus.
   b. the condylar process.
   c. the coronoid process.
   d. the alveolar process.

C. Which nerve exits via this foramen *(arrow 2)* and may be traumatized by a mandibular removable prosthesis?
   a. the mandibular nerve.
   b. the mylohyoid nerve.
   c. the facial nerve.
   d. the mental nerve.

207. A. The pontic used to replace the lateral incisor is *most* obviously:
   a. a custom pontic.
   b. a sanitary pontic.
   c. a ridge lap pontic.
   d. a cantilever pontic.

B. The decision to use this design was *most* likely due to:
   a. the generous root support of the canine.
   b. a desire to avoid preparing the central incisor.
   c. a desire to make the bridge as simple as possible.
   d. the poor positional relationship of the canine and central incisor, thus complicating bridge fabrication.
   e. a and b.
   f. c and d.

C. The rest on the incisor was included to:
   a. allow for easy cleansing of the pontic.
   b. avoid an open embrasure.
   c. provide additional support for the pontic.
   d. allow a crown on the central to be post-soldered.

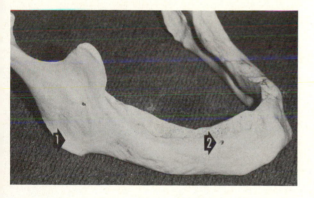

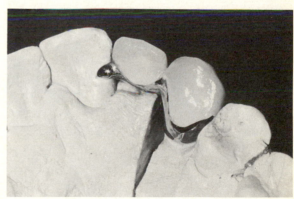

208. A. A three-unit porcelain-fused-to-metal bridge is to be fabricated and retained by the endodontically treated canine and central incisor. The darker areas on the prepared teeth are:
  a. the result of endodontic therapy.
  b. die spacer material painted on the preparations avoiding the marginal areas.
  c. copings to increase the crown length to enhance the retention and support of the bridge.
  d. a temporary procedure until the bridge is fabricated.

B. Copings are indicated in fixed prosthodontics:
  a. when little coronal structure remains after crown preparation.
  b. when abutment parallelism needs to be enhanced.
  c. often after endodontics.
  d. all the above.

209. A. This patient is to have a mandibular removable partial denture fabricated to replace all posterior teeth on the right side of the mandible. Tooth No. 19 is missing. Tooth No. 18 would be *best* treated by:
  a. a survey crown to retain the partial denture.
  b. doing a post buildup and survey crown to retain the partial.
  c. performing periodontal flap surgery and a survey crown to retain the partial.
  d. extraction.

B. Tooth No. 17 should be:
  a. retained to serve as an abutment.
  b. splinted to No. 18 so that both may serve as abutments.
  c. used as an abutment for a fixed bridge replacing teeth Nos. 19 and 18 that will also retain the partial denture via precision attachment.
  d. extracted.

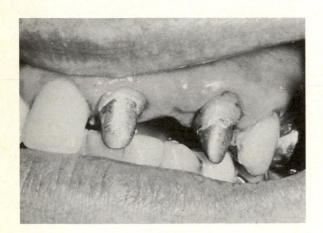

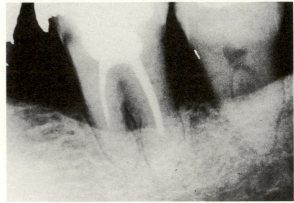

210. A. The pontic pictured is *best* termed:
   a. a cantilever pontic.
   b. a sanitary pontic.
   c. a custom pontic.
   d. a ridge lap pontic.
   B. This design was used to:
   a. promote gingival health.
   b. allow the patient to readily clean in the area of the bridge.
   c. prevent food from getting trapped under the bridge.
   d. reduce the cost of the metal needed for the bridge.
   e. all the above except d.
   f. b and c.

211. A. This blunt instrument is being used to palpate for an oral landmark involved in complete denture fabrication. This landmark is:
   a. the vibrating line.
   b. the semilunar notch.
   c. the hamular notch.
   d. the pterygomandibular notch.
   e. b and d.
   B. This landmark is important when determining:
   a. the size of the maxillary teeth.
   b. the posterior termination of maxillary dentures.
   c. the position of the posterior teeth.
   d. the need for a surgical tuberosity reduction.

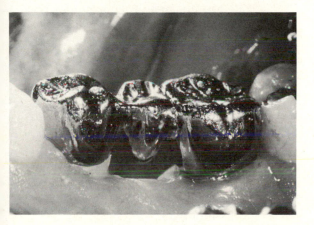

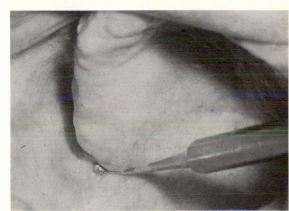

212. A. This 30-year-old woman has had a six-unit porcelain-fused-to-metal bridge replacing teeth Nos. 7 to 10 in place for at least 10 years. Recently she noticed that the bridge was loose and she sought dental care. On removal of the bridge, it was obvious that caries had involved the pulpal tissues of tooth No. 6. Radiographic examination showed the tooth to be well supported by alveolar bone and that the caries did not progress subgingivally. Treatment at this time should be:

a. extraction of No. 6, temporization of No. 11, and fabrication of a removable temporary partial replacing teeth Nos. 6 to 10.

b. pulpectomy of No. 6 and use of the current fixed prosthesis as a temporary until a removable partial replacing teeth Nos. 6 to 10 can be fabricated.

c. root canal therapy on No. 6 and use of the current bridge for a temporary.

d. pulpectomy of No. 16, fabrication of a post buildup that accommodates the current bridge, and recementing the bridge.

B. Definitive treatment for this patient might well include:

a. root canal therapy.

b. using the first premolars as abutment teeth along with the canines when a new fixed partial is fabricated.

c. a cast buildup procedure to enhance the success of a new fixed or removable partial denture.

d. a clasp or attachment retained removable partial denture to distribute functional forces to more teeth and oral tissues.

e. a and c.

f. b and d.

g. a, b, c, and d as all valid choices.

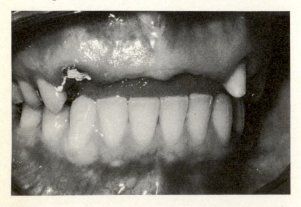

213. A. The most posteriorly located line on the master cast for a maxillary immediate complete denture represents:

a. the junction of the movable and immovable portions of the palate.

b. the pterygomaxillary raphae.

c. the vibrating line.

d. the pterygomandibular raphae.

e. a and c.

f. a and b.

B. A posterior palatal seal will be provided in this complete maxillary immediate denture. The case will be mechanically altered so that the denture may take advantage of the resilient tissues of the posterior portion of the palate and improve its retention. What types of tissue are located in the area of the posterior palatal seal that supplies this resilience?

a. loose connective tissue.

b. adipose tissue.

c. minor salivary glands.

d. periosteum.

e. all the above.

C. Why is a posterior palatal seal advantageous in complete maxillary dentures?

a. It provides a border seal along the posterior of the prosthesis.

b. It reestablishes tissue contact lost as a result of processing shrinkage of the denture base.

c. It prevents oral contents from getting under the denture.

d. It keeps the denture away from the dorsum of the tongue and prevents gagging.

e. a and b.

f. c and d.

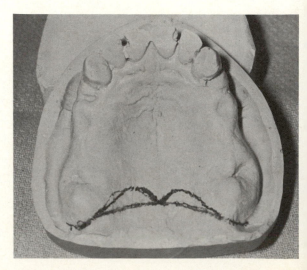

214. A. This recently processed denture has been reunited with its master cast so that a laboratory remount can be accomplished and the denture occlusion refined. This gap *(arrow)* was noticed along the posterior of the denture. The cause of this failure to seat ideally on the cast is:
   a. a foreign body (e.g., wax, plaster) under the denture.
   b. distortion of the denture base because of rapid cooling after processing.
   c. anticipated shrinkage of the base material.
   d. distortion of the denture base because of desiccation after processing.

B. The fact that the denture distorted during processing:
   a. will prevent this appliance from ever being used successfully.
   b. is one reason that posterior palatal seals are essential for complete maxillary dentures.
   c. will surely have affected the occlusion, and an occlusal correction via selective grinding will be required.
   d. will require that the denture be relined before it will ever fit ideally.
   e. a and d.
   f. b and c.

215. A. This waxup demonstrates:
   a. an extreme range of mandibular protrusion.
   b. an obvious retrognathic condition.
   c. a Class II jaw relationship.
   d. a prognathic mandible.
   e. b and c.
   f. a and d.

B. The opposite of this condition would be:
   a. an extreme range of mandibular retrusion.
   b. an obvious prognathic condition.
   c. a Class III jaw relationship.
   d. a retrognathic mandible.
   e. b and c.
   f. a and d.

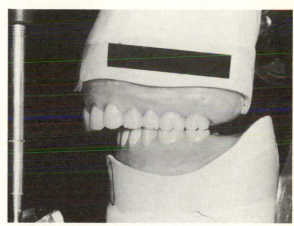

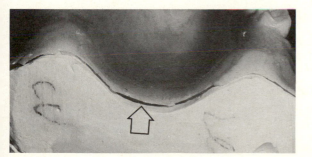

216. A. The rough, bumpy tissue on the palate is *most* likely:
   a. a yeast infection.
   b. smoker's stomatitis.
   c. epulis fissurata.
   d. benign papillary hyperplasia.
   B. Probable causes for the type of tissue reaction may be:
   a. poor oral hygiene.
   b. poorly fitting dentures.
   c. a suction-promoting area incorporated in the denture to enhance retention.
   d. prolonged or even continuous denture wearing for a long period.
   e. none of the above.
   f. all the above.
   C. Treatment might include:
   a. tissue conditioning.
   b. improved home hygiene habits.
   c. surgical removal.
   d. discontinuing or diminishing use of the denture.
   e. none of the above.
   f. all the above.

217. In this radiograph, the objects in the posterior area of the alveolar process of the mandible:
   a. are foreign objects, probably jewelry, superimposed on the radiograph.
   b. are commonly used to treat mandibular fractures.
   c. are dental implants to retain fixed partial dentures.
   d. may be used to retain fixed or removable partial dentures.
   e. c and d.

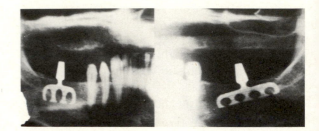

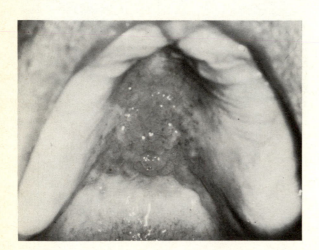

218. A. This 35-year-old patient has not undergone any restorative procedures for 7 years. From these radiographs it can be determined that:
   a. the margins of some of the restorations are irregular.
   b. periodontal health is satisfactory.
   c. the interproximal areas are constricted by the restorations.
   d. no pulpal pathology requiring endodontic therapy is indicated in any of the teeth.

   B. These dental restorations:
   a. in general have excellent marginal adaptation.
   b. allow for interproximal hygienic management.
   c. are contoured to promote gingival health.
   d. are obviously too large and will promote orofacial discomfort.
   e. all the above.
   f. a, b, and c.

219. A. These porcelain-fused-to-metal crowns have supported a removable partial denture for almost 5 years. This follow-up photograph shows that:
   a. a great deal of gingival recession has occurred since the crowns were placed.
   b. the margins have discolored on the crowns.
   c. the gingival tissues are quite healthy.
   d. the porcelain has stained.

   B. To promote gingival health and to enhance the prognosis of these three periodontally involved teeth:
   a. the crown margins were placed well away from the gingival tissues.
   b. the gingival embrasures were contoured to allow easy access for cleaning.
   c. the crowns have been made as one unit to splint the teeth.
   d. stress-breaking components may be considered for the design of the partial denture.
   e. a and b.
   f. all the above.

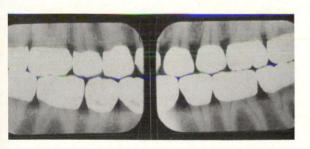

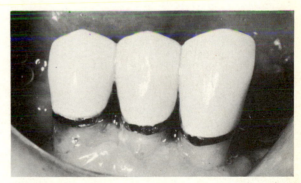

220. A. These processed dentures have just been recovered from their flasks and reunited with the articulator on which they were fabricated. The dentures:
   a. have severely warped and should be discarded.
   b. have the same occlusion they had before processing and can be given to the patient.
   c. must be occlusally refined to adjust for the fact that the bases distorted slightly during processing.
   d. should never be remounted until they have been placed in the mouth.

B. Occlusal correction and equilibration is indicated to:
   a. reestablish bilaterally balanced occlusion.
   b. eliminate any base-to-base or tooth-to-base contact that developed during processing.
   c. reestablish contact of all posterior teeth at the patient's centric relation position.
   d. eliminate premature tooth contacts that will prevent effective denture function or comfort.
   e. all the above.
   f. a and c.
   g. b and d.

221. A. The arrow points to a painful, whitish spot near the labial frenum. The *most* likely cause of the whitish area is:
   a. the natural appearance of the frenum.
   b. a denture irritation.
   c. a fungal infection.
   d. scarring from past surgical treatment.
B. Treatment of the whitish area should be:
   a. none.
   b. tissue conditioning.
   c. antifungal oral rinses.
   d. adjusting the denture.

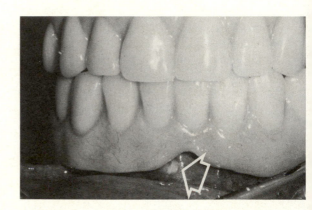

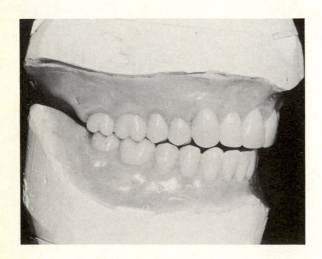

222. A. The lingual portion of this impression registered which area of the oral cavity?
 a. the vestibule.
 b. the oral pharynx.
 c. the alveolingual sulcus.
 d. the lingual shelf.
 B. A facial area that provides primary support for mandibular complete dentures is:
 a. the buccal shelf.
 b. the oral vestibule.
 c. the masseteric prominence.
 d. the mental protuberance.

223. A. This device is used mainly:
 a. for lateral jaw records.
 b. to determine the centric relation position.
 c. to relate the maxilla to the opening/closing axis of the mandible.
 d. to determine the rest vertical dimension.
 B. When using this device it is important that:
 a. it is centered on both trial bases so that it is stable when the record is made.
 b. it is adjusted to contact at the correct vertical dimension of occlusion.
 c. the patient be made aware of its experimental status.
 d. it be used in conjunction with a fully adjustable articulator.
 e. a and b.
 f. a and c.
 g. a and d.

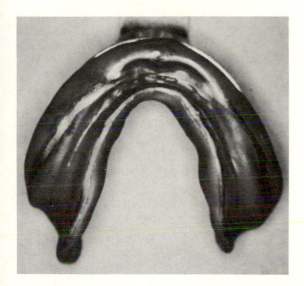

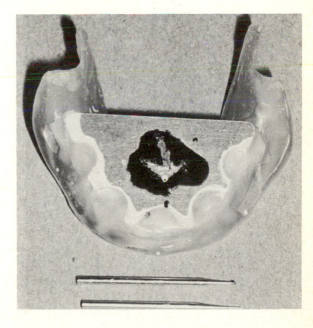

224. A. The record shown here is *most* likely:
   a. a centric occlusion record.
   b. a lateral check bite.
   c. a protrusive record.
   d. a centric relation record.
B. For this record to be reliable it *must* be made:
   a. on stable bases.
   b. with uniformly thick and consistently soft wax.
   c. at the correct vertical dimension of occlusion.
   d. on three separate bases and verified.
   e. a and b.
   f. a and c.
   g. all the above except d.
C. This record will be used to:
   a. set both condylar and incisal guidance.
   b. program Bennett movement on the articulator.
   c. relate the mandible to the maxilla on an acceptable articulator.
   d. relate the maxilla to the opening/closing axis of the mandible.

225. A. These processed dentures have been reunited on the articulator on which they were fabricated. It is now obvious that the anterior teeth do not overlap vertically and the premolars do not have any contact in centric relation. What can be done to correct this situation?
   a. Check for and eliminate any base-to-base or tooth-to-base contact.
   b. Equilibrate the new prostheses and reestablish the desired occlusion.
   c. Replace the anterior teeth so that a correct aesthetic condition exists.
   d. Reline the dentures to correct the situation.
   e. All the above.
   f. a and b.
   g. c and d.
B. When equilibrating dentures:
   a. fossae and embrasures are deepened so that cusps are maintained.
   b. maxillary buccal cusps are recontoured more often than mandibular buccal cusps.
   c. stamp cusps are recontoured only when they display gross premature contact at three or more occlusal positions.
   d. the procedure should continue until all teeth contact at centric relation except for the anterior teeth.
   e. all the above.

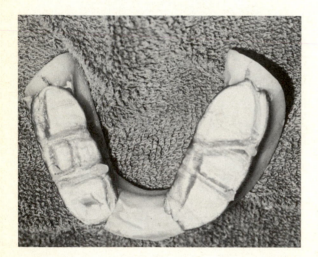

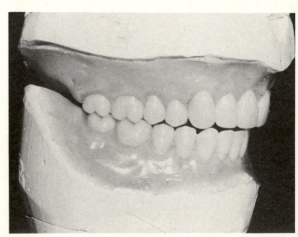

226. A. While this denture was being equilibrated, poor protrusive contact was observed. Improved contact will be correctly achieved by:
   a. grinding the mandibular buccal cusps.
   b. deepening the fossae on the maxillary teeth.
   c. reducing the maxillary buccal cusps.
   d. reducing the maxillary lingual cusps.
   e. a and b.
   f. c and d.

B. If no posterior protrusive contact was observed on this side, you would proceed by:
   a. rechecking the articulator settings.
   b. evaluating the other side.
   c. rechecking this side as the equilibration progressed.
   d. assuming that this contact will not be achieved.
   e. all the above except d.
   f. b and c.

227. A. While the complete dentures are equilibrated as shown in this figure, what statement(s) is/are correct regarding this situation?
   a. A balancing-side discrepancy exists.
   b. The triangular ridge of the distobuccal cusp of the mandibular second molar can be recontoured.
   c. The triangular ridge of the mesiolingual cusp of the maxillary second molar can be recontoured.
   d. Balancing contacts on the contralateral side might contribute to this discrepancy.
   e. All the above except d.
   f. b and c.

B. Contralaterally you would be:
   a. improving protrusive contacts at this time.
   b. improving working contacts at this time.
   c. improving balancing contacts at this time.
   d. refining centric occlusion.

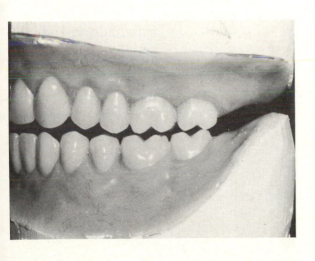

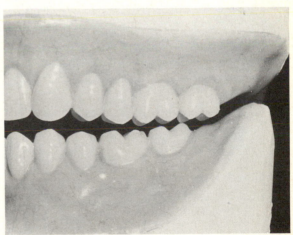

228. A. Which picture shows a correctly equilibrated working contact?
B. Which picture shows a correctly equilibrated balancing contact?
C. Which picture shows a correctly equilibrated protrusive contact?
D. Ideally, complete dentures will display which occlusal scheme?
   a. canine-protected occlusion.
   b. bilaterally balanced occlusion.
   c. group function.
   d. any of the above.

229. A. The working contact shown in this set of complete dentures can be improved by:
   a. recontouring the maxillary buccal cusps.
   b. deepening and widening the buccal grooves and embrasures of the mandibular teeth.
   c. recontouring the mandibular buccal cusps.
   d. deepening and widening the buccal grooves and embrasures of the maxillary teeth.
   e. all the above except c.
   f. a and b.
   g. c and d.
B. When making an interocclusal jaw relation record to clinically remount a set of complete dentures:
   a. a thin layer of softened recording material is indicated.
   b. the denture bases should have maximal contact with the denture-bearing areas.
   c. the patient is asked to bite heavily into the recording material to acquire a good registration.
   d. actual tooth contact should be avoided.
   e. all the above except c.
   f. a and b.
   g. a and d.

A

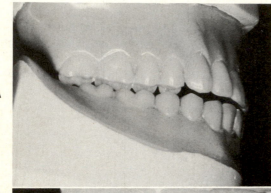

B

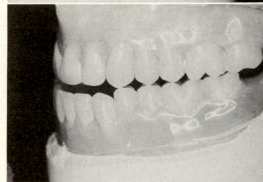

C

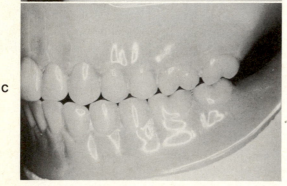

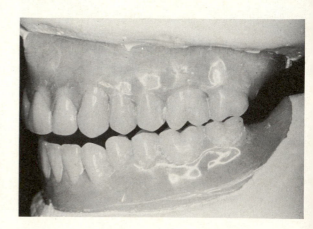

230. A. This patient has received the maximal dose of therapeutic radiation to the head and neck to treat oral cancer. The teeth show the result of:
   a. encroachment of the tumor.
   b. reduced salivary output due to the cancer therapy.
   c. the effect of radiation on tooth structure.
   d. diminished blood and lymphatic flow to the mandible.

B. Proper treatment of this patient at this time would be:
   a. surgical removal of the teeth.
   b. long-term antibiotic coverage after extractions to prevent postoperative infection.
   c. frequent recall examinations.
   d. root canal therapy followed by full crowns.
   e. all the above except d.

231. A. This prominent, firm area on the palate is *most* likely:
   a. torus palatinus.
   b. the result of poorly fitting dentures.
   c. not uncommon.
   d. a slowly progressive malignancy.
   e. a and c.

B. Upon discovery, recommended treatment would be:
   a. surgical removal prior to any dental treatment.
   b. surgical removal so that a more satisfactory denture can be made.
   c. tissue conditioning.
   d. fabricating the denture with minor alterations to accommodate the situation.

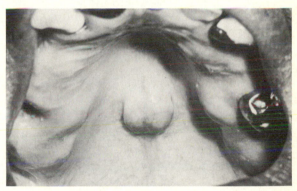

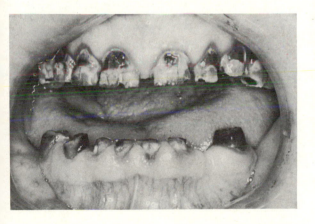

232. This extensive maxillary bridge has a portion of its occlusal surface fabricated in metal. This design is used to:
   a. reduce the possibility of the porcelain's fracturing.
   b. reduce the possibility of the porcelain abrading the opposing teeth.
   c. enhance the aesthetics of the restoration.
   d. control the cost of fabrication.
   e. all the above.
   f. a and b.
   g. c and d.

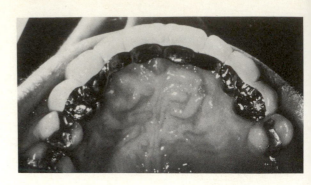

233. A. The holes shown in these prosthetic teeth **(A)** serve to:
      a. prevent fracture of the teeth.
      b. mechanically retain the teeth in a denture base.
      c. improve aesthetics by allowing base material to flow into the teeth.
      d. permit greater masticatory efficiency.
   B. These teeth **(B)** are made of:
      a. porcelain.
      b. acrylic.
      c. extensively crosslinked polymers.
      d. ivorine.

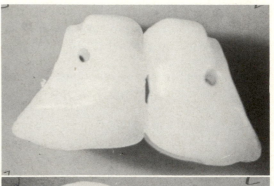

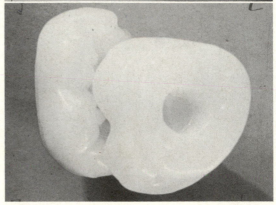

234. A. What is the Kennedy classification of this partially edentulous arch?
      a. Class I.
      b. Class II.
      c. Class II, modification I.
      d. Class III.
   B. What type of major connector is being used in this removable partial denture?
      a. palatal plate.
      b. palatal bar.
      c. palatal strap.
      d. horseshoe.

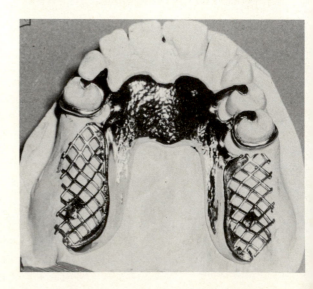

235. A. What is the Kennedy classification of this partially edentulous arch?
   a. Class I.
   b. Class II.
   c. Class III.
   d. Class III, modification I.
B. What type of major connector is being used in this removable partial denture?
   a. lingual strap.
   b. palatal plate.
   c. palatal bar.
   d. palatal strap.

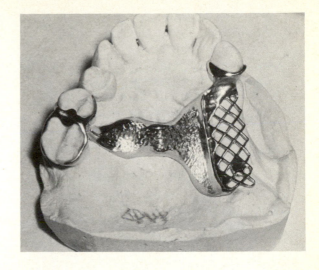

236. A. What is the Kennedy classification of this partially edentulous arch?
   a. Class I.
   b. Class II.
   c. Class III.
   d. Class IV.
B. What type of major connector is being used in this removable partial denture?
   a. horseshoe.
   b. lingual bar.
   c. lingual plate.
   d. lingual beam.
C. This major connector ideally should be how far from the dental-gingival border?
   a. 2 mm.
   b. 4 mm.
   c. 6 mm.
   d. 8 mm.

237. A. This major connector is:
   a. a lingual bar.
   b. a double lingual bar.
   c. a lingual plate.
   d. a Kennedy bar.
B. The portion of the metal posterior to the abutment teeth has many perforations in order to:
   a. enhance its flexibility.
   b. reduce the framework's weight.
   c. retain acrylic bases on the framework.
   d. permit recording bases to be added.

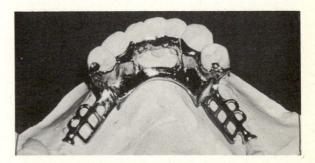

238. A. The type of clasp used on the molar could be called:
   a. a suprabulge clasp.
   b. a circumferential clasp.
   c. an infrabulge clasp.
   d. a bar clasp.
   e. a and b.
   f. c and d.

   B. The terminal portion of the clasp arm functions to:
   a. supply support for the partial.
   b. supply stability for the partial.
   c. supply retention for the partial.
   d. supply reciprocation for the retentive arm.

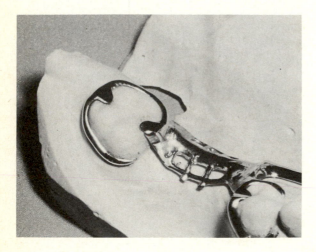

239. A. Surveying is an aid to designing partial dentures because it:
   a. locates potential retention areas.
   b. determines the best type of connector to use.
   c. determines whether indirect retention is needed.
   d. quickly determines the crown-to-root ratio.

   B. The carbon line scribed on the potential abutment teeth during surveying represents:
   a. the guide planes.
   b. areas of potential retention.
   c. the maximal circumference of the tooth.
   d. the height of contour of the tooth.
   e. a and b.
   f. c and d.

   C. The analyzing rod is being used here to:
   a. determine the path of insertion of the partial.
   b. evaluate the parallelism of the abutments.
   c. search for retention areas on the proximal surfaces of the teeth.
   d. locate a source for indirect retention.
   e. a and b.
   f. c and d.

   D. These proximal areas of the teeth will serve as:
   a. retentive areas.
   b. occlusal rests.
   c. guide planes.
   d. indirect retention.

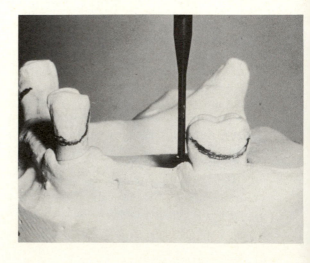

240. A. The mesio-occlusal rest on the first premolar serves to supply:

    a. stability to the appliance.

    b. indirect retention.

    c. a spare rest in case the rest on the second premolar fractures.

    d. extra strength for the major connector.

  B. Indirect retention acts:

    a. to minimize the risk of distal extension bases lifting away from the edentulous ridges.

    b. in lieu of a posterior direct retainer.

    c. to minimize torque on the primary abutment teeth.

    d. as a safety catch.

    e. all the above except d.

    f. a and c.

    g. b and c.

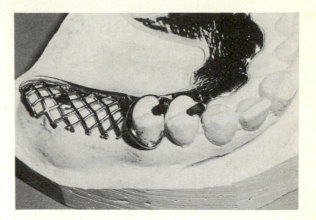

■ SECTION G

Pedodontics and orthodontics

241. What is the best way to manage the asymptomatic tooth with the short roots in this 16-year-old boy?

    a. Extract it immediately and replace with a three-unit bridge.

    b. Perform routine endodontic therapy.

    c. Follow it periodically until after the patient becomes 18 years old, and then when necessary extract it and place a bridge.

    d. Extract it immediately and place a space maintainer.

    e. Do nothing; the second premolar will very likely develop soon.

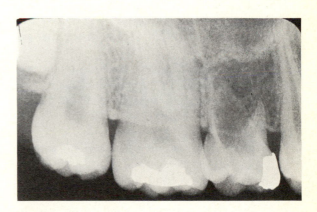

242. What is the indicated treatment for this quadrant if the remainder of the examination proves to be noncontributory?
  a. Do nothing; just keep it under periodic surveillance.
  b. Extract the carious deciduous molar only.
  c. Use the deciduous molar to support a fixed space maintainer.
  d. Use extensive fluoride therapy.
  e. Extract the deciduous molar and place a space maintainer.

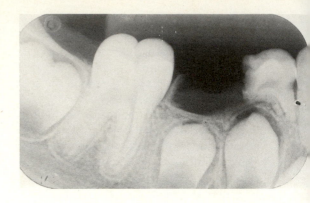

243. The mother of this patient is concerned about the space between her child's teeth. The remainder of the oral examination is unremarkable. The correct approach is to:
  a. refer the child immediately to an orthodontist for treatment.
  b. try to bring the centrals together with rubber bands.
  c. do an arch space–tooth width study.
  d. use an inclined bite plane fixed to the lower arch.
  e. advise the mother that the situation is normal and that the spaces will soon be reduced as normal development takes place.

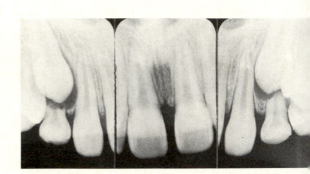

244. What is the correct treatment for this patient?
  a. Perform a complete pulpotomy on the second deciduous molar tooth.
  b. Do a complete root canal filling on the second deciduous molar tooth and observe.
  c. Extract the second deciduous molar tooth and observe.
  d. Extract the second deciduous molar tooth, place a space maintainer, and observe.
  e. Extract the second deciduous molar tooth, enucleate the area distal to the second premolar crown, submit tissue for microscopic study, and plan for a space maintainer.

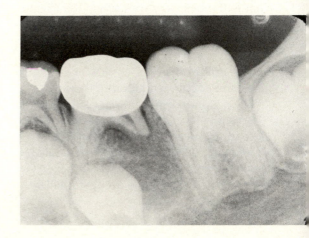

245. You should advise the mother of this child (**A** and **B**) that:

a. nothing need be done until the child reaches 12 years of age.

b. if the deciduous left central incisor is extracted, the permanent central incisors will likely erupt normally.

c. thyroid tests should be performed.

d. the thumb habit should be discontinued immediately.

e. you will refer them immediately to an orthodontist and oral surgeon for immediate steps to begin correction of the problem.

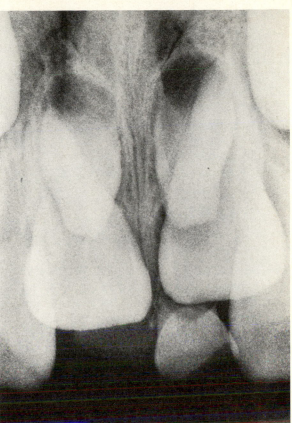

B

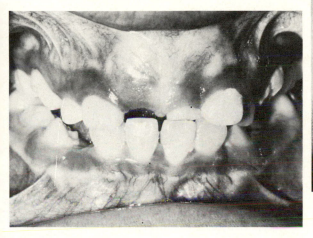

246. What is the proper management of the derangement in the dentition of this 9-year-old girl?

a. Advise the mother that no treatment is required at present.

b. The left mandibular incisor should be carefully scaled.

c. The child at age 12 should be referred to an orthodontist for treatment.

d. Immediate steps should be initiated to correct the problem.

e. The case should be evaluated again in 6 months to see if differential growth has rendered the problem less severe.

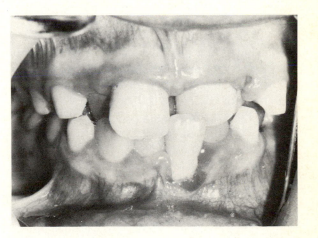

247. What is the *most* correct treatment for this 8-year-old boy, who has never seen a physician? The dental problem is seen only in the anterior regions of the arches.
   a. Work with a physician to eliminate the mouth-breathing habit.
   b. Request that the physician change the medication if possible.
   c. Prescribe antibiotics and carry out debridement procedures.
   d. Reinforce home-care instruction.
   e. a and d.

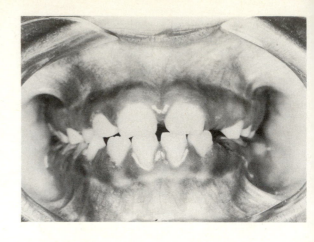

248. What is the correct treatment for this asymptomatic vital second deciduous molar tooth?
   a. Extract the tooth if it becomes painful.
   b. Place an MO restoration and perform a pulp-capping procedure if necessary.
   c. Plan a pulpotomy.
   d. Plan a pulpectomy.

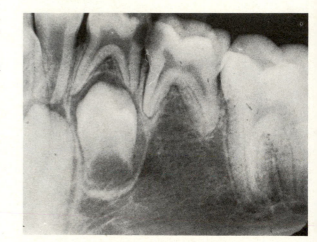

249. What is the *best* plan of treatment for this deciduous second molar tooth, which has been aching some recently? The boy says it has not been sore to bite on.
   a. Place an MO restoration only.
   b. Perform a pulpotomy procedure and place a stainless steel crown.
   c. Extract the tooth and place a fixed type of space maintainer.
   d. Extract the tooth and place a removable type of space maintainer.
   e. Do a root canal filling and place a stainless steel crown.

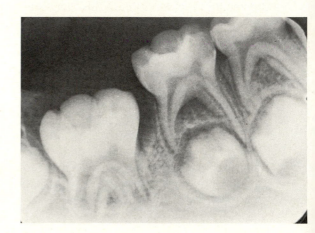

250. A physician's wife brings her 13-year-old daughter to you with this problem. The *best* advice you could give the mother is:

a. that no treatment is necessary.

b. to reevaluate the problem in 3 years to see if adequate growth has occurred to permit proper eruption of the second premolar tooth.

c. that one of the premolar teeth should be extracted.

d. that the third molar tooth on that side should be extracted.

e. to consult an orthodontist immediately.

251. The eruption of the second premolar tooth on this side of the arch (**A** and **B**) is found to be delayed compared with its counterpart on the other side of the arch. Correct management would be to:

a. keep the situation under surveillance for 6 months.

b. look for a history of this in the family.

c. perform available arch-length studies.

d. extract the crown of the deciduous molar now.

e. test the vitality of the second premolar to determine whether its pulp has died and thus root development may have been arrested.

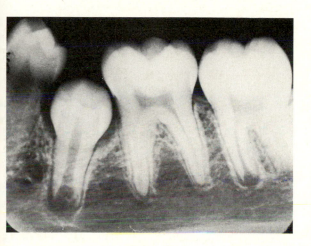

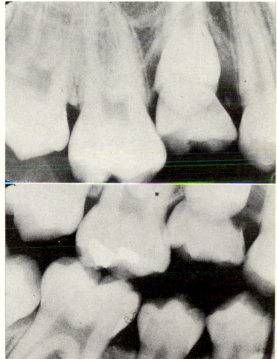

A

B

252. You should advise the mother of this 8-year-old child that:
   a. this is a normal situation.
   b. this is a common finding at this age and will be alleviated with growth of the arch.
   c. this is a common finding at this age and will be alleviated when the permanent canine teeth erupt.
   d. this condition is caused by the developing wisdom teeth.
   e. she should seek an orthodontic consultation soon.

253. This 22-year-old patient's upper left canine is impacted. The *most* desirable treatment, if the patient is willing, is to:
   a. place a large crown on the left central incisor, thus eliminating the diastema.
   b. move the left lateral and central incisor into correct position othodontically, and either bring the canine into correct position or build a bridge.
   c. extract the left canine and the lateral and central incisor, and place a fixed bridge.
   d. extract the left canine and the lateral and central incisor teeth, and place a removable partial denture.
   e. do nothing.

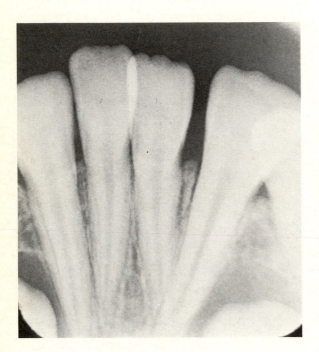

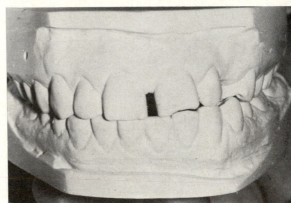

254. How would you advise this patient, who would like the diastema closed?
 a. Nothing can be done for the problem.
 b. When the maxillary canines erupt, this will close the diastema considerably.
 c. The eruption of the maxillary third molars will close the diastema considerably.
 d. The teeth can be brought together permanently by use of rubber bands around the two central incisors.
 e. Extensive orthodontic treatment will be required to close the space successfully, although acid etch bonding techniques could diminish the space considerably.

255. How should the eruption of the permanent central incisor *best* be facilitated in this 10-year-old boy?
 a. Give it another 6 months to erupt by itself.
 b. Send him for thyroid tests.
 c. Extract the deciduous central incisor.
 d. Leave it alone until the boy is 12 years of age and then refer him to an orthodontist.
 e. Immediately extract the deciduous incisor, remove the odontoma, and be prepared to bring the permanent incisor into the mouth by orthodontic means.

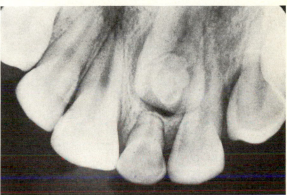

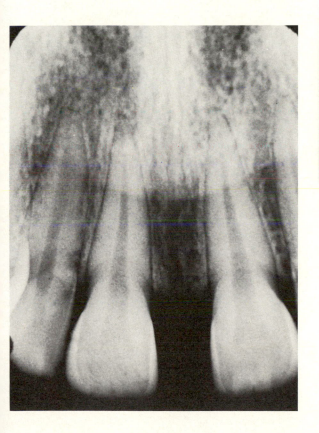

256. This asymptomatic, curious 35-year-old woman comes to your office to seek advice about the correct management of the extra-lateral incisor tooth on the right side. She says she can budget $500 over the next 3 years for her teeth. Her centric, working, lateral, and protrusive relationships are satisfactory. What advice would you give this patient?

a. Extract the more distal "lateral" incisor and move the other four incisors to the right, distributing space between each tooth to minimize the gaps.

b. Do nothing; the present situation provides suitable aesthetics, and the patient should be counseled to accept this.

c. Extract the two "lateral" incisors on the right side and replace with a five-unit bridge, shaping the crowns in such a way that the lateral incisor pontic will be of acceptable size.

d. Extract the extra tooth and have full banding orthodontics begun right away.

e. Extract the two right "lateral" incisors and construct a partial denture, using a tooth large enough to fill the gap.

257. What is the best treatment for this sensitive second deciduous molar tooth?

a. No treatment.

b. Perform a pulpotomy and place an MO restoration.

c. Perform conventional root canal therapy and place a stainless steel crown.

d. Extract the tooth only.

e. Extract the tooth and possibly the first deciduous molar, and place a space maintainer.

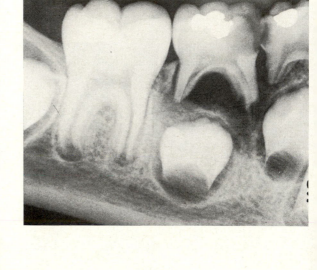

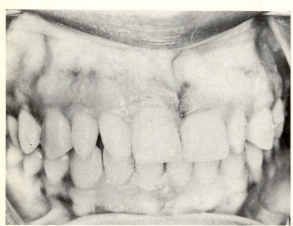

258. If the remainder of the examination yields noncontributory data, how should this problem be managed?

    a. Keep the patient under surveillance and refer to an orthodontist when the patient is at age 12.

    b. Keep the patient under surveillance and refer to an orthodontist when the patient is at age 10.

    c. Treatment is unnecessary.

    d. Extract the mesiodens immediately and follow carefully.

    e. Extract the mesiodens immediately and eliminate the diastema surgically.

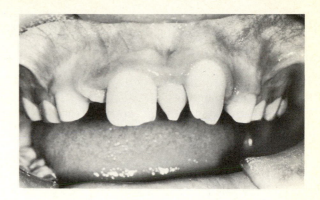

259. During the routine oral examination of a 10-year-old boy you observe this uneven resorption of the second deciduous molar tooth. The most correct approach is to:

    a. extract the deciduous tooth immediately.

    b. observe the situation in 6 months' time with new radiographs.

    c. order thyroid tests.

    d. extract the deciduous molar and orthodontically move the second premolar tooth now.

    e. extract the supernumerary tooth now.

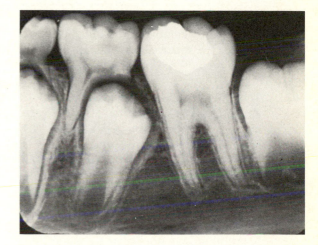

Dr. Roger Noonan authored questions 260 through 269.

260. The correct approach to the asymptomatic second deciduous molar in this 8-year-old girl is to:

    a. extract the tooth.

    b. open into the pulp to drain the periapical abscess.

    c. do nothing as the tooth will exfoliate within 3 to 4 months.

    d. remove caries, perform a pulpotomy if an exposure occurs, and place a stainless steel crown on the tooth.

    e. remove caries, do a pulp cap if an exposure occurs, and place an oversized amalgam restoration.

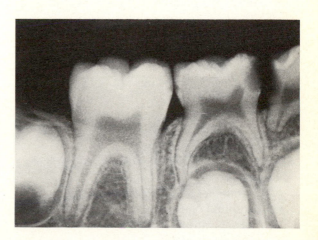

261. On routine initial visit examination of this 13-year-old boy, this radiograph was taken of the lower canine area. The patient has Class I occlusion with slight tipping of the mandibular right second premolar. He is without symptoms.

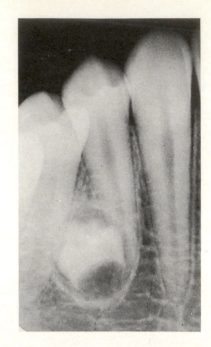

A. The diagnosis of this condition is:
   a. supernumerary tooth.
   b. dens in dente.
   c. compound odontoma.
   d. impacted first premolar.
   e. condensing osteitis.

B. The *best* treatment plan is to:
   a. do nothing; evaluate yearly.
   b. extract the canine so that the impacted tooth can erupt.
   c. extract the second premolar so that the impacted tooth can erupt.
   d. surgically remove the tooth.
   e. open the space orthodontically to allow the impacted tooth to erupt.

262. A. This 18-month-old child presents for examination. The mother had noticed "large bluish swellings on the gum tissues." The child is drooling more than usual and is somewhat fretful, but is having no trouble eating. The swellings are fluctuant and are nontender upon palpation. The most likely diagnosis is:

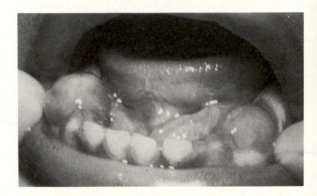

   a. giant cell granuloma.
   b. eruption hematoma.
   c. odontogenic cyst.
   d. bilateral ranuli.
   e. Bohn's nodules.

B. The best treatment plan is:
   a. none at this time.
   b. excisional biopsy.
   c. marsupialization.
   d. incision and drainage with placement of drains.
   e. antibiotic prophylaxis followed by surgical removal.

263. The condition noted in this photograph is an example of:

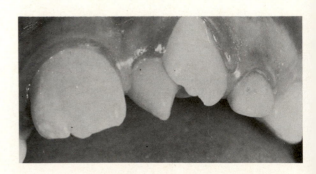

   a. a retained primary central causing ectopic eruption of the permanent central incisor.
   b. transposition of a lateral incisor and a central incisor.
   c. a talon cusp on the central incisor.
   d. a dilacerated central incisor.
   e. an erupted mesiodens causing displacement of the central incisors.

264. A. Examination of this asymptomatic 5-year-old boy shows poor oral hygiene with marginal gingivitis and a dark green stain in the gingival third of the upper anterior teeth. The stain is removable by scaling and pumicing. The diagnosis and cause of this stain is:
- a. tetracycline staining from administration of tetracycline as an infant.
- b. fluorosis from ingestion of excessive fluoride as an infant.
- c. green stain caused by chromogenic bacteria.
- d. early trauma with bleeding into the pulp chamber.
- e. lead lines from early ingestion of lead from paint.

B. Complete removal of this stain will disclose:
- a. smooth, normal enamel.
- b. decalcified enamel.
- c. darkened enamel.
- d. sclerotic dentin.

C. Examination of this same patient reveals that, as he occludes from the open position, the midline is aligned and the maxillary and mandibular cuspids are edge to edge. The patient then functionally shifts into the occlusion shown in the photograph as he closes completely. The proper diagnosis of this type of malocclusion is:
- a. unilateral crossbite.
- b. bilateral crossbite.
- c. normal occlusion.
- d. posterior open bite.

265. This 11-year-old boy presents to the office with intermittent and spontaneous pain in the mandibular left posterior quadrant. The right mandibular posterior segment is similar in development to the left side pictured in the radiograph. The *best* treatment plan is to:
- a. extract Nos. 19 and K and place a fixed space maintainer.
- b. restore No. K with a DO amalgam, extract No. 19, and let No. 18 drift mesially.
- c. extract No. K, perform root canal therapy on No. 19, and restore with a full gold crown.
- d. extract No. K, perform a pulpotomy on No. 19, and restore the tooth with amalgam.
- e. extract No. K, perform root canal therapy on No. 19, and restore it with a stainless steel crown.
- f. perform root canal therapy on No. 19, restore with stainless steel crown, and continue to observe an eruptive pattern on No. 20.

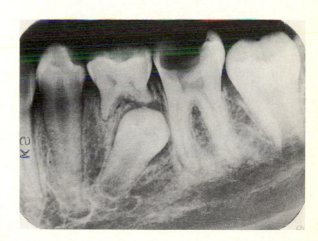

266. Examination of this asymptomatic, black 5-year-old boy shows a clean mouth, free of caries **(A)**. A radiograph was obtained of the upper right cuspid area **(B)**. Surgical removal of the radiopaque multiple mass over the primary cuspid was performed. Two fragments containing elements of enamel, dentin, and cementum were removed. The correct diagnosis is:

a. a supernumerary tooth.
b. condensing osteitis.
c. odontoma.
d. torus palatinus.

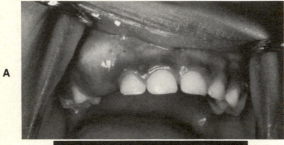

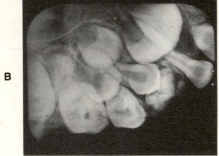

267. A. This 18-year-old youth is seen on routine examination. He has no complaint other than the stippled or pitted appearance of the enamel, which is present on all the teeth. He is caries free and has an angle Class I molar relationship. There is some plaque and stain in the cervical area, causing marginal gingivitis. The radiographs indicate thin enamel, normal pulp chambers, and a full complement of teeth. The correct diagnosis is:

a. acid decalcification of the teeth and anterior crossbite.
b. dentinogenesis imperfecta and Class III malocclusion.
c. ectodermal dysplasia and anterior crossbite.
d. amelogenesis imperfecta and anterior crossbite.
e. amelogenesis imperfecta and Class III malocclusion.

B. The *best* immediate treatment plan for this patient is:

a. prophylaxis and full coverage of all the teeth.
b. diet analysis, prophylaxis, and full coverage of the posterior teeth.
c. prophylaxis, genetic evaluation, and correction of the crossbite.
d. prophylaxis, placement of anterior veneers, and a night splint.

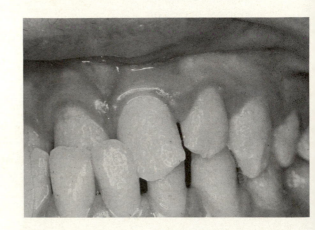

268. A. You examine this caries-free, 4-year-old girl, who is paying her first visit to the dentist. She has normal occlusion except for the diastemas between the maxillary incisors. The mother reports that the father has spaces here also and that one of his front teeth is very small. On a radiograph of the maxillary anterior you would expect normal development except for:

    a. impacted primary lateral incisors.

    b. supernumerary teeth blocking the eruption of the primary and permanent lateral incisors.

    c. congenitally missing primary and permanent lateral incisors.

    d. bilateral dens in dente.

    e. congenitally missing primary lateral incisors but normal permanent lateral incisors.

  B. An anterior film of a 3½-year-old child with a similar clinical presentation reveals that there are no primary lateral incisors and no development of the permanent lateral incisors. What is the *best* treatment plan?

    a. No treatment at this time; inform the parents of the missing teeth and the future need for tooth guidance and prosthetics.

    b. No treatment at this time; counsel the mother that the spaces will close with their eruption.

    c. Close the diastemas and wait for the development of the permanent lateral incisors.

    d. Orthodontically open the spaces in the region of the lateral incisors and wait for development and eruption of the permanent lateral incisors.

    e. Extract the central incisors and canines and place a temporary partial denture (flipper) for aesthetics.

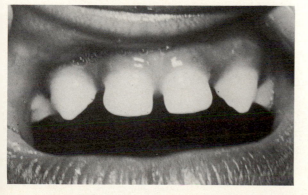

269. A. This radiograph of a 10½-year-old child reveals this asymptomatic condition. The *most* likely diagnosis is:

    a. radicular cyst.

    b. nasal chamber.

    c. globulomaxillary cyst.

    d. hyperplastic follicle of erupting canine.

    e. dentigerous cyst.

  B. The treatment of choice at this time is:

    a. extraction of the permanent lateral incisor to facilitate eruption.

    b. extraction of the primary canine followed by evaluation of surgical exposure and biopsy.

    c. continue to observe eruptive pattern.

    d. extraction of the primary canine and closure of the diastema to allow eruption of the permanent canine.

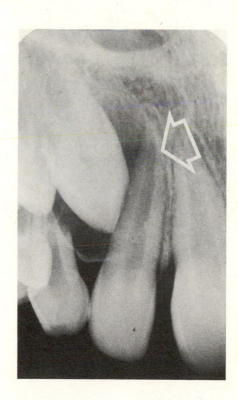

Dr. William McElroy authored questions 270 through 281.

270. This 5½-year-old girl presents for an emergency examination with "a double row of teeth." The right mandibular primary central incisor is mobile upon palpation. The *best* treatment plan for this patient is to:

a. extract the supernumerary tooth that is erupting lingual to the primary central incisor.

b. extract the mobile primary central incisor and place an active lingual arch to guide the permanent incisor into the arch.

c. advise the patient to wiggle the tooth out on her own and allow for the influence of the tongue to guide the tooth into the arch.

d. extract the primary canines and allow for the distal drifting of the primary lateral incisor in order to allow the erupting tooth to attain proper alignment.

271. This 12-year-old girl presents with a fractured incisor received in a bike accident. The account of the accident and the clinical presentation of the injury match appropriately, and you have therefore ruled out child abuse. The tooth upon examination exhibits a substantial pulp exposure. The correct treatment at this time is:

a. pulpotomy and temporization with zinc oxide eugenol.

b. placement of calcium hydroxide over the extraction site followed by a protective resin bandage over the exposed dentin.

c. pulpectomy and placement of a calcium hydroxide paste into the canal to stimulate closure of the immature root.

d. apicoectomy and reverse fill of the canal.

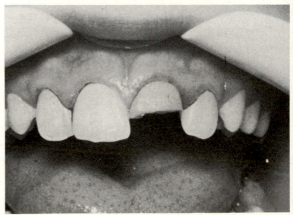

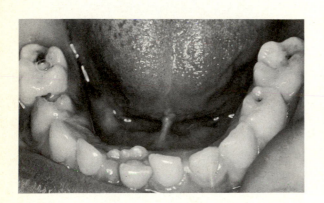

272. This radiograph was taken as a 3-month follow-up after trauma to the maxillary right primary incisor. The treatment of choice at this time is:

a. apexification.
b. root canal therapy.
c. extraction.
d. reverse-fill surgical approach.
e. no treatment.

273. Oral examination revealed the failure of tooth No. 3 to reach occlusion. Examination of these bite-wing radiographs shows that the *most* likely reason is:

a. chronic alveolar abscess of the second primary molar.
b. ectopic eruption of tooth No. 3.
c. supereruption of tooth No. 30.
d. distalization of the second primary molar.

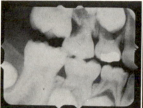
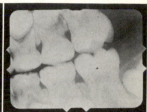

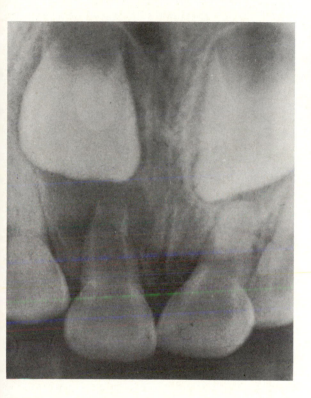

274. A. The spaces to the mesial of the maxillary canine and to the distal of the mandibular canine are commonly referred to as the:
   a. intercanine width.
   b. intracanine width.
   c. interdental spaces.
   d. primary spaces.
   e. primate spaces.

   B. The purpose of the appliance pictured in this photograph is:
   a. to maintain space for the developing first premolar.
   b. to maintain space for the developing first primary molar.
   c. distalization of the banded tooth to create additional space.
   d. to tip the maxillary canine into proper occlusion.

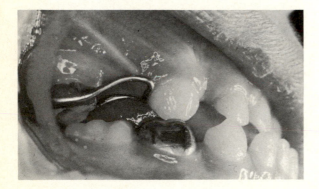

275. A. This 8-year-old boy has a history of a thumb habit. He is currently doing it "only at night or when tired." His mouth is caries free. The soft tissues are normal, except that when the upper lip is pulled up, the gingival tissues between the central incisors and palatally into the area of the incisive papilla blanch. The correct diagnosis of this condition is:
   a. anterior open bite caused by a prolonged digital habit.
   b. anterior open bite caused by an abnormal labial frenum attachment.
   c. anterior crossbite of the maxillary central and lateral incisors.
   d. posterior bilateral crossbite.
   e. normal occlusion for this age.

   B. The *most* correct treatment plan at this time is:
   a. observation until all the permanent teeth are in, then consultation with an orthodontist.
   b. frenectomy of labial frenum followed by tooth guidance to align the maxillary incisors.
   c. frenectomy of the labial frenum and allowing the teeth to self-align.
   d. placement of a habit appliance followed by frenectomy and observation.
   e. placement of a habit appliance followed by observation of the eruption of the permanent lateral incisors and canines to determine the need for frenectomy.

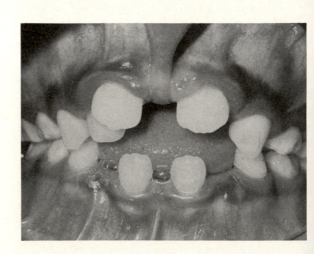

276. This 10½-year-old boy presents for examination. The appliance as shown:
a. has fulfilled its purpose and should be removed.
b. has fulfilled its purpose and should be removed and replaced with a Nance appliance.
c. should be left in to allow for proper root development of the premolar.
d. should be left in to guide the premolar distally.
e. should be left in and adjusted to allow the premolar to erupt within the confines of the wire loop.

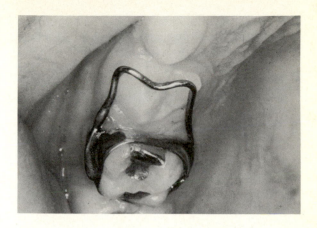

277. This 6-week-old infant has an ulceration on the ventral surface of the tongue. Examination reveals that the ulcer seems to be related to irritation from the hard, slightly raised, white area on the crest of the alveolar ridge. The *most* likely diagnosis of this white area is:
a. neonatal tooth.
b. bony sequestration.
c. Epstein's pearl.
d. Bohn's nodule.

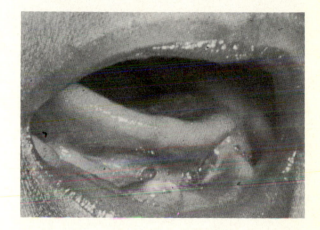

278. A. In the examination of this 5½-year-old child's occlusion, the terminal plane relationship is noted to be:
a. flush terminal plane.
b. mesial step.
c. distal step.
d. angle Class III.
B. Based on the terminal plane relationship of this patient, what occlusion is *most* likely to develop?
a. Class I.
b. Class II.
c. Class III.
d. Class II, division I.

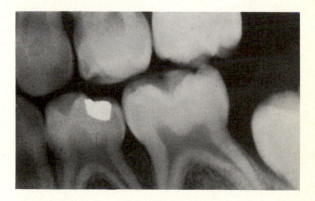

279. Assuming that the open coil spring in this orthodontic appliance was placed under compression, the *most* likely function of this preprosthetic appliance is:
   a. distalization and uprighting of the molars.
   b. mesialization and uprighting of the molars.
   c. mesialization and uprighting of the premolar.
   d. intrusion of the molars.
   e. extrusion of the molars.

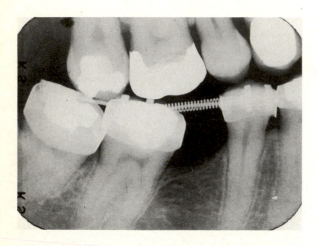

280. Hypoplasia of a crown of a tooth occurs during:
   a. initiation.
   b. proliferation.
   c. histodifferentiation.
   d. morphodifferentiation.

281. Congenital absence of the maxillary lateral incisors results from which stage of tooth development?
   a. initiation.
   b. proliferation.
   c. histodifferentiation.
   d. morphodifferentiation.

Dr. Edward Rothman authored questions 282 through 298.

282. The situation seen in this periapical radiograph is probably due to:
   a. a large perioendodontic abscess of the second primary molar.
   b. ectopic eruption of the first premolar into the root of the second primary molar.
   c. deep occlusal decay of the second primary molar, which has abscessed.
   d. idiopathic resorption of the second primary molar tooth.
   e. normal resorption of the second primary molar tooth.

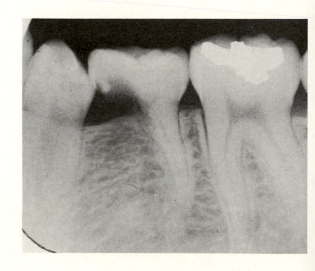

283. The following observation can be made regarding the periapical radiograph of this 3-year-old child:
    a. The patient is congenitally missing a second premolar.
    b. There is a carious lesion on the mesial of the second primary molar.
    c. The first primary molar has an unusually large pulp chamber.
    d. There is a radiolucency at the furcation of the first primary molar due to the deep caries.
    e. The enamel formation around these teeth is abnormal, indicating amelogenesis imperfecta.

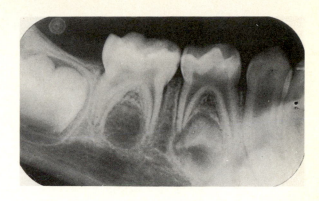

284. Upon reviewing the bite-wing radiograph of this 16-year-old patient, what observation do you make?
    a. The stainless steel crown is adequately placed.
    b. There is no interproximal decay.
    c. The maxillary first molar has undergone completed root canal therapy.
    d. There is an abnormal radiolucency around the periapical areas of the lower second molar.
    e. A periapical film is needed to further assess the condition of the upper first molar.

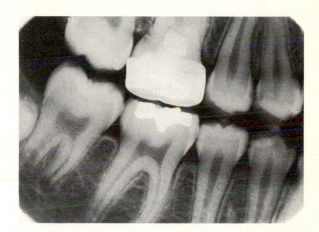

285. What is the correct management of the second primary molar?
    a. Do nothing at this time and observe for possible root remnant after normal exfoliation.
    b. Extract immediately and surgically remove the root remnant.
    c. Extract and place a lingual arch space maintainer.
    d. Extract and place a band loop space maintainer.
    e. Extract and place a Nance space maintainer.

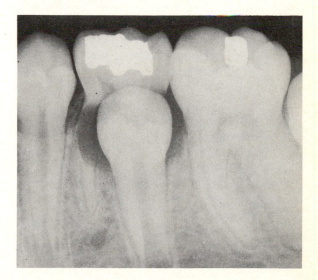

286. These teeth were extracted as one unit. They are joined by cementum only. This is an example of:
   a. fushion.
   b. gemination.
   c. concrescence.
   d. dilaceration.
   e. taurodontism.

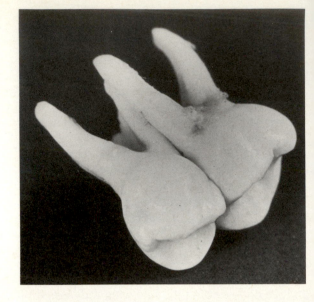

287. A. The patient seen in this photograph grew up in the western United States. The residents of his small community shared similar dental findings. The defects were most likely caused by:
   a. trauma to the primary dentition.
   b. congenital enamel defects.
   c. congenital dentin defects.
   d. poor oral hygiene.
   e. excessive amounts of fluoride in the drinking water.

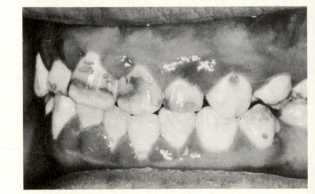

   B. The gingival conditions noted in this patient are probably due to:
   a. excessive fluoride intake.
   b. hereditary gingival fibromatosis.
   c. leukemic gingivitis.
   d. postorthodontic gingivitis.
   e. poor oral hygiene.

288. The condition of this child's teeth is a direct result of:
   a. trauma.
   b. enamel defects.
   c. dentin defects.
   d. prolonged nursing with sugar-containing liquids.
   e. hereditary soft teeth.

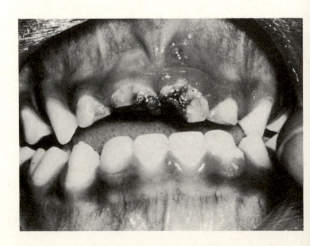

289. This 12-year-old boy comes to your office for a check-up. He has not seen a dentist since he traumatized the maxillary anterior teeth 3 years previously. On clinical examination you note some graying of the maxillary central incisors, but they are firm and asymptomatic. What is the *most* correct treatment?
   a. Extract the maxillary central incisors immediately and replace with a removable flipper appliance.
   b. Immediately place a bonded splint and observe for 1 week.
   c. Continue to monitor the teeth at 6-month recalls after telling the parents about the guarded prognosis for these teeth.
   d. Extract the teeth immediately and place a fixed Maryland Bridge because of the patient's young age.
   e. Continue to monitor every 6 months and tell the parents that the teeth should last a lifetime.

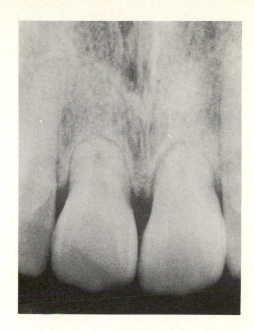

290. The patient whose Panorex is illustrated enters your office. You note that he has sparse hair and abnormal fingernails as well as a saddled nose. He reports that he is very uncomfortable in hot weather. He *most* likely has:
   a. amelogenesis imperfecta.
   b. dentinogenesis imperfecta.
   c. cleidocranial dysostosis.
   d. rickets.
   e. ectodermal dysplasia.

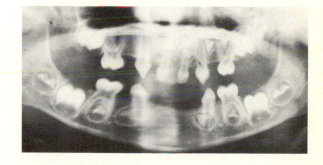

291. The open bite seen in the photograph of this healthy 3-year-old child is *most* likely due to:
   a. ankylosis of the central and lateral incisors.
   b. incomplete normal eruption of these teeth.
   c. a one-sided thumb-sucking habit.
   d. a fractured jaw that has healed incorrectly.
   e. trauma to the teeth, which caused intrusion.

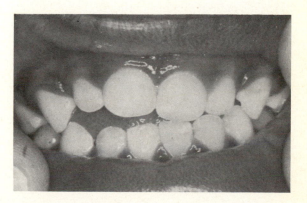

292. The radiograph seen below shows:
   a. splinting for periodontal conditions.
   b. lingual amalgam restorations.
   c. replantation and splinting of an evulsed central incisor tooth.
   d. an artifact caused by a crease in the film.
   e. a bonded lingual wire for postorthodontic stabilization.

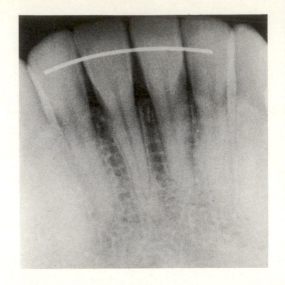

293. The appliance pictured:
   a. is most often used when a single tooth is lost, to maintain space.
   b. is most often used when there is a thumb habit that cannot be stopped by other methods.
   c. is most often used to correct posterior crossbite problems.
   d. is most often used to maintain space when one or more teeth are lost bilaterally and there is concern that opposing teeth will supererupt.
   e. is used to prevent further breakdown of teeth in a child with a bruxing habit.

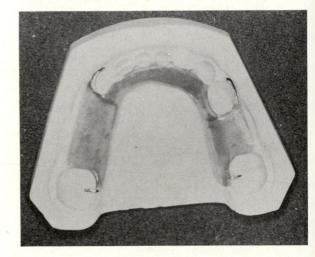

294. The patient in this photograph has an obvious open anterior bite. The appliance seen was probably placed to:
   a. interrupt an existing digital habit and allow the anterior teeth to close.
   b. mechanically force the anterior teeth to close down.
   c. prevent the child from aspirating foreign objects.
   d. prevent further movement of the teeth.
   e. allow permanent teeth to erupt in the proper positions.

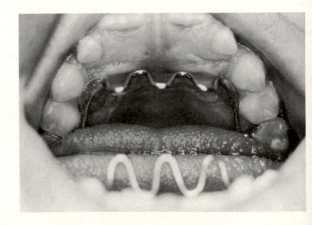

295. This appliance is known as:
   a. a band-loop space maintainer.
   b. a lingual arch space maintainer.
   c. a distal shoe space maintainer.
   d. a Nance space maintainer.
   e. a quadhelix appliance.

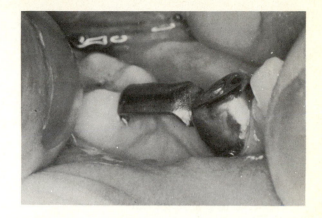

296. The periapical radiograph of this 12-year-old patient *most* likely suggests:
   a. that the patient is *congenitally* missing a premolar.
   b. that rapid orthodontic movement was performed.
   c. dens in dente of the canine.
   d. ectodermal dysplasia.
   e. a blood dyscrasia.

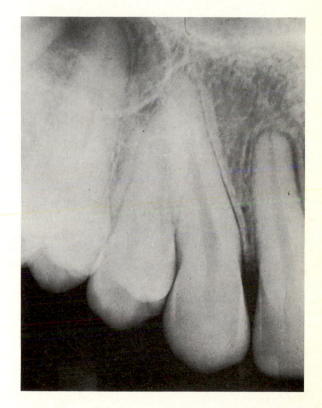

297. This 7-year-old patient presents for a routine 6-month recall. You note the lesions around the lips of this otherwise healthy child. They are apparently:
   a. herpetic lesions.
   b. bruises from a skateboarding accident.
   c. adolescent acne.
   d. chapped lips secondary to a lip-licking habit.
   e. *Candida albicans* (thrush).

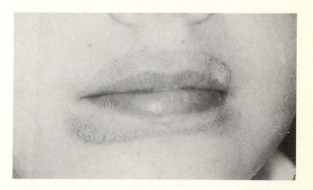

298. A. This picture shows:
    a. normal tonsillar tissue.
    b. hypertrophied tonsillar tissue.
    c. bifid uvula.
    d. macroglossia.
    e. cleft palate.
  B. This condition has been associated with mouth breathing. In patients who are chronic mouth breathers, what condition is most often seen?
    a. normal occlusion.
    b. an open anterior bite.
    c. a deep anterior bite.
    d. an excessive wearing of anterior teeth.
    e. an anterior crossbite.

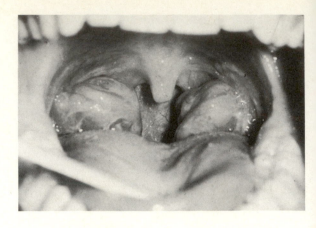

■ SECTION H

Cardiopulmonary resuscitation

Dr. Donald Doemling authored questions 299 through 320.

299. The initial pulse check should take a minimum of:
    a. 2 seconds.
    b. 5 seconds.
    c. 10 seconds.
    d. 15 seconds.
    e. 30 seconds.

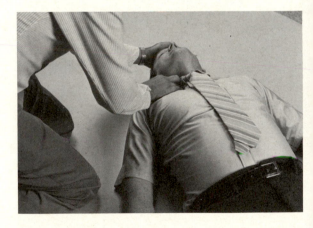

300. Which of the figures below depicts an incorrect procedure being performed on an infant?
  a. **A** only.
  b. **B** only.
  c. **C** only.
  d. **A** and **B**.
  e. **B** and **C**.

301. Propping the head up with a purse or other object as shown:
  a. will increase the likelihood of opening the airway.
  b. will increase the likelihood of aspiration of vomitus.
  c. should routinely be done for any unconscious victim.
  d. will make it more difficult to open the airway.
  e. is left to the discretion of the rescuer, inasmuch as the procedure has no significant effect on the effectiveness of resuscitation efforts.

A

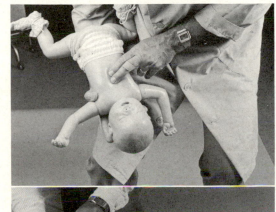

B

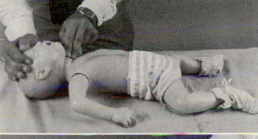

C

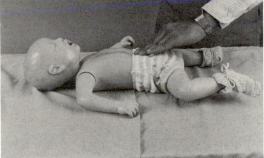

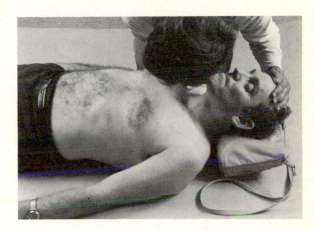

302. When performing chest compressions:
   a. the downstroke and the upstroke should be of approximately equal duration.
   b. at the end of the upstroke the heel of the hand should come off the chest slightly.
   c. the downstroke should be 2½ to 3 inches in adults.
   d. the rescuer should evenly press with the palm of the hand.
   e. the rate should be 60/min in adults for both one-rescuer and two-rescuer CPR.

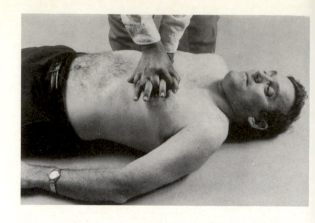

303. Ventilation performed as depicted in the figure will *not* be very effective because:
   a. a chin-lift is being used instead of a neck-lift.
   b. the head is not extended enough.
   c. the head is extended too much.
   d. the nose is not pinched closed.

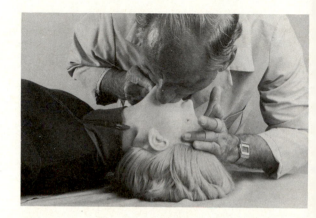

304. In cases of obstructed airway, back blows should be performed on:
   a. pregnant women.
   b. unconscious adults.
   c. conscious adults.
   d. infants.
   e. very obese individuals.

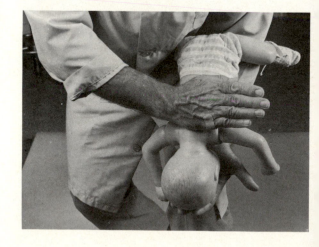

305. Generally, Heimlich maneuvers should *not* be performed on:

a. infants.
b. pregnant women.
c. very obese individuals.
d. all the above.
e. none of the above.

306. The jaw-thrust maneuver is used to:

a. remove a foreign body obstruction.
b. minimize the likelihood of the victim's vomiting.
c. remove dentures.
d. open the airway.
e. open the mouth.

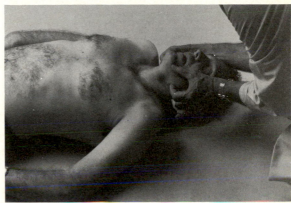

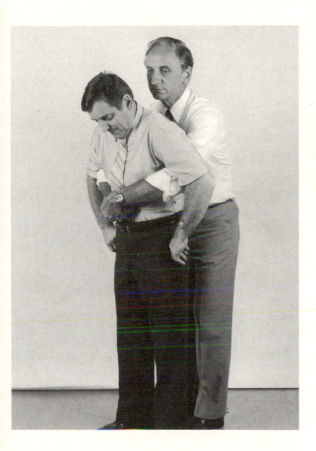

307. Which of the following is the correct sequence for resuscitating an unconscious adult victim with an obstruction?
1. Attempt to ventilate.
2. Establish unresponsiveness.
3. Check for a foreign body, using tongue-jaw lift and deep sweep.
4. Reposition the head and reattempt to ventilate.
5. Perform abdominal thrusts (Heimlich maneuver).
6. Open the airway and check for breathing.
   a. 2, 6, 1, 4, 5, 3.
   b. 2, 6, 3, 1, 4, 5.
   c. 6, 2, 1, 4, 3, 5.
   d. 2, 5, 6, 3, 1, 4.
   e. 2, 1, 6, 3, 4, 5.

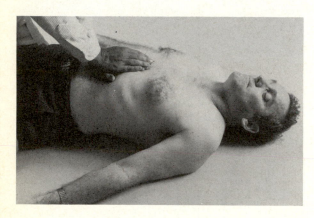

308. If an unconscious victim is not breathing, the trained rescuer should immediately:
a. check the carotid pulse.
b. check the brachial (arm) pulse.
c. phone for help.
d. ventilate the victim with two slow breaths.
e. ventilate the victim with four rapid breaths.

309. While performing chest compressions on an accident victim, the rescuer's second hand should:
a. be used to apply slight pressure on the abdomen.
b. be placed on top of the hand that is in contact with the chest.
c. be placed alongside the hand that is in contact with the chest.
d. continuously monitor the carotid pulse.
e. continuously monitor the brachial (arm) pulse.

310. If an unconscious adult victim is not breathing but has a pulse, the rescuer should continue resuscitation by ventilating:
a. once every 5 seconds.
b. once every 10 seconds.
c. twice every 15 seconds.
d. four times every 15 seconds.
e. four times every minute.

311. What is the correct position on the chest for compressions in an infant?
a. One finger should be placed on the sternum over an imaginary line between the nipples.
b. Two fingers should be placed on the sternum straddling an imaginary line between the nipples.
c. Two fingers should be placed on the sternum one fingerwidth toward the head from the notch at the lower end of the sternum.
d. Two fingers should be placed on the sternum one fingerwidth below an imaginary line between the nipples.
e. One finger should be placed on the middle of the sternum.

312. Chest compressions in an adult victim should be performed at the rate of about:
a. 60/min for two-rescuer CPR.
b. 90/min for one-rescuer CPR.
c. 120/min for one-rescuer CPR.
d. 90/min for both one-rescuer and two-rescuer CPR.
e. as fast as is practical for both one-rescuer and two-rescuer CPR.

313. When performing two-rescuer CPR:
   a. one ventilation should be given during the upstroke of every fifth compression.
   b. one ventilation should be given during a pause at the end of every fifth compression.
   c. one ventilation should be given every 5 seconds.
   d. two ventilations should be given during a pause at the end of every 15 compressions.
   e. four ventilations should be given during a pause at the end of every 15 compressions.

314. After completing the fourth set of compressions, i.e., after about 1 minute of one-rescuer CPR, the sequence for checking the pulse is as follows:
   a. one ventilation, check pulse, one ventilation, resume compressions.
   b. two ventilations, check pulse, resume compressions.
   c. two ventilations, check pulse, two ventilations, resume compressions.
   d. check pulse, one ventilation, resume compressions.
   e. check pulse, two ventilations, resume compressions.

315. Which of the following is the correct sequence for performing basic CPR on a suspected victim of cardiac arrest?
   1. Ventilate twice.
   2. Activate the EMS system if someone has responded to your call for help.
   3. Establish unresponsiveness.
   4. Palpate for pulse.
   5. Open the airway and check for breathing.
   6. Perform chest compressions.
      a. 3, 4, 6, 5, 1, 2.
      b. 3, 4, 5, 2, 1, 6.
      c. 3, 5, 1, 4, 2, 6.
      d. 5, 4, 3, 2, 6, 1.
      e. 3, 5, 4, 2, 6, 1.

316. After "opening the airway" of an unconscious infant and determining that there is no breathing, the next step should be to:
   a. check for a foreign body.
   b. attempt to ventilate.
   c. deliver four back blows.
   d. deliver four chest thrusts.
   e. reposition the head.

317. Resuscitation techniques for the obstructed small child (not infant) are similar to those for the adult with what exception?
   a. Back blows are substituted for abdominal thrusts.
   b. Thoracic thrusts are substituted for abdominal thrusts.
   c. Blind sweeps of the mouth and throat are not performed.
   d. The crossed-finger technique of opening the mouth is not used.
   e. The tongue-jaw technique of opening the mouth is not used.

318. Which of the following is *not* correct in regard to ventilating an adult victim?
   a. The inspiratory phase of each breath should take 1 to 1½ seconds.
   b. Two breaths are given both before and after the pulse check at the end of the first minute of CPR.
   c. The victim should be allowed to exhale passively between breaths.
   d. For one-rescuer CPR, breaths are always given two at a time.
   e. Four breaths are given when it is initially determined that the victim is not breathing.

319. When checking the carotid pulse after initially ventilating the victim:
   a. maintain the head-tilt with the hand on the forehead.
   b. use the hand that was used for the chin-lift to check the pulse.
   c. take 5 to 10 seconds for the diagnosis.
   d. all the above.
   e. none of the above.

320. If, when attempting to ventilate a nonbreathing, unconscious victim, the chest does not rise, the rescuer should:
   a. blow harder.
   b. open the mouth and check for a foreign body.
   c. reposition the head and again attempt to ventilate.
   d. roll the victim toward the rescuer and administer back blows.
   e. straddle the victim's legs and administer abdominal thrusts.

■ SECTION I

Medical considerations and emergencies

Dr. James Lehnert authored questions 321 through 373.

321. A. The *most* likely cause of hyperventilation syndrome as seen in the dental office is:
   a. acute anxiety.
   b. metabolic acidosis.
   c. obstructive lung disease.
   d. hyperactive airway disease.
   e. congestive heart failure.

B. Clinical manifestations of this syndrome would *least* likely include:
   a. tachypnea.
   b. paresthesia of the extremities.
   c. hypotension.
   d. dizziness.
   e. tachycardia.

C. Management of the dental patient with hyperventilation syndrome may include all of the following *except:*
   a. reassure and calm patient.
   b. cadence breathing.
   c. rebreathe expired CO_2.
   d. diazepam 5 to 15 mg, IM or orally.
   e. oxygen therapy.

322. A 39-year-old man presents for emergency treatment of tooth No. 19. His medical history is unremarkable. Pretreatment blood pressure measures 138/84, and heart rate is 88 and regular. While giving him an inferior alveolar block, you note that he is pale and diaphoretic. Afterward, the patient states that he is nauseated and feels dizzy. Moments later you find the patient as illustrated in the figure following Question "C" p. 333.

A. A differential diagnosis for loss of consciousness should include all the following *except*:
   a. drug overdose.
   b. angina pectoris.
   c. cerebrovascular accident.
   d. epilepsy.
   e. hypoglycemia.

B. The patient's vital signs are now as follows: blood pressure 60/40, heart rate 44 and regular. The respiratory rate is 16 with good air movement. He has *most* likely experienced:
   a. orthostatic hypotension.
   b. anaphylaxis.
   c. hysteria reaction.
   d. syncope.
   e. acute adrenal insufficiency.

C. Correct management of this patient includes:
   1. epinephrine, 0.2 to 1.0 mg, IM or IV.
   2. O_2 therapy.
   3. maintaining a patent airway.
   4. atropine, 0.4 mg, IV or subcutaneously.
   5. psychological counseling.
   6. placement of the patient in the supine position with legs slightly elevated.
   7. diphenhydramine, 25 to 50 mg, IM or IV.
   8. hydrocortisone, 100 mg, IM or IV.
      a. 1, 2, 3, and 6.
      b. 2, 3, 4 and 6.
      c. 2, 3, and 6.
      d. 2, 3, 6, 7, and 8.
      e. 2, 3, and 5.

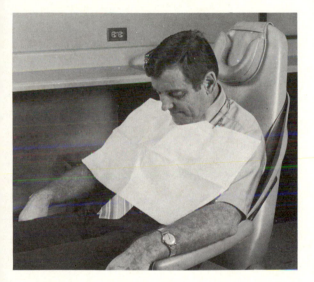

323. A 70-year-old patient states that 2 years ago he was hospitalized for "fluid in the lungs." Since then he has been taking digoxin, 0.25 mg q am; Lasix, 40 mg b.i.d.; and Slow-K, 1 tablet t.i.d. These drugs are used in combination in the medical mangement of:
   a. ventricular arrhythmia.
   b. congestive heart failure.
   c. emphysema.
   d. ischemic heart disease.
   e. sinus bradycardia.

324. Major determinants of myocardial oxygen demand include all the following *except*:
   a. coronary vasodilatation.
   b. preload.
   c. heart rate.
   d. contractility.
   e. afterload.

325. The patient in the figure below is simulating a reaction to the pain of an acute myocardial infarction. Which of the following statements regarding the pain of acute myocardial infarction is *incorrect*?
   a. may be described as a "crushing" or "vice-like" retrosternal pain.
   b. may be accompanied by sweating.
   c. is usually not relieved by sublingual nitroglycerin tablets.
   d. may radiate to the shoulder, neck, or mandible.
   e. is often relieved by sitting the patient up and leaning him forward.

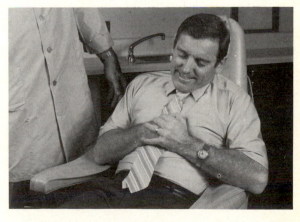

326. Proper management of a conscious patient who you suspect has had an acute myocardial infarction during dental treatment should include all the following *except*:
a. loosen restrictive clothing.
b. morphine, 4 to 8 mg IM as necessary.
c. place in a comfortable position.
d. personally drive the patient to the nearest hospital.
e. O_2 therapy.

327. *Elective* dental treatment should *not* be performed on a patient who has had a myocardial infarction for a period of:
a. 1 month.
b. 4 months.
c. 6 months.
d. 9 months.
e. 12 months.

328. In the spaces provided, write the antibiotic regimens recommended by the American Heart Association for prevention of bacterial endocarditis in dental patients as indicated.
A. Oral amoxicillin in an adult:

B. Oral erythromycin ethylsuccinate in an adult:

C. Oral erythromycin stearate in an adult:

D. Oral clindamycin in an adult:

E. Oral penicillin in an adult:

F. Oral amoxicillin in a child (in mg/kg):

G. Oral erythromycin (ethylsuccinate or stearate) in a child (in mg/kg):

H. Oral clindamycin in a child (in mg/kg):

I. Oral penicillin in a child weighing less than 60 pounds:

329. Which of the following conditions would *not* require prophylactic antibiotics before extraction of a tooth?
   a. ventricular septal defect.
   b. history of rheumatic heart disease 10 years previously.
   c. history of coronary artery bypass surgery 3 years previously.
   d. mitral valve prolapse with murmur.
   e. coarctation of the aorta.

330. Which of the following places the patient at *highest* risk for bacterial endocarditis?
   a. prosthetic heart valve.
   b. tricuspid insufficiency.
   c. atrial septal defect, primum type.
   d. mitral stenosis.
   e. transvenous cardiac pacemaker.

331. What is the AHA's recommended *loading dose* using parenteral antibiotics in an adult patient considered at high risk for bacterial endocarditis?
   a. penicillin G, 3 million units IV or IM.
   b. ampicillin, 2.0 g IV or IM.
   c. oral tetracycline, 1.0 g.
   d. gentamicin, 1.5 mg/kg IV or IM.
   e. b and d.

332. What is the corresponding *maintenance* dose for the preceding question?
   a. vancomycin, 1 g IV.
   b. oral penicillin V, 1.0 g.
   c. penicillin G, 1 million units IV or IM.
   d. oral amoxicillin, 1.5 g.
   e. no maintenance dose is required.

333. Drugs normally used in the medical management of asthmatic patients include all the following *except*:
   a. isoproterenol.
   b. prednisone.
   c. propranolol.
   d. aminophylline.
   e. cromolyn sodium.

334. Which clinical finding would be *most* indicative of impending respiratory distress in a patient having a severe asthma attack?
   a. sudden absence of wheezing.
   b. pulsus paradoxus.
   c. use of accessory muscles of respiration.
   d. tachycardia.
   e. dyspnea.

335. A 26-year-old man with a history of drug abuse presents for dental treatment complaining of malaise, nausea, a recent 10-pound weight loss, and right upper quadrant pain. The results of the serology tests you order are as follows:

   + anti-HAV (IgG)
   + HBsAg
   + HBeAg
   + anti-HBc

   These findings are *most* consistent with:
   a. acute hepatitis A.
   b. acute hepatitis B.
   c. acute hepatitis C.
   d. past hepatitis A infection.
   e. b and d.

336. The principal mode of transmission of which type of viral hepatitis is thought to occur via contaminated blood, blood products, and body secretions:
   a. hepatitis A.
   b. hepatitis B.
   c. hepatitis C.
   d. b and c only.
   e. a, b, and c.

337. Delta hepatitis is a potential complication of:
   a. hepatitis A.
   b. hepatitis B.
   c. hepatitis C.
   d. b and c only.
   e. a, b, and c.

338. The most likely cause of post-transfusion hepatitis currently is:
   a. hepatitis A.
   b. hepatitis B.
   c. hepatitis C.
   d. b and c only.
   e. a, b, and c.

339. The principal mode of transmission of which type of viral hepatitis is thought to occur by the fecal-oral route:
   a. hepatitis A.
   b. hepatitis B.
   c. hepatitis C.
   d. b and c only.
   e. a, b, and c.

340. A chronic viral hepatitis disease state may be associated with:
   a. hepatitis A.
   b. hepatitis B.
   c. hepatitis C.
   d. b and c only.
   e. a, b, and c.

341. A dentist with no serologic markers for viral hepatitis accidentally inoculates himself with a hepatitis B–contaminated needle. Postexposure prophylaxis in this case should include:
   a. no treatment.
   b. receiving immune globulin.
   c. receiving hyper B immune globulin.
   d. starting the hepatitis B vaccine regimen.
   e. c and d.

342. The *safest* time to treat a potentially threatening carious lesion in a pregnant patient is during which trimester?
   a. First.
   b. Second.
   c. Third.
   d. Absolutely no dental treatment should be performed on a pregnant patient.
   e. Treatment can be rendered with the same relative degree of safety during any trimester.

343. Midway through restoration of a symptomatic tooth on a healthy woman who is 8 months pregnant, she loses consciousness. The dentist's *first* action for the supine hypotensive syndrome should be to:
   a. elevate the patient's legs to increase blood flow to the brain.
   b. sit the patient up and administer oxygen.
   c. roll the patient onto her left side to increase venous return to the heart.
   d. administer aromatic spirits of ammonia.
   e. start an IV in case there is a need for vasopressor administration.

344. The use of which drug is contraindicated in a patient who is nursing?
   a. tetracycline.
   b. erythromycin.
   c. aspirin.
   d. 2% lidocaine with epinephrine 1:100,000.
   e. nitrous oxide.

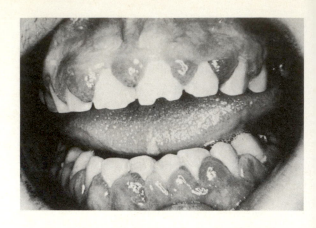

345. The 15-year-old patient pictured above presents for emergency dental treatment with swollen, bleeding gums. The intraoral examination also reveals palatal petechiae. The results of a CBC are as follows:

	Patient	Normal
RBC count	3.0	$4.6–6.2 \times 10^6$ cells/cu mm
WBC count	18,000	4,500–11,000/ cu mm
Differential:		
neutrophils	20%	50%–70%
lymphocytes	50%	20%–40%
monocytes	5%	0%–7%
blasts	25%	less than 1%
Platelet count	50,000	150,000–300,000/ cu mm

These findings are most consistent with:
   a. acute bacterial infection.
   b. aplastic anemia.
   c. acute viral infection.
   d. acute leukemia.
   e. idopathic thrombocytopenic purpura.

346. A patient has been taking high doses of aspirin every day because of arthritis. Which blood test would *best* screen for an associated *functional* platelet defect?
   a. platelet count.
   b. bleeding time.
   c. tourniquet test.
   d. prothrombin time.
   e. partial thromboplastin time.

347. A patient with chronic renal failure presents for emergency extraction of tooth No. 15 immediately after hemodialysis. Which test should be ordered to screen for a bleeding problem associated with heparin therapy?
a. bleeding time.
b. tourniquet test.
c. prothrombin time.
d. partial thromboplastin time.
e. thromboplastin generation time.

348. A 48-year-old woman with a history of thrombophlebitis is taking Coumadin, 5 mg every day. She needs to have several periodontally involved teeth extracted. Which test is generally ordered to screen for the effects of this drug on coagulation?
a. thromboplastin generation time.
b. venous clotting time.
c. prothrombin time.
d. partial thromboplastin time.
e. tourniquet test.

349. Which of the statements regarding prothrombin time (PT) is (are) correct?
a. Vitamin K injections may prolong the PT.
b. The PT must be in the normal range before any dental surgery can be done.
c. Dental surgery can generally be performed if the PT is within 1.5 to 2.0 times the control
d. Dental surgery can be performed as long as the PT is within the therapeutic range.
e. a and d.

350. Which bleeding tests might be abnormal in a patient with advanced liver disease and splenomegaly?
a. platelet count.
b. prothrombin time.
c. partial thromboplastin time.
d. a and b only.
e. a, b, and c.

351. Considerations in the dental management of a patient who is taking exogenous corticosteroids include all the following *except:*
a. need for supplemental steroids before dental treatment.
b. increased risk for infection.
c. returned normal adrenal function usually within 3 months after discontinuing the exogenous steroids.
d. decreased tolerance to stress.
e. delayed wound healing.

352. The relative anti-inflammatory potency of prednisone is how many times that of hydrocortisone?
a. one fourth.
b. one half.
c. two.
d. four.
e. seven.

353. Clinical manifestations of systemic hypertension would least likely include:
a. occipital headache.
b. dizziness.
c. clubbing of the digits.
d. easy fatigability.
e. visual disturbances.

354. Although there are many factors to consider, as a general rule elective dental treatment is contraindicated in an adult when the systolic blood pressure is greater than:
a. 140 mm Hg.
b. 160 mm Hg.
c. 180 mm Hg.
d. 200 mm Hg.
e. 220 mm Hg.

355. With the same qualifications as mentioned in the preceding question, elective dental treatment is contraindicated in an adult when the diastolic blood pressure is greater than:
a. 95 mm Hg.
b. 105 mm Hg.
c. 115 mm Hg.
d. 125 mm Hg.
e. 130 mm Hg.

356. The blood pressure of a 48-year-old man taken during the initial examination is 150/94. His medical history is unremarkable. This blood pressure *best* fits into the category of:
a. normotension.
b. borderline hypertension.
c. moderate hypertension.
d. secondary hypertension.
e. c and d.

357. What would be the proper management of the patient in the preceding question?
    a. Do nothing, as the blood pressure is within normal limits.
    b. Recheck blood pressure only at each appointment.
    c. Refer immediately for medical consultation.
    d. Refer for medical consultation if successive rechecks are in the same range.
    e. Recheck blood pressure at each appointment and, if the same, avoid anesthetics with epinephrine.

358. Potential complications of chronic hypertension include all the following *except*:
    a. atrophy of the left ventricle.
    b. stroke.
    c. peripheral vascular disease.
    d. congestive heart failure.
    e. kidney disease.

359. Dental patients can be categorized according to the American Society of Anesthesiologists physical status classification system. Using this system, a 60-year-old man with chronic obstructive lung disease who gets short of breath walking up two flights of stairs at a normal pace would be a:
    a. Class 1.
    b. Class 2.
    c. Class 3.
    d. Class 4.
    e. Class 5.

360. A 17-year-old patient with a history of a traumatic fracture of the left arm 5 years previously would be a:
    a. Class 1.
    b. Class 2.
    c. Class 3.
    d. Class 4.
    e. Class 5.

361. A 60-year-old patient with a long history of heart disease who states that he gets angina pectoris several times a day, sometimes while sitting, would be a:
    a. Class 1.
    b. Class 2.
    c. Class 3.
    d. Class 4.
    e. Class 5.

362. A 62-year-old patient who was diagnosed as having moderate hypertension 4 years previously, whose blood pressure is well controlled with a diuretic and a beta blocker, would be a:
    a. Class 1.
    b. Class 2.
    c. Class 3.
    d. Class 4.
    e. Class 5.

363. Stress reduction for a dental patient should include all the following *except*:
    a. avoiding local anesthetics containing epinephrine.
    b. special attention to postoperative pain control.
    c. a short appointment.
    d. nitrous oxide analgesia.
    e. appointments scheduled in the morning.

364. Daily dependence on exogenous insulin to maintain life is characteristic of the patient with:
    a. Type I diabetes.
    b. Type II diabetes.
    c. Type III diabetes.
    d. impaired glucose tolerance.
    e. b and c only.

365. Which of the following statements regarding diabetes mellitus is *incorrect*?
    a. Insulin requirements may increase with infection.
    b. It is a clinical syndrome characterized by hyperglycemia.
    c. Sulfonylureas act by stimulating insulin secretion.
    d. Diet is an important component of the medical management of this disease.
    e. All the above statements are correct.

366. Long-term diabetes is known to place the patient at increased risk for all the following *except*:
    a. blindness.
    b. pancreatic cancer.
    c. arteriosclerosis.
    d. kidney disease.
    e. peripheral neuropathy.

367. Clinical manifestations of insulin shock may include all the following *except*:
    a. tachycardia.
    b. abnormal behavior.
    c. sweet odor of ketone bodies.
    d. sweating.
    e. tremor.

368. This ECG strip shows:
  a. normal sinus rhythm.
  b. ventricular tachycardia.
  c. atrial fibrillation.
  d. Q waves.
  e. premature atrial contractions.

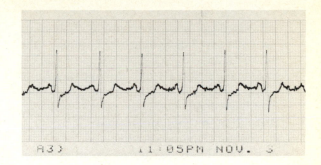

369. On an ECG strip, the T wave represents:
  a. atrial depolarization.
  b. ventricular depolarization.
  c. atrial repolarization.
  d. ventricular repolarization.
  e. atrial hypertrophy.

370. Sinus tachycardia refers to a heart rate greater than _____ per minute.
  a. 80.
  b. 90.
  c. 100.
  d. 110.
  e. 120.

371. The arrow on this ECG strip points to a:
  a. nodal escape beat.
  b. premature atrial contraction.
  c. ventricular flutter.
  d. run of trigeminy.
  e. premature ventricular contraction.

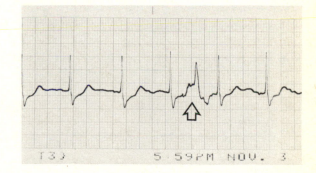

372. This ECG strip shows:
  a. heart block.
  b. ventricular fibrillation.
  c. premature ventricular contractions.
  d. ventricular tachycardia.
  e. atrial fibrillation.

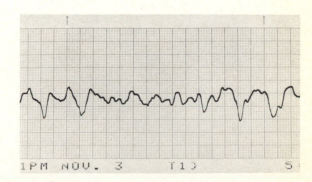

373. A 52-year-old woman comes to your office for diagnosis and treatment of a burning tongue as well as itching and burning of the labial mucosa in the incisor region. A clinical examination reveals that the appearance of these surfaces is within normal limits. After you have completed your examination, you should inform this patient that:
a. vitamin C therapy is indicated.
b. this condition will regress spontaneously.
c. this condition is referred to as postmenopausal burning mouth, the cause and treatment of which are not well understood.
d. antifungal therapy is indicated.
e. the vertical dimension should be increased.

374. A 32-year-old patient receives radiation treatment for cancer of the oral cavity. The patient might expect to experience all but *one* of the following as a result:
a. mucositis.
b. xerostomia.
c. an increased caries rate.
d. osteomyelitis (osteoradionecrosis).
e. short malformed roots.

■ SECTION J

Preventive dentistry

Dr. Kirk Hoerman authored questions 375 through 384.

375. The Y-axis of the depicted figure can be labeled:
a. Ca/P ratio.
b. enamel fluoride content.
c. DMFS.
d. plaque weight.
e. collagen.

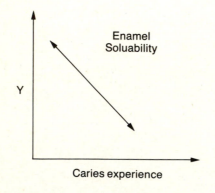

376. The epidemiology of dental caries reveals that:
a. the intensity is evenly spread worldwide.
b. the prevalence correlates negatively with consumption of refined sugar.
c. the incidence is highest in primitive populations.
d. the intensity decreases upon adoption of modern living conditions and standards.
e. the highest attack rate occurs in childhood and adolescence.

377. If your answer to Question 375 was "c. (DMFS)," the slope of the line in the depicted figure should be:
a. positive.
b. negative.
c. exponential.
d. horizonal.

378. Fixation of topically applied fluorides can be accomplished by:
a. increasing the concentration of solutions.
b. lowering the pH of solutions.
c. increasing the exposure time.
d. pretreatment of enamel with 0.5% phosphoric acid.
e. all the above.

379. A common factor in the etiology of coronal caries and gingivitis is:
  a. cell-mediated immunity.
  b. extracellular polysaccharide in plaque.
  c. *Streptococcus mutans.*
  d. *Actinomyces viscosus.*
  e. lipoteichoic acid.

380. Pellicle is believed to be:
  a. a positively charged film on enamel surfaces.
  b. of blood origin.
  c. composed of bacteria and their products.
  d. amphoteric.
  e. largely composed of salivary mucinous material.

381. Tetracycline can be an antibiotic of choice for the initial treatment of:
  a. aggressive osteolytic disease of alveolar bone processes.
  b. necrotizing ulcerative gingivitis.
  c. gram-positive streptococci in plaque.
  d. gram-negative aerobic bacteria in periodontal pockets.
  e. herpes zoster.

382. Below is shown a distribution curve of the number of persons in a population with regard to the prevalence of caries (DMFS). If the drinking water of the population were defluoridated, eventually the distribution curve should shift:
  a. because the number of caries-free persons would increase.
  b. not at all.
  c. to the right.
  d. to the left.
  e. none of the above.

383. Below is a diagram of one of the current theories to explain plaque adherence, namely, adsorption because of electrostatic forces. Which of the following actions might break that binding force?
  a. chelation.
  b. greater affinity for bound acidic groups.
  c. inorganic anions, reactive with Ca^{++}.
  d. all the above.

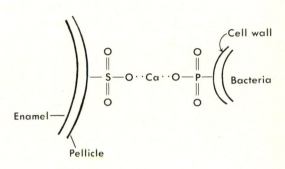

384. Which of the following sweeteners is synthetic and noncaloric?
  a. xylitol.
  b. dihydrochalcone.
  c. mannose.
  d. sorbitol.
  e. saccharin.

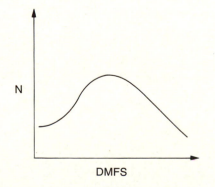

■ SECTION K

Forensic dentistry and ethics

Dr. E. Steven Smith and Dr. Larry Pierce authored questions 385 through 399.

385. This child is accompanied by her parents to your office. During the initial workup and evaluation, patterned injuries resembling bitemarks are observed on the patient's arm and leg *(arrows)*. What is the most appropriate course of action?
   a. Alert the parents to the injuries so that appropriate follow-up care can be instituted.
   b. Make an entry in your treatment record of "suspected child abuse" and evaluate the patient's physical condition at the next visit.
   c. Take the child to see the nearest emergency room and report the incident.
   d. Immediately report your findings to the child protective agency in your state.

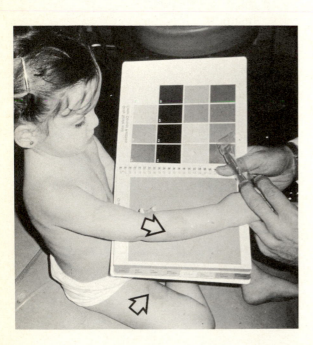

386. The morning news broadcast is interrupted to announce the crash of a commercial airliner. Later that day, the newspaper lists three of your patients as potential victims on the fatal flight. What action should you follow in an effort to assist the authorities?
   a. Immediately forward all patient records to the local authorities.
   b. Maintain patient confidentiality until the next of kin authorize the release of patient records.
   c. Duplicate all significant dental records and submit a copy to the appropriate authorities upon request.
   d. Communicate with the disaster team and offer your assistance, as you might be able to identify your patients' dental work.

387. The state's attorney in your county requests that you take dental impressions on a suspect charged with murder. Because the bitemark evidence is crucial in this case, accurate study models are essential for suspect evaluation. Before proceeding, it is important to:
   a. have the suspect sign a release form.
   b. make certain that a court order has been issued authorizing you to take the impressions.
   c. arrange to have an officer of the court present to witness the procedure.
   d. solicit permission from the defense attorney.

388. The state police believe that an unidentified female homicide victim is the missing secretary from your community. You are asked to compare one antemortem radiograph **(A)** with a postmortem film taken at the time of the autopsy **(B).** After careful evaluation, what do you conclude?

a. There are enough similarities to state that, within reasonable dental certainty, the murder victim is the missing secretary.

b. The antemortem radiograph is totally inconsistent with the postmortem film.

c. There are some points of similarity but not enough for a positive identification.

d. There are consistent points, but sufficient contradictory points to cast serious doubt on an identification based on the information provided.

389. You receive a telephone call from a coroner in an adjacent state. He requests your assistance in the dental identification of a victim of a mountain climbing accident. There is reason to believe that the deceased is one of your patients. The coroner asks you to describe the teeth and dental restorations of the patient in question. You should:

a. decline and request that the coroner forward all relevant dental information to your office for comparison prior to any report.

b. cooperate with the coroner and give your verbal report over the telephone, but request that all postmortem dental information be forwarded to your office for final comparison.

c. refuse to answer any questions until a court order is secured.

d. cooperate with the coroner and give your telephone report, then forward a copy of the patient record to his office upon request.

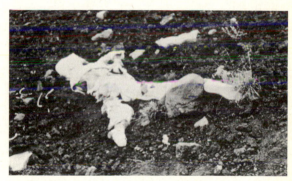

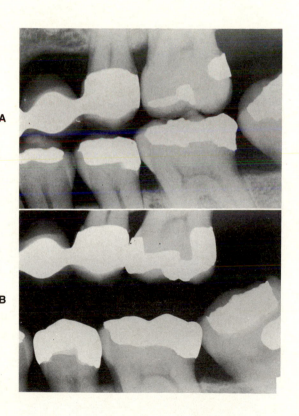

390. A partially incinerated human skeleton is found in a shallow grave just outside of town. The medical examiner dispatches the dentition to your laboratory for age determination. Which of the following factors should be considered during your examination?
a. root apical translucency and pulp chamber morphology.
b. cementum apposition and formation of secondary dentin.
c. periodontal condition, epithelial attachment, attrition and abrasion.
d. all the above.

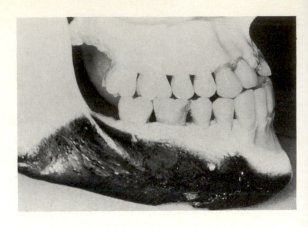

391. Which one of the following individuals is considered to be the "Father of Forensic Dentistry"?
a. G.V. Black.
b. William Morten.
c. Oscar Amoëdo.
d. Paul Revere.
e. A. Zsigmondy.

392. The first reported case of child abuse in the United States occurred in New York City in the year:
a. 1874.
b. 1905.
c. 1935.
d. 1960.
e. 1975.

393. A patient presents to your office complaining of pain in tooth No. 8 (maxillary right central incisor). A periapical radiograph shows a completed root canal, which the patient indicates was performed last year by a specialist. The tooth was subsequently restored by a general dentist. The radiograph shows that a commercial woodscrew has been used for retention beneath the crown. This case is an example of:
a. res ipsa loquitur.
b. malpractice.
c. malfeasance.
d. fraud.

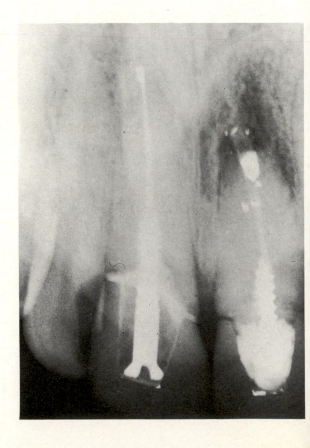

394. The legal time limit within which a civil suit must be filed is called the:
   a. time limitation.
   b. legal window.
   c. reasonable compensatory deadline.
   d. statute of limitations.

395. The literature states that 50% of child abuse victims have injuries inflicted to the head and neck regions. Dentists must be aware of the signs of child abuse, which include a torn labial frenum, fractured or avulsed teeth, and multiple areas of bruising at various stages of healing. All the following disease processes could produce physical findings that could be misread as child abuse *except*:
   a. idiopathic thrombocytopenic purpura.
   b. dentinogenesis imperfecta.
   c. epilepsy.
   d. Peutz-Jeghers syndrome.

396. A 25-year-old woman was raped under the threat of death. During the struggle she reported that she was bitten on her right shoulder, as shown in this photograph. Several days later, a suspect was apprehended. Which *one* of the following items would be of *minimal* importance to this case?
   a. dental impressions of the suspect.
   b. impressions of the bitemark.
   c. ABO blood typing from the saliva.
   d. photographs of the bitemark.

397. A 5-year-old black girl was taken to the emergency room for treatment of an injury reportedly resulting from, but not consistent with, a fall. During the clinical examination, a well-defined adult human bitemark was observed on the child's back **(A)**. A child abuse complaint was reported by the hospital. An investigation ensued that led to four possible suspects who could have caused the bitemark. In your opinion, which dentition caused the bitemark?
   a. **B.**
   b. **C.**
   c. **D.**
   d. **E.**

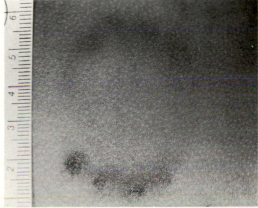

A

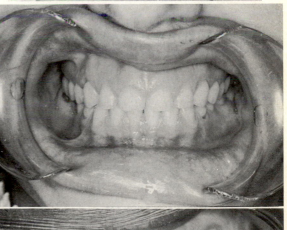

B

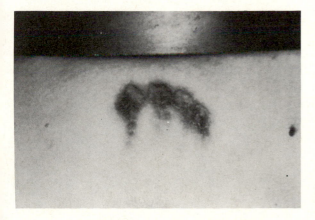

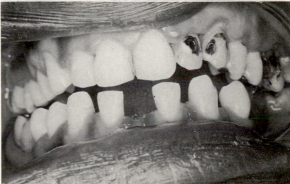

C

Continued.

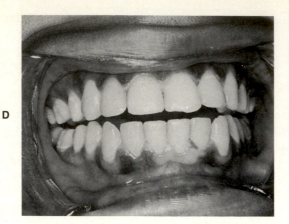

D

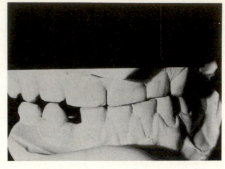

E

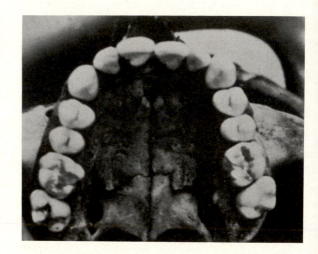

398. An American diplomat was kidnapped 2 years ago. The kidnappers claimed to have "executed" him, but no body was found. Recently, children playing in a mountainous area found a human skull. The figure shows a photograph that was returned to the United States for use in dental comparison. The diplomat had the following restorations:

Tooth No. 2: Occlusal-lingual amalgam.
Tooth No. 3: DO inlay that tips the distolingual cusp.
Tooth No. 8: Porcelain-fused-to-metal crown.
Tooth No. 14: MO inlay that tips the mesiolingual cusp.

Evaluate the photograph and compare it with the diplomat's record. You conclude that:
a. the deceased is the diplomat.
b. there are consistent points but insufficient evidence to establish an identification.
c. the deceased is not the diplomat.
d. there are consistent points but sufficient contradictory points to cast serious doubt on an identification based on the information provided.

399. As a general dentist you consider yourself to be proficient in root canal therapy. While instrumenting a canal, a file breaks, the tip of which you cannot remove. You should do the following:
a. complete the root canal and restore the tooth.
b. record the incident in the patient's folder and evaluate at a later date.
c. inform the patient and refer to a specialist.
d. extract the tooth, because the broken file is not retrievable.

Pitfalls in treatment planning

Dr. James M. Plecash authored questions 400 through 407. Questions 400 through 402 relate to this case.

400. "Mr. K," a 51-year-old man, presents with a chief complaint of gradual loss over the past 3 to 4 years of the "white plastic" from the front of the crowns on his lower front teeth. These crowns were placed approximately 20 years ago. Clinical examination of this region reveals that the crowns on all the mandibular incisors are splinted to each other. The fractured labial facings are plastic materials. There is a moderate degree of plaque on the lingual surfaces of the crowns. Also, the surrounding gingival tissues exhibit a slight erythema and edema, with resultant minor bleeding on periodontal probing, with sulci depths ranging from 3 to 4 mm. The prominences of the labial ridge are firm to palpation and the lingual surfaces of the crowns are normal. Periapical radiographs reveal that the left lateral incisor of this sextant has undergone endodontic therapy; there is an increased trabecular density at the middle third of the mandibular incisors but no other abnormalities. The opposing anterior dentition consists of a removable partial denture that replaces all the maxillary incisors, including the left canine. The partial denture is constructed of a cast metal with extension of the metal well up onto the cingulum of the artificial teeth, serving as occlusal stops for the mandibular incisor crowns. A review of the patient's medical history reveals that he has been hospitalized twice in the past 6 years: the first episode for 3 weeks after a myocardial infarction, and the second 2 years ago for "heart palpitations." Consultation with the patient's physician provides the information that Mr. K. did suffer an infarct of the ventricular anteroseptum and that the palpitations were a result of an episode of paroxysmal ventricular tachycardia. An angiogram performed during the second hospitalization revealed complete occlusion of the origin of the left anterior descending coronary artery, which caused the acute anteroseptal infarct. However, there was no other significant evidence of coronary artery disease nor of heart valve pathology. A beta-adrenergic blocking agent (sotalol hydrochloride) is being taken that has antianginal and antihypertensive action, blocks catecholamine-induced increase in heart rate, and decreases the velocity and extent of myocardial contraction. Other medications are a coated ASA tablet in a daily dosage of 325 mg and 400 IU of vitamin E daily. Measurement of heart rate and blood pressure shows both of these to be within normal limits. Before treatment on this patient is started, preparatory procedures should include (circle all correct answers):

a. Withdrawing the ASA at least 5 days before beginning treatment in order to avoid exacerbation of the existing gingival bleeding.

b. Prescribing amoxicillin in the dosage recommended by the American Heart Association to prevent endocarditis occurring at the septal defect produced by the infarct.

c. Contacting the physician to have the dosage of the beta-blocker increased so that there is no possibility of onset of tachycardia during the proposed treatment.

d. Contacting the physician to inform him of your treatment plan and the nature of the drugs you will be using to perform the proposed dental therapy.

e. Having the patient double his dosage of vitamin E so that he will be receiving maximal blood flow through the coronary arteries.

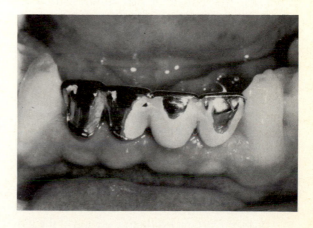

401. Your recommended dental treatment should consist of (circle all correct answers):

a. plaque control instructions with weekly follow-up until you are satisfied as to the effectiveness of the patient's home-care.

b. periodontal osseous surgery to reduce the labial exostoses.

c. extraction of the four anterior teeth with replacement by a fixed bridge or a partial denture, as splinted crowns make it impossible to maintain effective plaque control.

d. removing the crowns and remaking with well-contoured ceramometal crowns.

e. removing the remaining plastic material and repairing with one of the new adhesive-to-metal composite materials.

f. no matter what you elect to do for the mandibular incisors, redesign and remake the partial upper denture so that the incisal edges of the mandibular anterior crowns are in contact with acrylic rather than metal.

402. Precautions to observe during the delivery of dental care should include (circle all correct answers):

a. Because vital signs are within normal limits, there are no precautions with regard to any local anesthesia or any form of treatment.

b. Monitoring of blood pressure before, during, and after treatment.

c. Because post–myocardial infarct patients cannot tolerate the routine supine position for dental therapy, they must be treated at about a 45-degree position of the dental chair.

d. The use of epinephrine in local anesthesia for this patient is absolutely contraindicated.

e. If the patient is treated in the supine position, care should be exercised upon completion of treatment in returning him to the fully upright position.

f. All post–myocardial infarct patients must be premedicated with at least 5 mg of diazepam (Valium) or 10 mg of chlordiazepoxide (Librium) to reduce anginal attacks.

403. This 35-year-old man presents for a routine dental examination. The clinician observes a generalized, mild-to-moderate amount of plaque; extreme erythema; edema of the gingiva at the labial surface of the maxillary central incisors; and a thin knife-edge appearance of the labial marginal gingiva of the laterals as noted in the photograph. Bleeding with periodontal probing is observed at most interproximal locations, but no significant pocket depths are found except for a 5-mm probing measurement associated with the mesial and distal surfaces of the maxillary left first molar and the distal surfaces of the mandibular left and right second molars. The only significant finding noted in the full-mouth radiographic survey of this patient is the 1 to 1.5 mm of horizontal bone loss at areas with the 5-mm pocketing. In addition, it is noted that the incisal edges of the maxillary and mandibular anterior teeth exhibit wear facets. However, there is only a 1-mm overbite and a 2-mm overjet and in protrusive position, all the anteriors occlude first and prevent the posterior teeth from occluding. Canine guidance is observed in right and left lateral excursions, and nonworking side interferences are not present. The medical history is noncontributory and vital signs are within normal limits. Although retained bacterial plaque is the major factor responsible for the condition of the gingiva, the contributing factor *most* likely associated with the exaggerated response of the labial gingiva of the maxillary central incisors is (circle all correct answers):

a. traumatic occlusion.

b. overcontoured crowns.

c. a contact allergic response to the ceramic material.

d. nocturnal bruxism.

e. a defect in polymorph chemotaxis.

f. a combined endodontic-periodontic lesion.

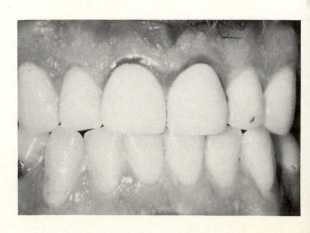

404. This 62-year-old man **(A)** presents for permanent replacement of a temporary crown on the maxillary left canine and a full crown on the mandibular right first premolar. Both these teeth received endodontic therapy about 6 to 8 months ago while the patient was living in another city. He also requests that missing teeth be replaced. Clinical and radiographic examinations reveal the following missing teeth in the maxilla: the right first premolar and first and third molars; and the first premolar and first, second and third molars on the left side. On the mandible, all right molars and left second and third molars are missing. The occlusal surfaces of all the remaining teeth have a Class II degree of attrition, resulting in the loss of 3 to 4 mm of vertical dimension owing to a nocturnal bruxing habit. The radiographs reveal that there is a successful endodontic fill of the left canine, and a considerable loss of distal crown structure can be observed through the acrylic crown. The premolar has an adequate occlusal restoration, but there is a 1-mm radiolucency at the root apex. In addition, there is a mild generalized gingivitis due to a moderate amount of plaque distributed evenly on the remaining teeth, and a mild generalized periodontitis accompanied by 1 to 2 mm of gingival recession associated with the canines and premolars of both arches. A review of the patient's medical history reveals that he is under the care of his physician for treatment and control of diabetes mellitus and hypertension. He also experienced a myocardial infarct 7 years ago. Consultation with his physician reveals that the patient's hypertension currently is adequately controlled with an antihypertensive agent. However, the diabetes is not under control despite twice-daily injections of insulin and a supposedly close adherence to a recommended diet. Further, the physician indicates that cardiac fitness tests are barely at a passing level, although the patient does not experience anginal pain. Please note that **C** and **D** are mirror images. The proposed dental treatment for this patient should include (circle all correct answers):

a. routine periodontal therapy sessions including oral home care.

b. placement of full-crown coverage on all the remaining dentition.

c. contacting the former dentist to obtain the radiographs showing obturation of the endodontically treated teeth.

d. placement of a fixed bridge from the right maxillary canine to the second premolar and onto the second molar, as well as a fixed bridge to replace the missing left first premolar, followed by a maxillary partial denture for replacement of missing left molars and a mandibular partial for replacement of the missing right molars.

e. placement of dowel cores in the endodontically treated left maxillary canine and right mandibular first premolar, followed by preparation and placement of full crowns if the obtained radiographs verify that healing has taken place.

f. placement of a dowel and crown on the left maxillary canine, construction and insertion of maxillary and mandibular partial dentures, and continued monitoring by radiography of the right mandibular first bicuspid.

g. construction of a night guard.

h. recalling the patient at 9-month intervals.

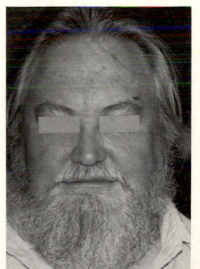

A

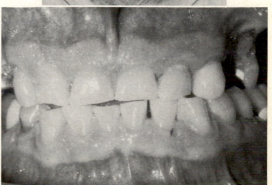

B

Continued.

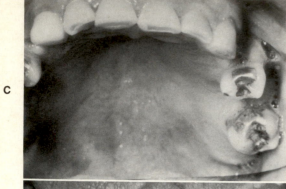

C

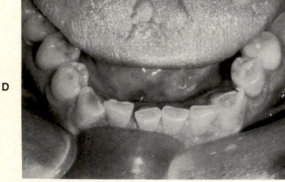

D

dictable result, one should (circle all correct answers):

a. make an occlusal assessment and correct any excessive centric contacts and any eccentric contacts.

b. have the patient demonstrate her current methods of personal plaque control, and if necessary provide corrective measures to your satisfaction.

c. place a composite on the buccal of the premolar, which has had minimal cavity preparation already.

d. perform a coronal repositioning–type procedure on the existing gingival tissue from the canine to the second premolar.

e. locate suitable donor palatal tissue and perform a gingival graft to include the canine through to the distal of the second premolar.

f. do a laterally positioned flap over the lateral incisor, using the tissue from the distal of the tooth.

405. This 54-year-old woman is aware of a progressive gingival recession associated with the mandibular incisors, canine, and premolars. Six years ago she underwent a surgical mandibular advancement to correct a retrognathism, which left her with paresthesia of the left mandible from the mental foramen forward. A year of orthodontic therapy followed this surgery, consisting of full banding of the maxillary and mandibular teeth. Fixed bridges, replacing both left first molars, were completed 2 years ago. Periodontal examination of the mandibular left side reveals recession of 3 to 5 mm on the labial and buccal surfaces of the incisors, canine, and first premolar. In addition, interdental papillae show blunting, probing depths are 2 to 4 mm, and the first premolar shows a Class I mobility. Attached keratinized gingiva on the labial surface is about 1 mm at the mandibular incisors, but inadequate at the canine and two premolars. The patient expresses a wish to have the recession corrected, particularly that associated with the canine and premolars. A review of the medical history reveals no contraindications to treatment. To obtain the most pre-

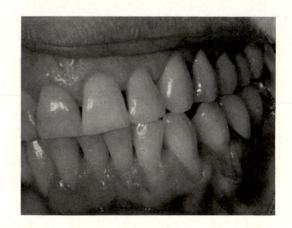

406. This 61-year-old woman recently had the maxillary right molar restored with a MOD inlay, which reveals wear facets, as do the right maxillary first premolar and the palatal surface of the lateral incisor on that side. When the patient taps her teeth together, fremitus is felt through a finger placed on the labial surface of the maxillary right lateral incisor. This tooth also exhibits a Class I mobility pattern. Radiographic examination and peridontal probing reveal no areas of significant bone loss or loss of gingival attachment. No other dental problems are present and a review of the medical history reveals no contraindications to dental treatment. Future dental treatment should include (circle all correct answers):

a. a maxillary partial denture to restore right side function.
b. occlusal reshaping of the maxillary right lateral to reduce occlusal forces.
c. removing the crown from the lateral and replacing with a provisional crown until other treatment is completed.
d. replacing the restorations in the maxillary right molar and premolar to restore the lost vertical of this side.
e. moving the right maxillary molar distally with orthodontics until it is in a more favorable position.
f. splinting the lateral incisor to the canine and the central incisor.
g. preparing the right maxillary molar and premolar for crowns, and constructing and cementing into place a fixed prosthodontic appliance to replace the missing second premolar.
h. replacing the crown on the right lateral, as well as placing a crown on the right canine.

407. As noted in this picture of the maxillary arch, this 62-year-old man recently had a crown cemented onto the right maxillary first premolar, and a fixed prosthodontic appliance onto the left first premolar and first molar, to replace a missing second premolar tooth. What are the major errors associated with these restorations (circle all correct answers):

a. improper location of the ceramometal junction on the maxillary right first premolar crown.
b. undercontouring of the pontic.
c. overcontouring of the crown on the left first premolar.
d. overcontouring of the crown on the left first molar.
e. improper location of the ceramometal junction on the pontic and left first molar crown.

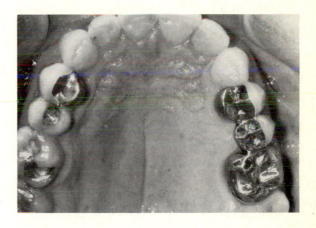

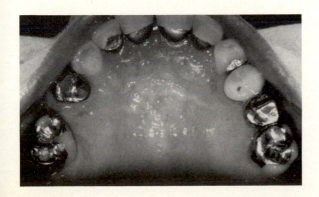

PART 3

AIDS and infection control

Dr. Danny Sawyer and Dr. Norman Wood authored questions 4 through 18.

The pictures associated with the first three questions are of patients who have seroconverted to HIV and also have been diagnosed as having AIDS.

1. A. The soft tissue gingival mass in the mandibular left canine region is *most* likely:
   a. inflammatory fibrous hyperplasia.
   b. Kaposi's sarcoma.
   c. melanoma.
   d. gingival cyst.
   e. squamous cell carcinoma.
   B. The condition observed on the margins of the free gingivae associated with the maxillary central incisors *most* likely represents:
   a. mouth-breathing gingivitis.
   b. acute necrotizing ulcerative gingivitis (ANUG).
   c. pregnancy gingivitis.
   d. drug-induced hyperplastic gingivitis.
   e. HIV-associated gingivitis.

2. This patient has experienced a moderately tender mouth for approximately 3 weeks. These whitish lesions are distributed bilaterally on the buccal mucosa and the labial mucosa. The lesions can be scraped off easily, leaving a raw, bleeding surface. The diagnosis *most* likely is:
   a. hairy leukoplakia.
   b. candidiasis.
   c. herpes simplex.
   d. Koplik's spots.
   e. speckled leukoplakia.

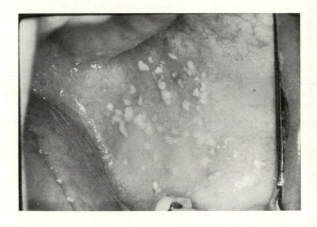

3. This painless condition on the lateral border of this man's tongue is becoming more apparent each week. The condition *most* likely is:
a. migratory glossitis.
b. erosive lichen planus.
c. erythroleukoplakia.
d. hairy tongue.
e. hairy leukoplakia.

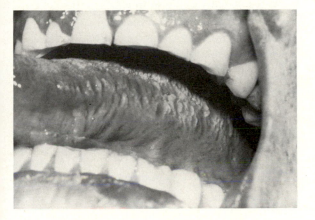

4. All of the following statements concerning AIDS dementia complex are correct but *one*:
a. It may precede the actual diagnosis of AIDS.
b. Initial symptoms include memory loss, difficulty in concentrating, and psychomotor deficiencies.
c. Early signs may be wrongly interpreted as depression.
d. These neurologic signs are caused by secondary opportunistic infections and are not due to direct HIV infection of neural tissue.
e. The first sign of motor disturbances is loss of coordination, and this may progress to severe ataxia and paraplegia.

5. All of the following statements concerning hairy leukoplakia are correct but *one*:
a. It occurs in a significant number of AIDS patients.
b. It occurs mostly on the lateral borders of the tongue.
c. The hairs (seen clinically) are diagnostic for this condition.
d. Epstein-Barr virus (EBV) is strongly associated with hairy leukoplakia.
e. Demonstration of EBV DNA by in situ hybridization is diagnostic for hairy leukoplakia.

6. All of the following statements concerning hairy leukoplakia are correct but *one*:
a. The persistence of nonremovable white lesions on the lateral border of the tongue after antifungal therapy is highly suggestive of hairy leukoplakia in HIV-positive individuals.
b. It is seen with considerable frequency in HIV-infected patients and has a propensity for malignant change.
c. It often has a corrugated appearance.
d. The hairs represent elongated projections of keratin, which are seen microscopically.
e. It may be seen in AIDS-related complex (ARC) patients.

7. All of the following represent high-risk groups for HIV infection, except *one*:
a. homosexuals.
b. IV drug users.
c. Americans or Canadians receiving blood transfusions in 1991.
d. newborn infants of HIV-positive mothers.
e. bisexual men.
f. individuals with multiple sex partners.

8. All of the following statements concerning the HIV virus are correct but *one*:
   a. It is an RNA retrograde virus.
   b. It is present in high numbers in semen of AIDS patients.
   c. It may occur in high numbers in serum of AIDS patients.
   d. It occurs in high numbers in saliva of AIDS patients.
   e. It is both lymphotropic and neurotropic.

9. All but *one* of the following oral conditions show a strong association with AIDS:
   a. squamous cell carcinoma.
   b. herpes lesions lasting more than 3 weeks in the absence of other immunocompetency states.
   c. Kaposi's sarcoma.
   d. hairy leukoplakia.
   e. prolonged candidiasis.

10. Which *one* of the following human viruses uses the enzyme reverse transcriptase as an important component in its pathogenesis?
    a. human HIV.
    b. herpes simplex.
    c. human papillomavirus.
    d. hepatitis B virus.
    e. EBV.

11. The *major* target cell of HIV is the:
    a. macrophage.
    b. T_4 helper lymphocyte.
    c. neutrophil.
    d. leukocyte.
    e. eosinophil.

12. *One* of the most suggestive findings indicating that a patient may very likely have AIDS is:
    a. microcytic hypochromic anemia.
    b. lymphocytosis.
    c. leukopenia.
    d. leukocytosis.
    e. reversed T_4/T_8 lymphocyte ratio.

13. All of the following are true about oral Kaposi's sarcoma in AIDS patients except *one*:
    a. It frequently occurs as multiple lesions.
    b. The most common site is the hard palate.
    c. The lesions may be red, blue, or purple.
    d. The lesions may be flat or raised.
    e. Spontaneous regression is a common occurrence.

14. Which *one* of the following agents would be the most successful in the treatment of hairy leukoplakia?
    a. nystatin.
    b. acyclovir.
    c. clotrimazole.
    d. methytrexate.
    e. ampicillin.

15. All the following oral lesions are strongly associated with AIDS except *one*:
    a. Kaposi's sarcoma.
    b. a special type of gingivitis.
    c. recurrent aphthous ulcer.
    d. a special type of periodontitis.
    e. hairy leukoplakia.

16. All the following statements except *one* are true of HIV-associated gingivitis:
    a. It may progress rapidly to HIV-associated periodontitis.
    b. Clinically, it mimics simple gingivitis of non-HIV patients in appearance and in response to scaling.
    c. It exhibits a high incidence of gram-negative rods.
    d. The drug of choice for treatment is 500 mg metronidazole b.i.d. for 5 days.

17. All the following statements about HIV-associated periodontitis are true but *one*:
    a. The associated gingival component resembles ANUG.
    b. There is rapid gingival recession and bone loss.
    c. There is acute pain and spontaneous bleeding.
    d. There is a high level of gram-negative rods.
    e. Amoxicillin is the agent of choice.

18. The interval between exposure of an individual and the manifestation of AIDS is approximately:
    a. 1 year.
    b. 4 years.
    c. 6 years.
    d. 10 years.
    e. 15 years.

19. All the following statements concerning the standard of "Universal Precautions" are correct except *one*:
    a. It is required because the health care worker is unable to identify who is HIV infectious or not.
    b. It is necessary except when a patient has recently tested negative for HIV infection.
    c. It is the standard of care that OSHA requires.
    d. It requires dental employers to establish and implement a written infection control plan for their employees.
    e. It includes routine use of masks, gloves, and eye protectors.
    f. It is necessary except in extraordinary circumstances: e.g., you detect a puncture in your glove while you are attempting to control threatening hemorrhage.

20. All the following statements concerning needles are true except *one*:
    a. They should be bent after use before they are discarded.
    b. They may be recapped safely by holding caps with forceps.
    c. They should not be left on the dental tray uncovered during the dental procedure.
    d. They should not be removed from the syringe with fingers; pliers can be used to accomplish this process.
    e. Needles and other sharp devices should be discarded into puncture-resistant containers.

21. All the following statements concerning sterilization and disinfection are correct except *one*:
    a. Instruments used to penetrate soft tissue or bone must be sterilized (i.e., autoclave, dry heat, or ethylene oxide is used).
    b. Plastic instruments that come into contact with oral tissues should be sterilized after each use, but may be placed in a chemical disinfectant instead.
    c. Impressions should be rinsed to remove saliva, blood, and debris, but under no circumstances should they be treated with disinfectants.
    d. The handpiece should be flushed by running water through it for 20 to 30 seconds, scrubbed thoroughly, and then sterilized or disinfected.
    e. Instruments should be bagged before sterilizing and kept in these sealed packages until used.

22. All the following statements concerning sterilization and disinfection are correct except *one*:
    a. Biologic monitoring should be done on a periodic basis to ensure the validity of sterilization.
    b. Ethylene oxide is an acceptable agent for sterilizing plastic instruments.
    c. Ethylene oxide is expensive, very penetrating (prone to leak from the apparatus), and toxic to breathe.
    d. Sterilization is the process by which all forms of microorganisms are destroyed, whereas disinfection refers to elimination of practically all known pathogenic organisms but not necessarily all microorganisms.
    e. Because sterilization is a more lethal process it is not necessary to clean instruments before sterilization; conversely, it is necessary to clean instruments before disinfection.

23. All the following statements concerning x-ray equipment and films are correct except *one*:
    a. Individual film packets should be sterilized or disinfected before use.
    b. Parts of the x-ray machine that are routinely handled by the operator should be disinfected or a protective covering should be placed.
    c. Exposed films should be opened in the darkroom with gloves.
    d. In the darkroom the film should be separated from the packets without being touched by the operator.
    e. After the operator has opened all the film packets in the darkroom the used packets and contaminated gloves should be discarded.

24. Tenets of "instrument recirculation" engage all of the following except *one*:
    a. "Maintenance" of instruments until further use is necessary.
    b. "Containment" of contaminated instruments is necessary.
    c. "Decontamination" is best achieved in the operatory.
    d. "Decontamination" basically refers to the gross and ultrasonic cleaning of instruments.
    e. "Renewal" involves the process of disinfection and sterilization.

25. All of the following are classified as "medical waste" except *one*:
a. blood-soaked gauze.
b. used masks.
c. used needles.
d. extracted teeth.
e. blood-stained x-ray packets.
26. All of the following statements are true except *one*:
a. Operators or assistants may use food handlers' gloves as overgloves when performing some procedures such as answering an unprotected telephone or working an unprotected switch.
b. Ancillary staff should use latex utility gloves when washing dental instruments.
c. Operators wearing gloves may avoid contamination by using tongue blades to operate light switches.
d. The best chemical sterilizing solution is 2% gluteraldehyde because it destroys all life.

27. All the following statements concerning disinfection of surfaces are true except *one*:
a. The spray and wipe-spray technique is advocated.
b. Sodium hypochlorite in 0.05 to 0.5% solutions is a suitable surface disinfectant. Sodium hypochlorite, once prepared in solution, has a shelf life of approximately 2 weeks.
d. Sodium hypochlorite solution is corrosive to metals and destroys fabric.

PART 4

Case analysis

CASE 1
Chief complaint

A 46-year-old woman presents (**A–F**) with a request to have her dentition cared for. She has not experienced recent dental pain but has suffered from intermittent bouts of such in the recent past.

Medical history

This patient is currently taking 20 mg of prednisone a day for the treatment of pemphigus. This condition was diagnosed 2 years ago, and she has responded well to the prednisone treatment.

Dental history

The patient says she had a great deal of dental work done during her teens and twenties, but has not been able to afford continued care since that time because of financial limitations. She has never worn dentures of any type.

Behavioral considerations

The patient says she has always been interested in maintaining her natural dentition, but because of the aforementioned financial limitations was unable to circumvent the extraction of some teeth. The fact that she has maintained basically a clean mouth even in the absence of routine dental visits lends credence to her statement.

Financial considerations

This patient has recently inherited a legacy of moderate size. She explains that she will be able to pay a "reasonable" amount for dental services but could not spare more than $2,000.

Clinical findings

The examination of the face, head, and neck basically yielded nonsignificant findings. There was what appeared to be a nevus in front of the left ear and also a firm, small, freely movable mass in the left submandibular space. The soft tissue examination of the oral tissues failed to reveal any significant pathosis. The accompanying illustrations show the clinical and radiographic features.

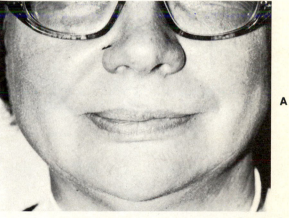

A

Continued.

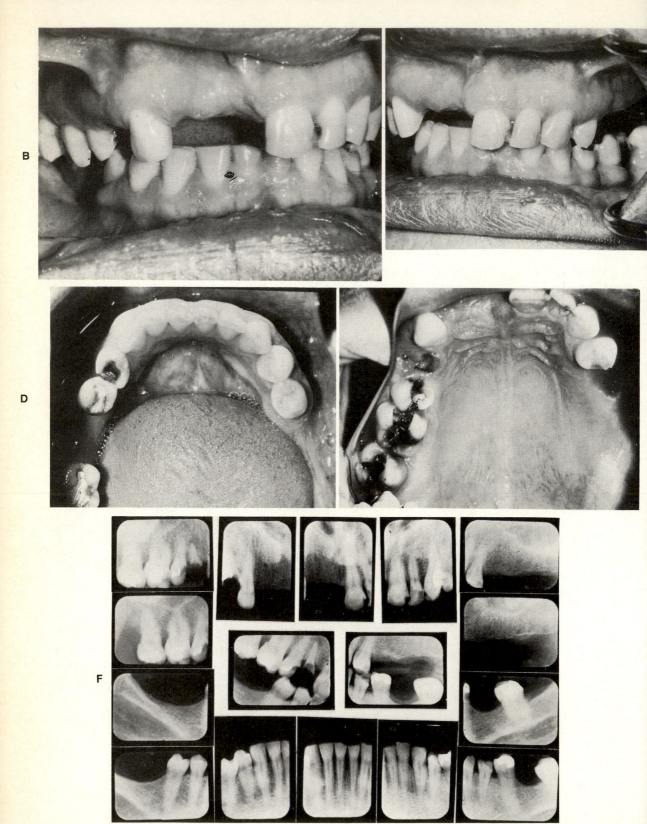

Patient management

Place a **T** or **F** at the beginning of each statement.

_____ 1. It will be necessary to consult with the patient's physician before any dental treatment is begun.

_____ 2. The major concern is that the institution of dental treatment may precipitate an exacerbation of the pemphigus.

_____ 3. There is a real possibility that the patient will suffer a cardiovascular collapse during dental treatment if prevention measures are not taken.

_____ 4. The possibility mentioned in No. 3 could be prevented by discontinuance of the prednisone for 12 hours before the dental appointment.

_____ 5. Ten milligrams of Valium taken one-half hour before the beginning of dental treatment is the preventive measure of choice.

_____ 6. Doubling the usual dosage of prednisone before the dental appointment will likely be recommended by the consulting physician.

_____ 7. Because of the drug-induced xerostomia, the patient should be warned of the likelihood of experiencing an increased caries rate soon.

_____ 8. It is necessary to hospitalize this patient for major oral surgical procedures.

_____ 9. It would be advisable to provide suitable antibiotic coverage when teeth are removed from this patient.

_____ 10. It is particularly important that this patient practice strict birth control measures because of the possibility of an increased risk of congenital defects in her offspring.

Specifics of diagnosis and treatment

Place an X in the appropriate boxes in the following tables.

CASE 1 ANALYSIS
Diagnosis

Tooth number	Apparently normal	Missing	Caries or chipped	Defective restoration	Overhanging margin	Calculus	Periapical pathosis	Periodontally involved
1								
2								
3								
4								
5								
6								
7								
8								
9								
10								
11								
12								
13								
14								
15								
16								
17								
18								
19								
20								
21								
22								
23								
24								
25								
26								
27								
28								
29								
30								
31								
32								

Treatment plan

Tooth number	Endodontics	Restoration	Periodontics	Extraction	Abutment crown	Pontic
1						
2						
3						
4						
5						
6						
7						
8						
9						
10						
11						
12						
13						
14						
15						
16						
17						
18						
19						
20						
21						
22						
23						
24						
25						
26						
27						
28						
29						
30						
31						
32						

Alternative treatment plan

Tooth number	Endodontics	Restoration	Periodontics	Extraction	Abutment crown	Pontic
1						
2						
3						
4						
5						
6						
7						
8						
9						
10						
11						
12						
13						
14						
15						
16						
17						
18						
19						
20						
21						
22						
23						
24						
25						
26						
27						
28						
29						
30						
31						
32						

CASE 2
Chief complaint

This 26-year-old man (**A–F**) presents with the chief complaint of several painful teeth.

Medical history

This patient is currently taking 40 units of NPH insulin daily for the treatment of diabetes. The diabetic condition was diagnosed when he was 21 years of age. He had rheumatic fever when he was 7 years old and has a resultant mild murmur of the mitral valve. He says he experiences bouts with hay fever and asthma and has suffered from several nosebleeds recently.

Dental history

The patient says he has visited a dentist only once, when he was 12 years old. The visit was for the purpose of extracting a painful mandibular left first permanent molar tooth, which was abscessed. He says the extraction was very painful and frightening and as a result he has not been to see a dentist since. He has never had any restoration placed and has never received a professional cleaning. He relates that he was in an automobile accident 2 years ago and the crown of his upper front tooth was fractured off at that time.

Behavioral considerations

The patient says he received a toothbrush for his tenth birthday and that he used to brush his teeth regularly for a while. He indicates that he mislaid his toothbrush after about 2 months and that he has not brushed his teeth since. He states that both his father and mother had poor teeth. His father received full dentures on his twenty-first birthday, and his mother wore partial dentures for a few years but had full dentures by the time she was 25 years old.

The patient realizes that his dentition is in a really degenerated state and partially relates his failure to seek early dental treatment to his fear of dentists. He says he is willing to accept whatever treatment plan you advise as long as he can afford it.

Financial considerations

The patient works as a laborer for a construction company and makes about $22,000 per year. He is married and has three children. His wife is now carrying their fourth child. He says his company provides hospitalization insurance, but he does not have a dental insurance policy. He indicates that he could not afford a treatment plan that would be over $1,000 even if the work was scheduled to extend over 1 year.

Clinical findings

Examination of the head, neck, and face failed to reveal any significant pathosis. A ragged scar was seen in the skin surface of the upper lip. Other than the presence of a generalized moderate gingivitis, the examination of the soft tissues of the oral cavity was basically negative. The accompanying illustrations show the clinical and radiographic features.

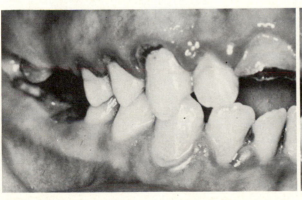
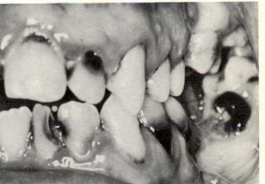

A B

Continued.

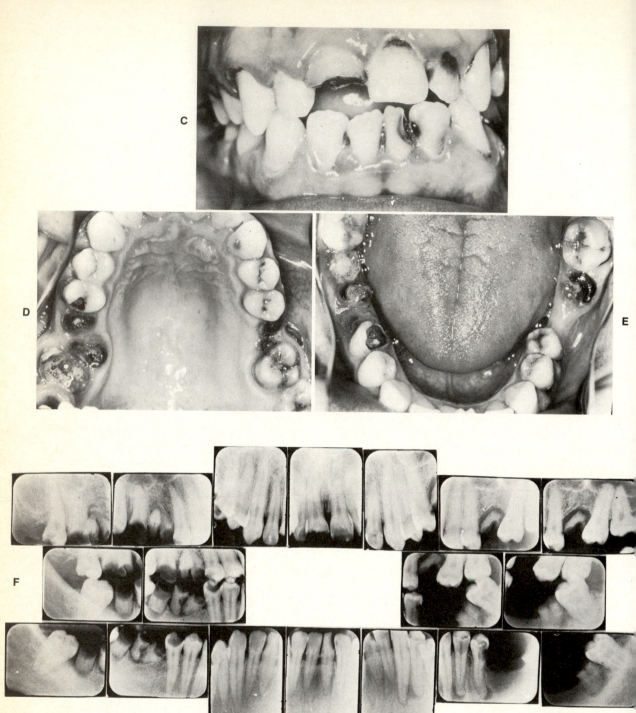

Patient management

Place **T** or **F** at the beginning of each statement.

_____ 1. In consideration of the various aspects of the case, it would be expedient to hospitalize the patient for the necessary extractions.

_____ 2. If the patient desires to have the teeth removed on an outpatient basis, thiopental sodium would be the intravenous agent of choice to use for sedation or general anesthesia.

_____ 3. If the dental work is to be done under a local anesthetic, you should advise the patient to partake of his regular meal before coming for the dental appointment.

_____ 4. You should advise the patient to double his insulin dosage before his dental appointment.

_____ 5. You can correctly advise the patient that his gross carious experience is mostly attributable to his diabetic condition.

_____ 6. If the urine test is negative for glucose on the day of a scheduled extraction and the teeth are not abscessed, he need not be covered with antibiotics presurgically or postsurgically.

_____ 7. Because of his heart condition, you should have nitroglycerin tablets readily available during the dental work.

_____ 8. It is necessary to supply suitable antibiotic coverage 1 hour before gingival scaling and 6 hours after the initial dose.

_____ 9. Oral amoxicillin is the antibiotic of choice if the patient is not allergic to it.

_____ 10. It would be advisable to order bleeding and clotting times before institution of surgery because patients on insulin therapy frequently have a prolonged prothrombin time.

Specifics of diagnosis and treatment

Place an X in the appropriate boxes in the following tables.

CASE 2 ANALYSIS
Diagnosis

Tooth number	Apparently normal	Missing	Caries or chipped	Defective restoration	Overhanging margin	Calculus	Periapical pathosis	Periodontally involved
1								
2								
3								
4								
5								
6								
7								
8								
9								
10								
11								
12								
13								
14								
15								
16								
17								
18								
19								
20								
21								
22								
23								
24								
25								
26								
27								
28								
29								
30								
31								
32								

Treatment plan 1

Tooth number	Endodontics	Restoration	Periodontics	Extraction	Abutment crown	Pontic
1						
2						
3						
4						
5						
6						
7						
8						
9						
10						
11						
12						
13						
14						
15						
16						
17						
18						
19						
20						
21						
22						
23						
24						
25						
26						
27						
28						
29						
30						
31						
32						

Treatment plan 2

Tooth number	Endodontics	Restoration	Periodontics	Extraction	Abutment crown	Pontic
1						
2						
3						
4						
5						
6						
7						
8						
9						
10						
11						
12						
13						
14						
15						
16						
17						
18						
19						
20						
21						
22						
23						
24						
25						
26						
27						
28						
29						
30						
31						
32						

Treatment plan 3

This patient has recently inherited $200,000 and expresses a desire to save as many teeth as is feasible. You instruct him in proper home care. When you evaluate the effects in 3 months, you find satisfactory hygiene. What would your treatment plan be now?

Treatment plan 3

Tooth number	Endodontics	Restoration	Periodontics	Extraction	Abutment crown	Pontic
1						
2						
3						
4						
5						
6						
7						
8						
9						
10						
11						
12						
13						
14						
15						
16						
17						
18						
19						
20						
21						
22						
23						
24						
25						
26						
27						
28						
29						
30						
31						
32						

Answer key

PART 1

Diagnosis, oral medicine, and radiology

1A. b	24. b	60. a
1B. b	25A. c	61. e
1C. c	25B. b	62A. c
2A. a	26. a	62B. a
2B. b	27. c	62C. d
2C. b	28A. c	62D. b
2D. c	28B. a	63. b
3A. a	29. e	64. d
3B. d	30. a	65. c
3C. e	31. c	66. c
4A. b	32. b	67. a
4B. d	33. a	68. e
4C. c	34. b	69A. d
4D. d	35. d	69B. c
5A. d	36A. a	70. b
5B. e	36B. e	71A. b
5C. a	37. b	71B. b
6A. d	38. c	71C. c
6B. c	39. e	72. e
6C. b	40. a	73. c
7A. e	41. d	74. d
7B. b	42. d	75. a
7C. e	43. a	76. d
8A. a	44. c	77. c
8B. b	45. d	78A. b
9A. c	46. d	78B. c
9B. c	47. c	79A. c
10. d	48. a	79B. d
11. e	49. b	79C. a
12. c	50. a	80. a
13. b	51. d	81. b
14. b	52. d	82. b
15. c	53. e	83. a
16. a	54. b	84. d
17. b	55. c	85A. e
18. a	56A. b	85B. b
19. d	56B. d	86. e
20. d	56C. e	87A. c
21. c	56D. a	87B. d
22A. d	57. e	88. c
22B. b	58. c	89. c
23. b	59. e	90A. a

90B. c	146. b	201. b
91. a	147. a	202A. a
92. d	148. a	202B. b
93. a	149. b	202C. e
94. b	150. a	203. d
95A. c	151A. c	204. d
95B. a	151B. a	205. c
96. d	152. b	206. b
97A. c	153. d	207. d
97B. b	154. d	208. b
98. e	155. c	209. a
99. c	156. d	210. c
100. d	157. c	211. a
101. b	158. a	212. b
102A. c	159. a	213. d
102B. a	160. a	214A. d
103. c	161. e	214B. b
104. a	162. d	215. c
105. a	163. c	216. a
106. d	164. e	217. c
107. d	165. e	218. c
108. c	166. d	219. d
109. b	167. c	220A. c
110. c	168. c	220B. b
111. d	169. b	221. a
112. d	170. b	222. e
113. d	171. c	223. d
114. b	172. b	224. b
115. a	173. b	225. c
116. b	174. c	226. a
117. c	175. e	227. c
118. a	176. a	228. d
119. a	177. a	229. a
120. b	178A. d	230. b
121. c	178B. d	231. d
122. d	179. c	232. c
123. d	180. b	233. b
124. a	181. c	234. c
125. a	182A. a	235. c
126. b	182B. e	236. b
127. d	183. b	237. e
128. c	184. a	238A. a
129. c	185. d	238B. e
130. d	186. b	239. b
131. d	187. d	240. b
132. b	188. d	241. d
133. a	189. e	242A. a
134. a	190. b	242B. d
135. e	191. d	243. b
136. b	192. a	244. a
137. b	193. a	245. c
138. b	194. b	246A. b
139. e	195. a	246B. d
140. c	196. a	247. a
141. c	197. a	248. e
142. a	198. c	249. b
143. b	199. d	250. a
144. d	200A. d	251. e
145. d	200B. c	252. c

253A. c	306. e	361. a	411. d	446B. d	463B. e
253B. e	307. b	362. e	412A. b	447. c	464A. c
254. c	308. a	363. b	412B. a	448. e	464B. d
255. e	309. c	364. c	413. d	449A. c	465. c
256. a	310A. c	365. d	414. e	449B. c	466A. c
257. b	310B. b	366. d	415. e	449C. a	466B. a
258. a	311. c	367. b	416. c	450A. a	466C. d
259. d	312. b	368. d	417. e	450B. b	466D. d
260. c	313. a	369. c	418A. b	450C. d	467A. e
261. b	314. b	370. e	418B. e	450D. e	467B. a
262. a	315A. b	371. c	419. a	451A. c	468. d
263. c	315B. d	372. e	420. d	451B. d	469. e
264. a	316. c	373. b	421. a	451C. a	470. c
265. c	317. b	374. c	422. d	451D. c	471. b
266. e	318A. e	375. e	423. a	452A. d	472. c
267. d	318B. c	376. b	424. b	452B. e	473. d
268. d	319. b	377. c	425. d	453A. b	474. e
269. b	320. c	378. c	426. c	453B. e	475. b
270A. e	321. e	379. b	427. d	454A. a	476. d
270B. b	322. b	380. b	428. a	454B. d	477. c
270C. b	323. a	381. c	429. e	455A. d	478. a
271A. d	324. b	382. b	430. c	455B. b	479. d
271B. a	325. c	383. a	431. d	456A. c	480. c
272. c	326. e	384. a	432. d	456B. c	481. c
273. a	327. b	385. d	433. c	457A. a	482. a
274. c	328A. d	386A. a	434. e	457B. d	483. c
275. d	328B. c	386B. e	435. c	458A. a	484A. b
276. c	329. c	387A. d	436. b	458B. c	484B. a
277. b	330. e	387B. c	437. b	458C. a	485. d
278A. c	331. e	388. a	438. e	459A. b	486. b
278B. b	332. c	389. b	439. b	459B. c	487A. d
279. a	333. d	390. a	440. a	460A. b	487B. c
280. d	334. b	391A. b	441. a	460B. e	487C. b
281. b	335. d	391B. d	442. a	461A. d	487D. d
282. a	336. b	392A. d	443. a	461B. a	488. a
283. b	337. e	392B. c	444. b	461C. a	489. a
284. a	338. b	393A. e	445. d	462. c	490. a
285. d	339. c	393B. e	446A. d	463A. b	
286. b	340. c	394. b			
287. a	341. b	395A. d			
288. e	342. d	395B. b			
289. a	343. c	396A. b			
290. b	344. d	396B. c			
291. d	345. e	397. d			
292. c	346. b	398. b			
293. b	347. d	399. d			
294. d	348. c	400. a			
295. a	349. b	401. d			
296. d	350. b	402. d			
297. b	351. a	403A. d			
298. c	352. e	403B. d			
299. b	353. a	404. b			
300. c	354. d	405. e			
301. d	355. c	406A. b			
302. c	356. e	406B. c			
303A. d	357. c	407. a			
303B. b	358. a	408. d			
304. a	359. d	409. d			
305. d	360. d	410. b			

PART 2

Comprehensive treatment planning

1. c	14. b	25B. c
2. b	15. a	26. d
3. d	16. b	27. d
4. a	17. c	28. e
5. a	18. c	29. b
6. a	19. e	30. d
7. d	20. d	31. c
8. a	21. c	32. a
9. d	22A. d	33. e
10. b	22B. b	34. b
11. b	22C. b	35. e
12A. b	23. c	36. c
12B. c	24. a	37. e
13. d	25A. b	38. a

39. b	94. b	144B. e	196A. a	222A. c	257. e
40. c	95. c	145. d	196B. c	222B. a	258. d
41. c	96. c	146. c	197A. c	223A. b	259. b
42. d	97. b	147A. b	197B. b	223B. e	260. d
43. c	98. a	147B. e	197C. a	224A. d	261A. a
44. c	99. c	148A. b	198A. a	224B. g	261B. d
45A. e	100. e	148B. a	198B. d	224C. c	262A. b
45B. a	101. b	149A. d	198C. b	225A. f	262B. a
46. c	102. c	149B. c	199A. d	225B. e	263. e
47. b	103. a	150A. e	199B. b	226A. c	264A. c
48. a	104. c	150B. c	199C. a	226B. e	264B. a
49. d	105. c	151. a	200A. b	227A. e	264C. a
50. b	106. a	152A. d	200B. d	227B. b	265. f
51. c	107. c	152B. c	200C. a	228A. C	266. c
52. a	108. d	153. e	201A. d	228B. A	267A. d
53. d	109. d	154. d	201B. c	228C. B	267B. c
54. e	110. c	155. d	202A. d	228D. B	268A. c
55A. c	111. b	156. a	202B. f	229A. e	268B. a
55B. d	112. c	157. b	203A. c	229B. e	269A. d
56. b	113. c	158. c	203B. d	230A. b	269B. c
57. b	114. a	159. e	204A. b	230B. e	270. c
58. e	115A. d	160. c	204B. a	231A. e	271. a
59. e	115B. b	161. a	205A. a	231B. d	272. c
60. d	116. d	162. d	205B. b	232. f	273. b
61. d	117. d	163. e	206A. d	233A. b	274A. e
62. b	118. a	164. a	206B. c	233B. a	274B. a
63. b	119. b	165. c	206C. d	234A. a	275A. a
64. e	120. c	166. d	207A. d	234B. d	275B. c
65. b	121. a	167. a	207B. e	235A. b	276. a
66. d	122. b	168. b	207C. c	235B. d	277. a
67. e	123. a	169. c	208A. c	236A. c	278A. b
68. b	124. c	170. b	208B. d	236B. b	278B. a
69. e	125. d	171. c	209A. d	236C. b	279. a
70. e	126. d	172. d	209B. d	237A. d	280. d
71. a	127. c	173. a	210A. b	237B. c	281. a
72. c	128. a	174. d	210B. e	238A. e	282. b
73. b	129. c	175. c	211A. c	238B. c	283. b
74A. b	130. d	176. c	211B. b	239A. a	284. e
74B. c	131. c	177. c	212A. c	239B. f	285. a
75A. e	132. d	178. c	212B. g	239C. e	286. c
75B. d	133. d	179. a	213A. e	239D. c	287A. e
76. a	134. c	180. c	213B. e	240A. b	287B. e
77. e	135. c	181. a	213C. c	240B. e	288. d
78. d	136. c	182. c	214A. c	241. c	289. c
79. a	137. d	183. c	214B. f	242. e	290. e
80. c	138. b	184. c	215A. e	243. e	291. c
81. b	139. c	185. b	215B. e	244. e	292. e
82. b	140A. b	186. d	216A. d	245. e	293. d
83. b	140B. e	187. b	216B. f	246. d	294. a
84. a	141. d	188. d	216C. f	247. e	295. c
85. c	142A. b	189. c	217. e	248. b	296. b
86. b	142B. e	190. c	218A. b	249. b	297. d
87. e	142C. d	191. b	218B. f	250. e	298A. b
88. a	143A. d	192. c	219A. c	251. d	298B. b
89. e	143B. b	193. b	219B. f	252. e	299. b
90. b	143C. c	194A. a	220A. c	253. b	300. e
91. a	143D. d	194B. b	220B. e	254. e	301. d
92. b	143E. a	195A. c	221A. b	255. e	302. a
93. d	144A. b	195B. e	221B. d	256. b	303. d

304. d
305. d
306. d
307. a
308. d
309. b
310. a
311. d
312. d
313. b
314. c
315. c
316. b
317. c
318. e
319. d
320. c
321A. a
321B. c
321C. e
322A. b
322B. d
322C. c
323. b
324. a
325. e
326. d
327. c
328.

A. Oral amoxicillin in an adult:
  *Amoxicillin, 3 g 1 hour before the procedure and then
  1.5 g 6 hours after the initial dose.*
B. Oral erythromycin ethylsuccinate in an adult:
  *Erythromycin ethylsuccinate, 800 mg 2 hours before
  the procedure and then 400 mg 6 hours after the initial
  dose.*
C. Oral erythromycin stearate in an adult:
  *Erythromycin stearate, 1.0 g 2 hours before the pro-
  cedure and then 500 mg 6 hours after the initial dose.*
D. Oral clindamycin in an adult:
  *Clindamycin, 300 mg 1 hour before the procedure
  and then 150 mg 6 hours after the initial dose.*
E. Oral penicillin in an adult:
  *Penicillin V, 2.0 g 1 hour before the procedure and
  then 1 g 6 hours after initial dose.*
F. Oral amoxicillin in a child (in mg/kg):
  *Amoxicillin, 50 mg/kg 1 hour before the procedure
  and then 25 mg/kg 6 hours after the initial dose.*
G. Oral erythromycin (ethylsuccinate or stearate) in a
  child (in mg/kg):
  *Erythromycin (ethylsuccinate or stearate), 20 mg/kg
  2 hours before the procedure and then 10 mg/kg 6
  hours after the initial dose.*
H. Oral clindamycin in a child (in mg/kg):
  *Clindamycin, 30 mg/kg 1 hour before the procedure
  and then 15 mg/kg 6 hours after the initial dose.*

I. Oral penicillin in a child weighing less than 60
  pounds:
  *Penicillin V, 1.0 g 1 hour before the procedure and
  then 500 mg 6 hours after the initial dose.*

329. c	356. b	383. d
330. a	357. d	384. b
331. e	358. a	385. d
332. b	359. c	386. c
333. c	360. a	387. b
334. a	361. d	388. a
335. e	362. b	389. d
336. d	363. a	390. d
337. b	364. a	391. c
338. c	365. e	392. a
339. a	366. b	393. b
340. d	367. c	394. d
341. e	368. a	395. d
342. b	369. d	396. c
343. c	370. c	397. c
344. a	371. e	398. a
345. d	372. b	399. c
346. b	373. c	400. d
347. d	374. e	401. a, e, f
348. c	375. b	402. a, e
349. c	376. e	403. b
350. e	377. a	404. a, c, f, g
351. c	378. e	405. a, b, e
352. d	379. b	406. b, e, g, h
353. c	380. e	407. b, c, d
354. d	381. a	
355. c	382. c	

PART 3

AIDS and infection control

1A. b	10. a	20. a
1B. e	11. b	21. c
2. b	12. e	22. e
3. e	13. e	23. a
4. d	14. b	24. c
5. c	15. c	25. b
6. b	16. b	26. d
7. c	17. e	27. c
8. d	18. d	
9. a	19. b	

PART 4
Case analysis
Case 1

1. T	6. T
2. F	7. F
3. T	8. T
4. F	9. T
5. F	10. T

CASE 1 ANALYSIS

Diagnosis

Tooth number	Apparently normal	Missing	Caries or chipped	Defective restoration	Overhanging margin	Calculus	Periapical pathosis	Periodontally involved
1		X						
2								X
3			X	X				
4			X	X				
5			X			X		
6	X							
7		X						
8		X						
9			X	X				
10			X	X				
11			X	X				
12				X				
13		X						
14		X						
15		X						
16		X						
17		X						
18	X							
19		X						
20	X							
21			X					
22	X							
23			X					
24			X					
25			X					
26	X							
27	X							
28	X							
29	X							
30		X						
31		X						
32		X						

Treatment plan

Tooth number	Endodontics	Restoration	Periodontics	Extraction	Abutment	Pontic
1						
2		X	X			
3		X				
4		X				
5				X		X
6					X	
7						X
8						X
9		X				
10		X				
11		X				
12					X	
13						X
14						X
15						X
16						
17						
18		X			X	
19						X
20					X	
21		X				
22						
23		X				
24		X				
25		X				
26						
27						
28						
29					X	
30						X
31						X
32						

By permission of Northeast Regional Board of Dental Examiners, Inc., Washington, D.C.

Alternative treatment plan

Tooth number	Endodontics	Restoration	Periodontics	Extraction	Abutment	Pontic
1						
2				X		
3		X				
4		X				
5				X		X
6					X	
7						X
8						X
9		X				
10		X				
11		X				
12		X			X	
13						X
14						X
15						X
16						
17						
18		X			X	
19						X
20		X			X	
21		X				
22						
23						
24						
25						
26						
27						
28					X	
29					X	
30						X
31						
32						

Case 2

1. T
2. F
3. T
4. F
5. F
6. F
7. F
8. T
9. T
10. F

CASE 2 ANALYSIS

Diagnosis

Tooth number	Apparently normal	Missing	Caries or chipped	Defective restoration	Overhanging margin	Calculus	Periapical pathosis	Periodontally involved
1			X					
2			X				X	
3			X				X	
4			X				X	
5			X					
6	X							
7	X							
8			X					
9			X				X	
10			X					
11			X					
12	X							
13			X					
14			X				X	
15			X					
16			X					
17			X					
18			X				X	
19		X						
20			X				X	
21			X				X	
22	X							
23			X			X		
24			X			X		
25						X		
26						X		
27	X							
28	X							
29			X					
30			X				X	
31			X				X	
32			X					

Treatment plan 1

Tooth number	Endodontics	Restoration	Peridontics	Extraction	Abutment crown	Pontic
1				X		
2				X		X
3				X		X
4				X		X
5		X				
6						
7						
8				X		X
9				X		X
10				X		X
11						
12						
13		X				
14				X		X
15				X		X
16				X		
17				X		
18				X		X
19						X
20				X		X
21				X		X
22						
23		X	X			
24		X	X			
25			X			
26			X			
27						
28						
29				X		X
30				X		X
31				X		X
32				X		

Treatment plan 2

Tooth number	Endodontics	Restoration	Periodontics	Extraction	Abutment crown	Pontic
1				X		
2				X		X
3				X		X
4				X		X
5				X		X
6				X		X
7				X		X
8				X		X
9				X		X
10				X		X
11				X		X
12				X		X
13				X		X
14				X		X
15				X		X
16				X		X
17				X		
18				X		X
19						X
20				X		X
21				X		X
22						
23		X	X			
24		X	X			
25			X			
26			X			
27						
28						
29				X		X
30				X		X
31				X		
32				X		

Treatment plan 3

Tooth number	Endodontics	Restoration	Periodontics	Extraction	Abutment crown	Pontic
1		X			X	
2				X		X
3				X		X
4	X				X	
5					X	
6						
7						
8	X	X				
9	X	X				
10		X				
11		X				
12						
13		X			X	
14				X		X
15		X			X	
16						
17		X			X	
18				X		X
19						X
20	X	X			X	
21	X	X			X	
22						
23		X	X			
24		X	X			
25			X			
26			X			
27						
28						
29		X			X	
30						X
31						X
32		X			X